W9-CFQ-616

Arthroscopic Rotator Cuff Surgery

Arthroscopic Rotator Cuff Surgery

A Practical Approach to Management

Edited by

Jeffrey S. Abrams, MD

Clinical Associate Professor, Department of Orthopaedic Surgery, Seton Hall University, School of Graduate Medical Education, Orange, New Jersey; Associate Director, Princeton Orthopaedic and Rehabilitation Associates, Princeton, New Jersey

Robert H. Bell, MD

Associate Professor, Northeastern Ohio Universities School of Medicine, Rootstown, Ohio; Division Chief Shoulder and Elbow, Department of Orthopaedics, Summa Health System, Akron, Ohio; Crystal Clinic, Inc., Akron, Ohio

DVD
INCLUDED

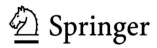

Jeffrey S. Abrams, MD
Clinical Associate Professor
Department of Orthopaedic Surgery
Seton Hall University
School of Graduate Medical Education
Orange, NJ
and
Associate Director
Princeton Orthopaedic and
  Rehabilitation Associates
Princeton, NJ 08540
USA

Robert H. Bell, MD
Associate Professor
Northeastern Ohio Universities
  School of Medicine
Rootstown, OH
and
Division Chief Shoulder and Elbow
Department of Orthopaedics
Summa Health System
Akron, OH
and
Crystal Clinic, Inc.
Akron, OH 44333
USA

Figures 11.3, 11.5A, 11.5B, 15.4, 15.5, 15.6, 17.5C, 22.5, 22.6, 24.1, 24.5, 25.1, and 25.3 were prepared by Alice Y. Chen.

Library of Congress Control Number: 2006932958

ISBN: 978-0-387-39340-7   e-ISBN: 978-0-387-39343-8

Printed on acid-free paper.

To Iris and Murry Abrams for their generosity and vision in providing me the opportunity of becoming a physician; to Kathleen for her untiring support for me as a surgeon; and to Kimberly and Matthew for sharing their childhood and love with me.

Jeffrey S. Abrams

To Ginger for enduring those endless years of medical school, residency, and practice building; to Kelly, Annie, and Brandon for their unconditional love and support for an often-absent Dad; and to Bob and Dorothy, parents who combined a wonderful mix of support, encouragement, and challenge to help me achieve my best.

Robert H. Bell

Foreword

It is a privilege and honor to write the foreword for this book. The contributors to *Arthroscopic Rotator Cuff Surgery: A Practical Approach to Management* are a national and international *Who's Who* of arthroscopic shoulder surgery. They are to be congratulated on presenting the most up-to-date, scientific, clinical, and, particularly, technical aspects of arthroscopic cuff surgery. The subject of this text is very timely given the current enthusiasm of arthroscopic and shoulder surgeons for achieving rotator cuff repairs through the arthroscope.

This book is carefully structured, organized, well written, and expertly illustrated. The inclusion of video footage that demonstrates selected procedures greatly enhances the textbook descriptions. The video is in DVD format, which is the ideal medium to help the reader understand the principles of arthroscopic cuff surgery.

I have been blessed to be able to grow with the evolution of shoulder surgery, and it is pleasing to see the current state of arthroscopic cuff surgery. Not too many years ago, we made rather large incisions in taking the deltoid off the acromion for exposure to achieve a rotator cuff repair. Some surgeons, particularly in Europe, osteotomized the acromion for exposure. We then slowly migrated to utilizing a mini approach that allowed arthroscopic inspection of the glenohumeral joint and subacromial space allowing decompression, if desired. We are now learning, particularly through focused texts such as this and expert teachers such as the authors, to achieve rotator cuff repair arthroscopically. I am reminded of the time when we did open incisions for partial meniscectomies in the knee. Today that would rarely be done. The day will soon come when the majority of repairs of the rotator cuff will be done arthroscopically.

On a personal note, let me share my pride in seeing Jeffrey Abrams and Rob Bell spearhead this publication. The three of us, as teacher and students, went through the evolution from open, to mini-open, to arthroscopic cuff repair. Now these individuals and the contributors to this book, many of whom have authored papers and books on this subject, have become world leaders in pioneering this type of surgery. The individuals who have contributed to this book have not only advanced the techniques described but have also developed instrumentation to help us get the job done.

Richard Hawkins, MD
Founding Member and Former President of the American
Shoulder and Elbow Surgeons
Team Physician, Denver Broncos and Colorado Rockies

Preface

Rotator cuff tears are recognized as a common disabling problem among athletes and active individuals. For decades, the common approach to tears of the rotator cuff tendon was an open repair often complicated by postoperative stiffness, the potential for infection, and by a limited capability to address coexistent glenohumeral pathology. With the advent of arthroscopic applications for the shoulder, much of this changed. The arthroscope provided the ability for concomitant examination and treatment of associated problems at the time of tendon repair; it lessened the postoperative morbidity, and offered an attractive option to open rotator cuff surgery. However, the technical limitations of performing an all-arthroscopic rotator cuff repair are daunting and the learning curve steep, which has prevented many general orthopedists from making the commitment to learn the procedure. Nevertheless, because of the rapidly growing patient demand for less invasive approaches to this common problem, more and more orthopedists are taking on the challenge and learning the nuances of this technique. This book is a tool to help facilitate this learning process and make the transition from an open to an all-arthroscopic repair possible.

To achieve that end, an international group of experts has been assembled to reveal the state of the art in this exciting area of minimally invasive surgery. These individuals are pioneers in arthroscopic repair who have made contributions to technique, implant design, and engineering principles that help to make this surgery reproducible and more beneficial to patients. Each contributor has been asked to describe the indications and technical steps to successfully perform an arthroscopic repair of a torn rotator cuff and to manage associated lesions. Controversies on the best techniques to reattach the torn cuff, tissue augmentation, implant and instrumentation options, and surgical options for biceps pathology are presented by these experts. To complement the text, a video has been created and indexed by the contributors to further illustrate their technique, with narration to add technical pearls and to avoid complications. Though the emphasis is on different repair techniques, the book also addresses setup, portal placement, rehabilitation, and advancements in the biology of tendon healing.

We hope that *Arthroscopic Rotator Cuff Surgery: A Practical Approach to Management* will help the novice gain the knowledge and confidence to venture further into this exciting new area of shoulder work and that it will provide helpful clues for advanced surgeons to refine their technique. This book can be valuable to orthopedic surgeons, orthopedic residents and fellows, sports medicine arthroscopists, and shoulder specialists.

We wish to acknowledge Dr. Richard Hawkins, who taught us to continue to question current techniques and encouraged us to explore new technology. Special thanks to Linda Dreyer and Linda Squires for their administrative assistance.

Jeffrey S. Abrams, MD
Robert H. Bell, MD

Contents

Foreword by *Richard Hawkins* vii

Preface... ix

Contributors xv

CHAPTER 1
Surgical Indications and Repairability of Rotator
Cuff Tears 1
Ken Yamaguchi and Robert Tashjian

CHAPTER 2
Making the Transition from Mini-Open to
All-Arthroscopic Repair 15
Benjamin S. Shaffer

CHAPTER 3
Patient Positioning, Anesthesia Choices, and Portals 25
Richard L. Angelo

CHAPTER 4
Suture Anchor Options 34
F. Alan Barber

CHAPTER 5
Suture Management and Passage 55
Richard K.N. Ryu

CHAPTER 6
Arthroscopic Knot Tying 68
Ian K.Y. Lo

CHAPTER 7
Role of Arthroscopic Decompression and Partial
Clavicle Resection   83
John S. Rogerson

CHAPTER 8
Tendon-to-Tuberosity Repair: Medial Footprint Fixation   105
Stephen J. Snyder, Aaron A. Bare, and Mark J. Albritton

CHAPTER 9
Tendon-to-Tuberosity Repair: Lateral Footprint Fixation   118
Gary M. Gartsman

CHAPTER 10
Tendon-to-Tuberosity Repair: Double Row Fixation   127
James C. Esch and Sarah S. Banerjee

CHAPTER 11
Partial Articular-Sided Tendon Avulsion Transtendon
Rotator Cuff Repair   143
Jeffrey S. Abrams

CHAPTER 12
Suture Anchor Repair of Small and Medium
Supraspinatus Tears   159
Robert H. Bell

CHAPTER 13
Arthroscopic Repair of Subscapularis Tears   174
Laurent Lafosse and Reuben Gobezie

CHAPTER 14
Tendon Mobilization in Large Rotator Cuff Tears   195
Felix H. Savoie III and Larry D. Field

CHAPTER 15
Arthroscopic Rotator Cuff Repair with Interval Release
for Contracted Rotator Cuff Tears   208
Joseph C. Tauro

CHAPTER 16
When and How to Do Margin Convergence Repair Versus
Interval Slides 218
Stephen S. Burkhart and David P. Huberty

CHAPTER 17
Repair of Large Anterosuperior Cuff Tears 228
Jeffrey S. Abrams

CHAPTER 18
Natural Extracellular Matrix Grafts for Rotator
Cuff Repair 246
Joseph P. Iannotti, Michael J. DeFranco, Michael J. Codsi,
Steven D. Maschke, and Kathleen A. Derwin

CHAPTER 19
Biceps Tenotomy: Alternative When Treating the Irreparable
Cuff Tear 269
E. Peter Sabonghy, T. Bradley Edwards, and Gilles Walch

CHAPTER 20
Biceps Soft Tissue Tenodesis 276
Alessandro Castagna, Raffaele Garofalo, Marco Conti, and
Victor M. Naula

CHAPTER 21
Biceps Tenodesis with Interference Screw 290
Pascal Boileau and Christopher R. Chuinard

CHAPTER 22
Biceps Subpectoral Mini-Open Tenodesis 306
Stephen C. Weber, Jeffrey I. Kauffman, and
Deanna L. Higgins

CHAPTER 23
Endoscopic Release of Suprascapular Nerve Entrapment
at the Suprascapular Notch 318
Laurent Lafosse and Tony Kochhar

CHAPTER 24
Mechanics and Healing of Rotator Cuff Injury   332
Miltiadis H. Zgonis, Nelly A. Andarawis, and
Louis J. Soslowsky

CHAPTER 25
Postoperative Rehabilitation Following Arthroscopic Rotator
Cuff Repair   348
Jonathan B. Ticker and James J. Egan

CHAPTER 26
How to Avoid and Manage Complications in Arthroscopic
Rotator Cuff Repair   363
Wesley M. Nottage

Index   375

Contributors

Jeffrey S. Abrams, MD
Clinical Associate Professor, Department of Orthopaedic Surgery, Seton Hall University, School of Graduate Medical Education, Orange, NJ; Associate Director, Princeton Orthopaedic and Rehabilitation Associates, Princeton, NJ 08540, USA

Mark J. Albritton, MD
Resurgens Orthopaedics, Fayettville, GA 30214, USA

Nelly A. Andarawis, PhD (candidate)
Bioengineering and Orthopedic Surgery, University of Pennsylvania, Philadelphia, PA 19104, USA

Richard L. Angelo, MD
Assistant Clinical Professor, Department of Orthopedics, University of Washington, Evergreen Orthopedic Clinic, Kirkand, WA 98034, USA

Sarah S. Banerjee, MD
Clinical Assistant Professor, Department of Orthopaedics, Texas Tech University, El Paso, TX 79965, USA

F. Alan Barber, MD
Plano Orthopedic and Sports Medicine Center, Plano, TX 75093, USA

Aaron A. Bare, MD
OAD Orthopaedics, Warrenville, IL 60555, USA

Robert H. Bell, MD
Associate Professor, Northeastern Ohio Universities School of Medicine, Rootstown, OH; Division Chief Shoulder and Elbow, Department of Orthopaedics, Summa Health System, Akron, OH; Crystal Clinic, Inc., Akron, OH 44333, USA

Pascal Boileau, MD
Professor, Orthopaedic Surgery and Sports Traumatology, University of Nice-Sophia Antipolis, L'Archet 2 Hospital, Nice 06200, France

Stephen S. Burkhart, MD
Director of Medical Education, The Orthopaedic Institute, San Antonio, Texas 78216, USA

Alessandro Castagna, MD
Unità di Chirurgia della Spalla, IRCCS Istituto Clinico Humanitas, Rozzano, Milan 20124, Italy

Christopher R. Chuinard, MD, MPH
Shoulder and Elbow Surgeon, Great Lakes Orthopaedic Center, Munson Medical Center, Traverse City, MI 49684, USA

Michael J. Codsi, MD
Staff Surgeon, Cleveland Clinic, Cleveland, OH 44195, USA

Marco Conti, MD, PhD
MedSport, Sports Medicine Center, Milan 20100, Como, Varese, Italy

Michael J. DeFranco, MD
Cleveland Clinic, Cleveland, OH 44195, USA

Kathleen A. Derwin, PhD
Assistant Staff Scientist, Biomedical Engineering, Cleveland Clinic Lerner College of Medicine, Cleveland, OH 44195, USA

T. Bradley Edwards, MD
Clinical Instructor, The University of Texas at Houston, Texas Orthopedic Hospital, Houston, TX 77030, USA

James J. Egan, PT
Island Orthopaedics and Sports Medicine, Massapequa, NY 11758, USA

James C. Esch, MD
Assistant Clinical Professor, University of California, San Diego, Tri City Orthopaedics, Oceanside, CA 92056, USA

Larry D. Field, MD
Co-Director, Upper Extremity Service, Mississippi Sports Medicine and Orthopaedic Center; Clinical Instructor, Department of Orthopaedic Surgery, University of Mississippi School of Medicine, Jackson, MS 39202, USA

Raffaele Garofalo, MD
Unità di Chirurgia della Spalla, IRCCS Istituto Clinico Humanitas, Rozzano, Milan 20124, Italy

Gary M. Gartsman, MD
Clinical Professor, University of Texas Health Science Center, Texas Orthopedic Hospital, Houston, TX 77030, USA

Reuben Gobezie, MD
Assistant Professor, Case Western Reserve University School of Medicine, Cleveland, OH 44106, USA

Deanna L. Higgins, CMA, LVN
Sacramento Knee and Sports Medicine, Sacramento, CA 95816, USA

David P. Huberty, MD
Oregon Orthopedics and Sports Medicine Clinic, Oregon City, OR 97045, USA

Joseph P. Iannotti, MD, PhD
Madden Professor and Chairman, Cleveland Clinic, Cleveland, OH 44195, USA

Jeffrey I. Kauffman, MD
Sacramento Knee and Sports Medicine, Sacramento, CA 95816, USA

Tony Kochhar, MBBS, MSc, FRCS (Tr & Orth)
Clinical Fellow, Alps Surgery Institute, Clinique General D'Annecy, Annecy 74000, France

Laurent Lafosse, MD
Alps Surgery Institute, Clinique Generale D'Annecy, Annecy 74000, France

Ian K.Y. Lo, MD, FRCSC
Assistant Professor, Department of Orthopaedic Surgery, The University of Calgary, Calgary, AB T2N IN4, Canada

Steven D. Maschke, MD
Cleveland Clinic, Cleveland, OH 44195, USA

Victor M. Naula, MD
Director, Centro de Perfeccionamiento Artoscòpico, Clinica Milenium, Guayaquil, Ecuador

Wesley M. Nottage, MD
Clinical Professor, University of California at Irvine; The Sports Clinic Orthopedic Medical Associates, Inc., Laguna Hills, CA 92653, USA

John S. Rogerson, MD
Assistant Clinical Professor, University of Wisconsin Medical School, Meriter Hospital, Madison, WI 53711, USA

Richard K.N. Ryu, MD
Orthopedic Surgeon, Santa Barbara, CA 93103, USA

E. Peter Sabonghy, MD
The University of Texas at Houston, Texas Orthopedic Hospital, Houston, TX 77030, USA

Felix H. Savoie III, MD
Mississippi Sports Medicine and Orthopaedic Center, Jackson, MS 39202, USA

Benjamin S. Shaffer, MD
Director, DC Sports Medicine Institute, Washington, DC 20006, USA

Stephen J. Snyder, MD
Medical Director of the CLASroom at Southern California Orthopaedic Institute, Van Nuys, CA 91405, USA

Louis J. Soslowsky, PhD
Professor of Orthopaedic Surgery and Bioengineering, Director of McKay Orthopaedic Research Laboratory, Philadelphia, PA 19104, USA

Robert Tashjian, MD
Assistant Professor, Department of Orthopaedics, University of Utah School of Medicine, Salt Lake City, UT 84180, USA

Joseph C. Tauro, MD
Assistant Clinical Professor of Orthopedic Surgery, New Jersey Medical School, and Director of Ocean County Sports Medicine Center, Toms River, NJ 08755, USA

Jonathan B. Ticker, MD
Assistant Clinical Professor, College of Physicians and Surgeons of Columbia University, New York, NY; Island Orthopaedics and Sports Medicine, PC, Massapequa, NY 11758, USA

Gilles Walch, MD
Centre Orthopédique Santy, Lyon 69003, France

Stephen C. Weber, MD
Sacramento Knee and Sports Medicine, Sacramento, CA 95816, USA

Ken Yamaguchi, MD
Sam and Marilyn Fox Distinguished Professor, Orthopaedic Surgery, Washington University School of Medicine at Barnes-Jewish Hospital, St. Louis, MO 63110, USA

Miltiadis H. Zgonis, MD
McKay Orthopaedic Research Laboratory, University of Pennsylvania, Philadelphia, PA 19104, USA

1
Surgical Indications and Repairability of Rotator Cuff Tears

Ken Yamaguchi and Robert Tashjian

Among those conditions causing shoulder pain, rotator cuff disease is the most common pathology; the prevalence of full-thickness rotator cuff tears in the elderly population ranges from 5% to 40%. Because rotator cuff surgical treatment is such an important and common procedure, it surprising that the surgical indications remain nonstandardized and controversial.[1,2] Surgical indications, at a fundamental level, involve a comparison of the relative risks and benefits of two different treatment alternatives. In the case of rotator cuff repair, we are dealing primarily with the risks of operative cuff repair versus nonoperative measures. The risks and benefits of both nonoperative and operative treatment have to be considered in order to fully consider treatment indications. Although the benefits of successful operative and nonoperative treatment are well known, the risks of conservative treatment are less apparent but also important to consider.

Operative treatment must be considered in the context of the reasonable expectations for success (benefits) as well as likelihood of adverse consequences (risks). In this context, *repairability*, or the potential of a surgical construct to heal is an important consideration in surgical indications. The concept of tendon reparability encompasses several different ideas. First, reparability refers to the physical ability, utilizing current surgical techniques, to appose a torn tendon back to bone. With advances in arthroscopic surgical skills and techniques, tears that once could not be repaired because of size, location, tendon retraction, or strength of repair construct are now reparable. However, surgical replacement of a torn tendon edge to the tuberosity bone does not ensure healing or restoration of dynamic muscle function. These issues can potentially affect both functional and symptomatic outcome. Thus, a surgical repair should also be considered in the context of the likelihood of obtaining healing. In this chapter, we will review the indications for surgery, including issues related to the risks of nonoperative treatment, the repairability of the cuff, and the potential for healing.

1.1. Assessing Rotator Cuff Tear Repairability

1.1.1. Incidence and Natural History of Partial- and Full-Thickness Rotator Cuff Tears

Information about the natural history and incidence of rotator cuff disease is fundamental to understanding treatment indications. The exact incidence overall of rotator cuff tears varies; however, there are two considerations that are well accepted. First, rotator cuff tears are relatively common with overall rates estimated at around 30% of the population.[3] Second, there is a significant correlation between increasing age and the frequency of rotator cuff tearing.[3-6] Lehman found an overall 17% incidence of full-thickness rotator cuff tears in cadaveric dissections, with as high as a 30% incidence over the age of 60.[6] Ultrasound, magnetic resonance imaging (MRI), and arthrography have all been utilized in asymptomatic patients and have found full-thickness tears in 4% to 13% of individuals between 40 and 60 years old, 20% between 60 and 70 years old, 31% to 50% between 70 and 80 years old, and between 50% and 80% over 80 years old.[3,4,7] Partial-thickness tears have been found in 4% of individuals younger than 40 years old and over 25% of individuals over 60 years of age.[3]

In a recent review of 586 consecutive patients with atraumatic rotator cuff disease, there were multiple findings regarding the demographics of cuff tears.[5] The data confirmed a strong relationship of rotator cuff tears with age. There was almost a perfect 10-year difference between patients with no tear, a unilateral tear, and bilateral tears. The average age of patients presenting with rotator cuff–derived pain with no tear was 48.7 years old; unilateral tear, 58.7 years old; and bilateral tears, 67.8 years old. Rotator cuff disease was not only age related, but also bilateral. Additionally, there was a strong relationship to family history. Interestingly, the many of these tears were initially asymptomatic on presentation (Figure 1.1).

Despite a relatively high percentage of individuals with asymptomatic rotator cuff tears, a number of these are at risk for the development of symptoms over time. Over 51% of patients with a previously asymptomatic rotator cuff tear and a contralateral symptomatic tear will develop symptoms in the nonsymptomatic tear over an average of 2.8 years.[8] Fifty percent of the newly symptomatic tears will progress in size while only 20% of those remaining asymptomatic will progress. No tears were found to decrease in tear size. This data suggests that a significant percentage of patients with asymptomatic tears are at risk for symptom development. Symptom development also correlated with enlargement of the tear. These data suggested a limited intrinsic healing potential for the rotator cuff if left unrepaired. Just as important, there was a significant risk for tear progression that would lead to the development of significant deterioration of function and symptoms.

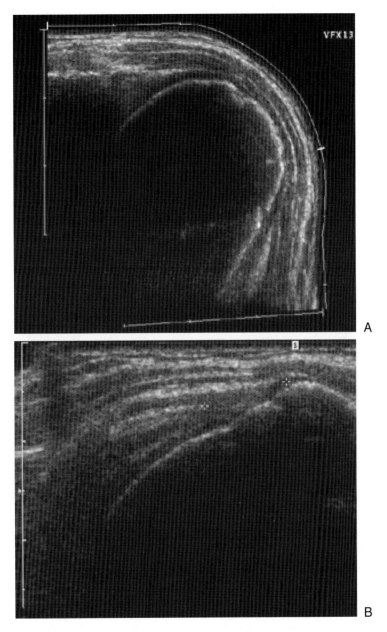

FIGURE 1.1. Ultrasound images from a representative patient with bilateral rotator cuff tears with only one side painful. (A) A massive cuff tear with no visible tendon seen on ultrasound image, indicating a tear greater than 3 cm in transverse dimension. This was the patient's symptomatic side. (B) Ultrasound images from the contralateral left side. This shoulder had a much smaller 1.5-cm tear, as shown between the two markers. This side was asymptomatic.

As in full-thickness tears, clinical evidence of spontaneous healing of partial-thickness tears appears limited. In a series of 40 articular-sided partial thickness tears diagnosed by arthrography, 80% of tears either progressed in size or became full-thickness tears at approximately 2 years.[9] Another series evaluated tear progression after open acromioplasty for impingement syndrome with no full-thickness tears and found 12.5% of shoulders went on to full-thickness tears even after decompression.[10] Also, no evidence of healing of partial-thickness tears was observed in another study on second-look arthroscopy for failed arthroscopic subacromial decompressions for partial-thickness tears.[11] Therefore, Codman's assumptions that partial-thickness cuff tears "may heal in whole or in part, p. 132" without repair is not likely to be true.[12] Nevertheless, the possibility that these tears will progress to the point where irreversible changes, such as muscle atrophy, fatty infiltration, or significant retraction, occur that may affect reparability or final outcome is likely to be much less than in acute, full-thickness tears.

1.1.2. Tendon Healing Potential

Several investigators have evaluated spontaneous rotator cuff healing utilizing both animal models and human tissue specimens. Both partial- and full-thickness tears have been evaluated in attempts to discover if spontaneous healing is possible. It appears that in both situations, an active but inadequate repair response is present, leading to persistence in tendon defects.

Tendon healing in full-thickness tears in a rat supraspinatus tear model was evaluated, and it was found that persistent defects were present in 78% of specimens, with disorganized and poor-quality tissue at the attempted repair site.[13] Similarly, no evidence of tendon healing was found in 12-mm tears at 3 weeks in a rabbit supraspinatus tear model.[14] Another group examined full-thickness tears in a rat model and found only scar tissue adhesions around the tendon stump.[15] Partial-thickness tears have also been evaluated in human surgical samples taken at the time of surgical repair, and no active spontaneous tendon repair was found in any portion of en bloc histological sections examined.[16] Consequently, evidence suggests that healing without repair in most tears is unlikely.

Healing of the rotator cuff with surgical intervention is also difficult to obtain. Historically, surgical repair has been associated with reliable, durable clinical outcome and, not surprisingly, healing of the tendon has been assumed for the majority of cases. Recently, several reports have suggested that healing of the surgical tendon–bone construct may be far less common than previously thought.[17–20] For example, in patients with two tendon tears, Galatz and colleagues demonstrated a

94% incidence of recurrent tear defect despite excellent clinical outcome.[17]

Multiple factors are probably important in maximizing the healing potential of surgical repair of the rotator cuff. While surgical technique is probably important and the focus of most surgeons, many other factors deserve consideration that may, in fact, be more important. These include multiple biological issues such as age of the patient, size of the tear, chronicity of the tear, general health of the patient, and genetic factors (family history). Environmental factors such as work activity, rehab protocol, use of nonsteroidal anti-inflammatory drugs (NSAIDs), and smoking also are likely to be important. Recently, we reported on a strong association between smoking and rotator cuff disease.[21]

Based on the natural history information, biological factors may be the most important in dictating the healing potential of a repair. In particular, patient age may be the most important factor. The important consideration here is that younger patients (below 65 years old) may have reasonable capacity to heal and a low rate of healing should be expected for physiologically older individuals.

Given the above discussion, there are three general categories of factors that help predict the healing potential of a rotator cuff tear. These include surgical technique, biology, and environmental issues. From a practical standpoint, surgeons can control all three issues, including biology. The control of biology comes from careful operative indications. Once a decision has been made for operative intervention, surgeons can only control for technique and environmental issues.

It should be emphasized that one important corollary of this line of reasoning is that when biological issues are favorable, surgeon control of technique and environmental factors become much more important. Thus, the best mechanical construct (perhaps double-row fixation), conservative rehabilitation, and control of smoking are more important in the younger individual with smaller tears. They are less important in the older individual with a large or massive tear where the best repair and rehabilitation will still most likely lead to a failure in healing. These considerations are also important in formulating indications as discussed below.

1.2. Indications and Timing for Surgical Repair

The decision to proceed with operative treatment of rotator cuff disorders requires an evaluation of the risks and benefits associated with both surgical and nonsurgical treatment. If surgery is to be chosen, good results are generally well established. The overall long-term clinical results of both arthroscopic and open rotator cuff repairs are durable, with over 90% good or excellent results at 10 years.[22,23] Similarly, results of treatment of partial- and full-thickness rotator cuff tears without repair have shown moderate success with 45% to 82% satisfactory results.[11,24–26] Nevertheless, most people consider both repairability and healing of the tear to be important for the best outcome.[20,27] Thus, these issues are important in considering indications.

In considering nonoperative treatment, Rowe was an advocate of non-operative treatment of rotator cuff disorders, stating that a majority of lesions would respond to exercises, occasional corticosteroid injections, and avoidance of repetitive motions. Indications for surgical treatment included a complete tear in an elderly patient with pain unresponsive to conservative treatment and a documented tear in a young patient.[28] However, data on the natural history of tears have shown that there could be important risks to certain individuals associated with non-operative treatment. These include the likelihood of symptom resolution, lack of spontaneous tendon healing, maintenance of shoulder function, tear progression, fatty degeneration, difficulty with tendon mobiliza-tion, and potential for rotator cuff arthropathy. Tear progression has been found in a significant number of these patients followed non-operatively. Increasing tear size has been shown to have a negative overall effect on rotator cuff repair outcome.[29] Therefore, repairing tears prior to significant progression will likely improve clinical outcomes (see Figure 1.2).

In addition to tear progression, fatty degeneration may occur with con-servative treatment of cuff tears. Fatty infiltration and atrophy of the rotator cuff muscles have also been described as important factors in deter-mining reparability of rotator cuff tears. Fatty infiltration increases with the size of tear and also with the time elapsed after a tear has occurred. Both clinical and experimental evidence suggests that fatty infiltration may be limited by tendon repair but not reversed.[30,31] More important, increased infiltration preoperatively predicts poorer postoperative results and increased re-tear rates.[21] Consequently, repairing tears prior to fatty infil-tration and atrophy will likely improve overall clinical results. All of these issues may significantly decrease the benefits of operative care, thus alter-ing the risk-to-benefit analysis.

The risk for the above-mentioned chronic changes to the rotator cuff provides the basis for an organized approach to operative indications.[32] Taking into consideration the natural history of partial- and full-thickness tears, the potential for repair healing, the repairability of the tear, and prognostic factors associated with functional outcomes, patients with rotator cuff tears can be divided into three categories: Group I includes patients with minimal risk for chronic changes in the near future; Group II consists of patients with significant risk for chronic, irreversible changes to the rotator cuff with prolonged nonsurgical treatment; and Group III consists of patients in whom chronic changes are already present. Based

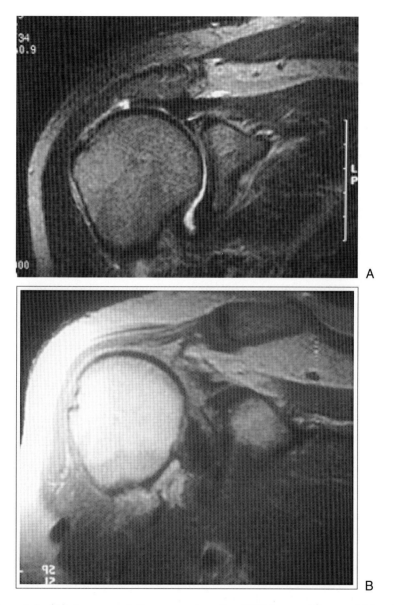

A

B

FIGURE 1.2. (A) A representative coronal section MRI from a 55-year-old female patient with a relatively small, supraspinatus tear. This tear with a good tendon edge and healthy muscle belly would be relatively easier to repair and have a high likelihood of healing. This is a typical Group II patient. (B) A representative coronal section MRI from a 70-year-old patient with a massive, chronic rotator cuff tear. If the patient in Figure 1.2A is treated with lengthy conservative treatment, she runs the risk of returning years later with this type of chronic progression. This MRI, typical of a Group III patient, shows a tear for which surgical prognosis for healing and repairability are limited. Good symptomatic improvement is still possible; however, functional improvement is unpredictable.

upon this classification, a decision for early arthroscopic reparability of a tear can be made.

1.2.1. Group I: Rotator Cuff Tendinitis and Partial-Thickness Tears

Group I patients have intact rotator cuffs or only partial-thickness tears. They can and should be treated with a relatively long course of physical therapy without significant risk to the patient. Irreversible, chronic changes, including fatty infiltration, tendon retraction, and glenohumeral arthritis, are unlikely with nonoperative treatment; prolonged therapy is safe. Recommending prolonged nonoperative treatment is further substantiated by its relative success in the treatment of impingement syndrome, with 67% of patients experiencing a satisfactory result.[33] It has been found, when looking specifically at partial-thickness tears, that bursal-sided tears do not respond as well to physical therapy and subacromial decompression as well as articular-sided tears.[16,34] Therefore, prolonged nonoperative treatment is recommended for tendonitis or partial-thickness tears, yet earlier repair may be indicated in bursal-sided partial tears due to treatment failure.

1.2.2. Group II: Full-Thickness Tears with Risk for Early Irreversible Rotator Cuff Changes

Patients in this Group II include individuals younger than 65 years old with small- or medium-sized tears, acute tears of any size, or tears with a recent loss of function. Wirth further suggested the indications for surgical treatment to include highly competitive athletes with tears involved in overhead throwing, 20- to 50-year-old patients with an acute tear secondary to a specific event, and all patients who have a tear and otherwise fail conservative treatment.[24] In acute complete tears, Cofield recommended surgical repair within 3 weeks of injury to obtain maximal recovery of shoulder function.[35]

These patients all have cuff disease that has not accrued significant chronic changes. Concern exists in this group of patients regarding the potential for tear extension with increasing fatty changes of the cuff leading to large and massive tears. Once a tear has advanced to the large/massive category, arthroscopic repair becomes increasingly difficult, with increased risks for re-tear and poorer functional outcomes.[17] Also, narrowing of the acromiohumeral interval occurs in three quarters of patients within 5 years with nonoperative treatment of full-thickness tears.[36] Consequently, these irreversible changes can be prevented by early surgical repair in this patient population.

In this group of people, early surgical intervention is warranted. There may be significant risks associated with nonoperative treatment.

1.2.3. Group III: Full-Thickness Tears with Irreversible Rotator Cuff Changes

The patients in Group III include individuals with either large or massive rotator cuff tears or elderly individuals over the age of 70 with full-thickness tears. Irreversible changes have already occurred to the cuff or the articular cartilage of the glenohumeral joint in a majority of these patients; therefore, attempting prolonged nonsurgical therapy is safe. These patients in effect do not have many risks of nonoperative care as chronic changes have already occurred. As healing in this group is relatively unlikely, the goal of any operative treatment, if necessary, may be to change a symptomatic cuff tear to an asymptomatic cuff tear. Arthroscopic rotator cuff repairs in elderly patients is feasible; one group demonstrated that 80% of patients over 60 years of age had a satisfactory result after arthroscopic rotator cuff repair independent of tear size or the ability to completely repair the tear by only performing margin convergence.[37] Complete repair was not required for a satisfactory result in this age group; consequently, tear progression may be of less importance and a prolonged trial of therapy is likely to be safe.

In large and massive tears, duration of symptoms prior to repair has not been found to correlate with postoperative outcome. In one series of operatively treated massive tears, the duration of symptoms prior to repair was over 2 years in those repairs that remained intact on postoperative evaluation.[19]

Finally, it may not be feasible to repair some very large or massive tears. A prolonged trial of therapy in these cases is very reasonable prior to considering surgical procedures such as tendon transfers or a reverse total shoulder replacement.

1.3. Enhancing Rotator Cuff Tear Repairability

1.3.1. Double-Row Anchor Fixation

As noted previously, failure of rotator cuff repairs secondary to re-tears has been shown to be a significant problem after both arthroscopic and open repairs. Although good symptomatic relief is possible without healing, final functional outcomes have been correlated with repair integrity.[20,27] Re-tear rates have been shown to increase with tear size in both open and arthroscopic repairs, approaching 55% and 94% in massive tears, respectively.[20,22] Small- and medium-sized tears have been shown to have re-tear rates between 10% and 20% after both open and arthroscopic repairs.[18,20]

Once the decision has been made to surgically fix a tear, the repairability, or ability to physically reattach the tendon so that it heals, may be enhanced with improved fixation techniques. As stated before, this consideration is most important in Group II individuals with a good biological potential to heal. One proposed technique for enhanced fixation is the creation of a double-row suture anchor construct.

The rotator cuff footprint is the insertion site for the supraspinatus from the edge of the humeral articular surface to the lateral edge of the greater tuberosity and has been found to be approximately 1.7 cm in width.[38] Suture anchor repair constructs using a single row of lateral anchors has been shown at best to restore only 67% of the original footprint of the rotator cuff.[39] Double-row suture anchor constructs have been described placing one anchor adjacent to the articular cartilage and one laterally at the edge of the tuberosity. The normal medial-to-lateral width of the rotator cuff insertion can therefore be re-established, increasing the area of contact for potential healing and potentially improving clinical outcomes.

Double-row fixation constructs have been described for both complete arthroscopic and mini-open repairs utilizing a mattress stitch medially and a simple stitch laterally.[40,41] In open repairs, modified Mason–Allen stitches are preferred because their strength is superior to simple stitches.[42] Attempts to recreate a locking-style stitch arthroscopically have been made with placement of a horizontal suture loop combined with a simple stitch placed medial to the horizontal loop, termed the *Mac stitch*.[43] The horizontal loop prevents pullout of the simple stitch. Biomechanical evaluation has confirmed its ultimate tensile load to be significantly stronger than the simple stitch, similar to the Mason–Allen stitch.[44] While the clinical utility of these constructs remains to be proved, it makes sense to maximize the mechanical construct when there is a high biological potential to heal.

1.3.2. Environmental Factors

Recently, two important environmental factors have been implicated that potentially affect rotator cuff healing. First, smoking has been shown to be highly correlated with the presence of full-thickness rotator cuff disease (Table 1.1).[21] The association of smoking with negative outcomes in other surgical procedures also supports the biological plausibility of this concern. It is our practice to insist on a cessation of smoking prior to and for 6 months following a rotator cuff procedure. Table 1.1 shows data on the risks factors for the presence of rotator cuff tears in a group of 586 patients evaluated by ultrasound for atraumatic, unilateral shoulder pain. The presence of a rotator cuff tear was significantly correlated with age, hand dominance, and smoking status.

Second, NSAID medication may alter bone-to-tendon healing. It has been suggested that NSAIDs decrease the healing response of the rotator cuff in an animal model.[45] It is also our practice to generally withhold

TABLE 1.1. Comparison of Risk Factors for Rotator Cuff Tears.

Factor	Rotator cuff tears	No rotator cuff tears	Significance (p value)
Age (years)	62.6	49.2	<0.001
Symptomatic dominant extremity (%)	66.4	54.2	0.004
History of smoking (%)	61.9	48.3	0.002
History of smoking within 10 years of presentation (%)	35.2	29.9	0.0006
Mean packs per day of tobacco use	1.25	1.1	0.004
Mean years of smoking tobacco	23.4	20.2	0.05
Mean pack-years of smoking tobacco	30.1	22	0.002

Source: Data from Baumgarten KM et al. (21) and from Yamaguchi et al. (5)

NSAIDs for the first 6 to 8 weeks following a cuff repair until motion exercises are initiated.

1.3.3. Postoperative Management

The high occurrence of persistent defects following repair has pushed many surgeons to be more conservative following repair procedures. We generally employ sling immobilization for 6 to 8 weeks following cuff repair. Patients are then started on passive motion exercises, including forward elevation in the scapular plane, supine external rotation in adduction, and pendulum exercises. We generally also employ continous passive motion (CPM) as a means to limit inadvertent or subconscious muscle activity. Active motion above shoulder level is allowed at 8 to 10 weeks, and resistive exercises are only started after 12 weeks.

1.4. Conclusions

The decision to proceed with early surgical treatment for rotator cuff tears depends on tear size and acuity, patient age, and the presence of irreparable changes to the rotator cuff and glenohumeral joint. Early repair should be undertaken for tears at significant risk for development of chronic changes such as fatty infiltration, tear extension, humeral head migration, and arthritic changes. Prolonged therapy may be undertaken safely in patients with pre-existing irreparable rotator cuff changes or in patients with tendon disorders with minimal risk for rapid development of irreparable changes.

In those patients taken to surgery, repairability or healing may be maximized by appropriate early intervention, maximizing the strength of repair (double-row construct), cessation of smoking and NSAIDs, and, finally, conservative rehabilitation.

References

1. Dunn WR, Shackman BR, Walsh C, et al. Variation in orthopaedic surgeons' perceptions about the indications for rotator cuff surgery. J Bone Joint Surg 2005;87A:1978–1984.
2. Mantone JK, Burkhead WZ, Noonan J. Non-operative treatment of rotator cuff tears. Orthop Clin North Am 2000;31:295–311.
3. Sher JS, Uribe JW, Posada A, Murphy BJ, Zlatkin MB. Abnormal findings on magnetic resonance images of asymptomatic shoulders. J Bone Joint Surg 1995;77A:10–15.
4. Tempelhof S, Rupp S, Seil R. Age-related prevalence of rotator cuff tears in asymptomatic shoulders. J Shoulder Elbow Surg 1999;8:296–299.
5. Yamaguchi K, Baumgarten K, Gerlach DJ, Ditsios K, Teefey SA, Middleton WD. The demographic and morphological features of rotator cuff disease: a comparison of asymptomatic and symptomatic shoulders. J Bone Joint Surg Am 2006;88:1699–1704.
6. Lehman C, Cuomo F, Kummer FJ, Zuckerman JD. The incidence of full thickness rotator cuff tears in a large cadaveric population. Bull Hosp Jt Dis 1995;54:30–31.
7. Milgrom C, Schaffler M, Gilbert S, van Holsbeeck M. Rotator cuff changes in asymptomatic adults. The effect of age, hand dominance and gender. J Bone Joint Surg 1995;77B:296–298.
8. Yamaguchi K, Tetro AM, Blam O, Evanoff BA, Teefe SA, Middleton WD. Natural history of asymptomatic rotator cuff tears: a longitudinal analysis of asymptomatic tears detected sonographically. J Shoulder Elbow Surg 2001;10: 199–203.
9. Yamanaka K, Matsumoto T. The joint side tear of the rotator cuff. A follow-up study by arthrography. Clin Orthop 1994;304:68–73.
10. Hyvonen P, Lohi S, Jalovaara P. Open acromioplasty does not prevent the progression of an impingement syndrome to a tear. J Bone Joint Surg 1998; 80B:813–816.
11. Weber SC. Arthroscopic debridement and acromioplasty versus mini-open repair in the treatment of significant partial-thickness rotator cuff tears. Arthroscopy 1999;12:126–131.
12. Codman EA. The shoulder: rupture of the supraspinatus tendon and other lesions in or about the subacromial bursa. Reprint ed. Malabar, FL: Robert E. Krieger; 1984.
13. Carpenter JE, Thomopoulos S, Flanagan CL, DeBano CM, Soslowsky LJ. Rotator cuff defect healing: a biomechanical and histologic analysis in an animal model. J Shoulder Elbow Surg 1998;7:599–605.
14. Hirose K, Kondo S, Choi HR, Mishima S, Iwata H, Ishiguro N. Spontaneous healing process of a supraspinatus tendon tear in rabbits. Arch Orthop Trauma Surg 2004;124:374–377.
15. Gimbel JA, Mehta S, Van Kleunen JP, Williams FR, Soslowsky LJ. The tension required at repair to reappose the supraspinatus tendon to bone rapidly increases after injury. Clin Orthop 2004;426:258–265.
16. Fukada H, Hamada K, Nakajima T, Yamada N, Tomonaga A, Goto M. Partial-thickness tears of the rotator cuff; a clinicopathological review based on 66 surgically verified cases. Int Orthop 1996;20:257–265.

17. Galatz LM, Ball CM, Teefey SA, Middleton WD, Yamaguchi K. The outcome and repair integrity of completely arthroscopically repaired large and massive rotator cuff tears. J Bone Joint Surg 2004;86A:219–224.
18. Bishop J, Lo I, Klepps S, Bird J, Gladstone JN, Flatow EL. Cuff integrity following arthroscopic versus open rotator cuff repair: a prospective study. Paper presented at: Annual Meeting of the American Academy of Orthopaedic Surgeons, San Francisco, CA, March 2004. Paper 216.
19. Gerber C, Fuchs B, Hodler J. The results of repair of massive tears of the rotator cuff. J Bone Joint Surg 2000;82A:505–515.
20. Harryman DT 2nd, Mack LA, Wang KY, Jackins SE, Richardson ML, Matsen FA 3rd. Repairs of the rotator cuff: correlation of functional results with integrity of the cuff. J Bone Joints Surg 1991;73A:982–989.
21. Baumgarten KM, Gerlach D, Galatz LM, et al. Smoking increases the risk for rotator cuff tears. Paper presented at: Annual Meeting of the American Academy of Orthopaedic Surgeons, Washington, DC, February 2005. Paper 333.
22. Galatz LM, Griggs S, Cameron BD, Iannotti JP. Prospective longitudinal analysis of postoperative shoulder function: a ten-year follow-up study of full-thickness rotator cuff tears. J Bone Joint Surg 2001;83A:1052–1056.
23. Wolf EM, Pennington WT, Agrawal V. Arthroscopic rotator cuff repair: 4- to 10-year results. Arthroscopy 2004;20:5–12.
24. Wirth MA, Basamania C, Rockwood, CA. Nonoperative management of full-thickness tears of the rotator cuff. Orthop Clin North Am 1997;28:59–67.
25. Itoi E, Tabata S. Conservative treatment of rotator cuff tears. Clin Orthop 1992;275:165–173.
26. Bartolozzi A, Andreychik D, Ahmad S. Determinants of outcome in the treatment of rotator cuff disease. Clin Orthop 1994;308:90–97.
27. Gazielly DF, Gleyze P, Montagnon C. Functional and anatomical results after rotator cuff repair. Clin Orthop 1994;304:43–53.
28. Rowe CR. Ruptures of the rotator cuff: selection of cases for conservative treatment. Surg Clin North Am 1975;43:1531–1540.
29. Cofield RH, Parvizi J, Hoffmeyer PJ, Lanzer WL, Ilstrup DM, Rowland CM. Surgical repair of chronic rotator cuff tears. J Bone Joint Surg 2001;83A: 71–77.
30. Gerber C, Meyer DC, Schneeberger AG, Hoppeler H, von Rechenberg B. Effect of tendon release and delayed repair on the structure of the muscles of the rotator cuff: an experimental study in sheep. J Bone Joint Surg 2004;86A: 1973–1982.
31. Goutallier D, Postel JM, Gleyze P, Leguilloux P, Van Driessche S. Influence of cuff muscle fatty degeneration on anatomic and functional outcomes after simple suture of full-thickness tears. J Shoulder Elbow Surg 2003;12:550–554.
32. Lashgari CJ, Yamaguchi K. Natural history and nonsurgical treatment of rotator cuff disorders. In: Norris TR, ed. Orthopaedic knowledge update 2: shoulder and elbow. Rosemont: AAOS; 2002:155–162.
33. Morrison DS, Frogameni AD, Woodworth P. Non-operative treatment of subacromial impingement syndrome. J Bone Joint Surg 1997;79A:732–737.
34. Cordasco FA, Backer M, Craig EV, Klein D, Warren RF. The partial-thickness rotator cuff tear: is acromioplasty without repair sufficient? Am J Sport Med 2002;30:257–260.

35. Bassett RW, Cofield RH. Acute tears of the rotator cuff: the timing of surgical repair. Clin Orthop 1983;175:18–24.
36. Walch G, Edwards TB, Boulahia A, Nove-Josserand L, Neyton L, Szabo I. Arthroscopic tenotomy of the long head of the biceps in the treatment of rotator cuff tears: clinical and radiographic results of 307 cases. J Shoulder Elbow Surg 2005;14:238–246.
37. Rebuzzi E, Coletti N, Schiavetti S, Giusto F. Arthroscopic rotator cuff repair in patients older than 60 years. Arthroscopy 2005;21:48–54.
38. Ruotolo C, Fow JE, Nottage WM. The supraspinatus footprint: an anatomic study of the supraspinatus insertion. Arthroscopy 2004;20:246–249.
39. Apreleva M, Ozbaydar M, Fitzgibbons PG, Warner JJP. Rotator cuff tears: the effect of the reconstruction method on three-dimensional repair site area. Arthroscopy 2001;18:519–526.
40. Fealy S, Kingham TP, Altchek DW. Mini-open rotator cuff repair using a two-row fixation technique: outcomes analysis in patients with small, moderate, and large rotator cuff tears. Arthroscopy 2002;18:665–670.
41. Lo IK, Burkhart SS. Double-row arthroscopic rotator cuff repair: re-establishing the footprint of the rotator cuff. Arthroscopy 2003;19:1035–1042.
42. Gerber C, Schneeberger AG, Beck M. Mechanical strength of repairs of the rotator cuff. J Bone Joint Surg 1994;76B:371–380.
43. MacGillivray JD, Ma CB. An arthroscopic stitch for massive rotator cuff tears: the Mac stitch. Arthroscopy 2004;20:669–671.
44. Ma CB, MacGillivray JD, Clabeaux J, Lee S, Otis JC. Biomechanical evaluation of arthroscopic rotator cuff stitches. J Bone Joint Surg 2004;86A:1211–1216.
45. Cohen DB, Kawamura S, Ehteshami J, Rodeo SA. Indomethacin and Celecoxib impair rotator cuff tendon-to-bone healing. Am J Sports Med 2006;34:1–8.

2
Making the Transition from Mini-Open to All-Arthroscopic Repair

Benjamin S. Shaffer

Many challenges confront the surgeon contemplating transition from the established mini-open approach to an all-arthroscopic rotator cuff repair. Perhaps the greatest hurdle is philosophical rather than technical: Why convert? After all, mini-open repairs are cosmetically acceptable, provide adequate exposure, permit secure fixation via trans-osseous tunnels or anchors, can be performed expeditiously, and pose little risk of deltoid injury. Clinical results are well established, durable, and provide a consistently high rate of patient (and surgeon) satisfaction. In contrast, arthroscopic repairs take longer, are more equipment intensive, more expensive, and have long learning curves, even among reasonably experienced arthroscopists. For those without considerable arthroscopic expertise or sufficient rotator cuff tear patient volume, the prospect of transitioning to arthroscopic repair may seem more imprudent than daunting.

Yet despite such disincentives, arthroscopic repairs have increased sixfold in recent years and stand to eclipse the "gold standard" mini-open approach in the near future.[1] Some of this enthusiasm undoubtedly reflects market economics, in which patient demand and physician peer pressure have encouraged pursuit of the "latest" technology. But the more important motivation behind this trend is that the arthroscopic approach has permitted evolution in our understanding and ability to anatomically repair rotator cuff tears. When compared to the mini-open technique, arthroscopic repairs of even small-to-medium tears pose less morbidity, pain, stiffness, and risk of deltoid injury. In larger, retracted, and/or massive cuff tears, an arthroscopic technique may be the only means by which a torn cuff can be successfully repaired.

2.1. General Approach to the Transition

Although the learning curve for arthroscopic cuff repair can be steep, transitioning from a mini-open approach presents a fairly easy platform from which to develop your skills and gain confidence. Ideally, this

transition consists of the best of both worlds in which you start arthroscopically, carrying out as many steps as your skills and the patient's tear permit,
followed by a mini-deltoid split. By committing to a mini-open repair from
the outset, you can comfortably try to accomplish each step arthroscopically, but bail out at anytime to confirm the adequacy of your efforts and/or
complete the repair. With experience, the mini-deltoid safety net can be
abandoned in favor of an all-arthroscopic approach. This chapter provides
strategies to help you comfortably transition at your own pace from mini-
open to all-arthroscopic repair.

2.2. Indications and Contraindications

Although nearly any rotator cuff tear pattern can be arthroscopically
repaired, I would suggest starting out with simple tears. The ideal
transition repair case would be a patient with a small (1–2 cm in length),
nonretracted, mobile, crescent-shaped, single-tendon (supraspinatus) tear
(Figure 2.1). Patients with larger, retracted, or massive tears are probably
poor candidates for initial all-arthroscopic repair attempts. Patients with
significant motion restriction (e.g., from adhesive capsulitis or previous
surgery), subscapularis and/or biceps tendon involvement, or significant
intratendinous or delaminating cuff pathology may be too challenging
early on. Revision repairs with deficient tissue or requiring tendon transfer
are inappropriate for arthroscopic repair attempts.

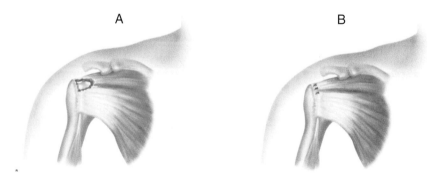

FIGURE 2.1. (A) A small crescent-shaped tear involving the supraspinatus tendon,
an ideal pattern for transitioning to arthroscopic cuff repair. (B) The tear after a
tendon-to-bone suture anchor repair. (From Parten PM, Burkhart SS. Arthroscopic
repair of full-thickness tears of the rotator cuff. In: Tibone JE, Savoie FH, Shaffer
BS, (eds). Shoulder Arthroscopy. New York: Springer, 2003. Reprinted with
permission.)

2.3. Preoperative Planning

Preoperative evaluation is important to identify adhesive capsulitis and muscle atrophy (suggestive of larger tear). Despite the trend away from routine decompression, radiographic workup should include an outlet view to assess acromial morphology. Preoperative magnetic resonance imaging (MRI) images should be reviewed for tear size, pattern, location, and extent of intratendinous involvement.

Candid preoperative discussion regarding your surgical approach is an important consideration as you transition to arthroscopic repairs. When beginning cuff repairs arthroscopically, you might inform your patients that some of the procedure will be done arthroscopically, with the final repair and assessment likely carried out through a mini-open approach. Patients may **prefer** an arthroscopic approach, but they will likely most depend upon your best-quality repair.

2.4. Surgical Procedure

2.4.1. Positioning and Setup

Patient positioning is surgeon preference. Conversion from arthroscopic to mini-open repair can be easily achieved from either the lateral decubitus or the beach chair position.

2.4.2. Instrumentation

Arthroscopic repair requires special instrumentation. Preoperative familiarity with arthroscopic instruments will facilitate efficient intra-operative use.

1. **Arthroscopic Cannulae.** Cannulae help maintain soft tissue portals and are especially useful during suture passage and knot tying (when soft tissue interposition can otherwise thwart well-placed sutures). Cannulae must accommodate the sometimes larger diameter suture passing instruments, whose dimensions must be known preoperatively.

2. **Tissue Grasper.** Loose body graspers permit grasping and manipulating tissue but can crush or damage already friable tendons. Specific tools for grasping and manipulating tissue during assessment of cuff tear patterns are preferable and widely available.

3. **Anchors/Inserters/Sutures.** Anchors vary considerably, and one must be familiar with the steps necessary for insertion and deployment. Double-loaded (two sutures per implant) anchors are increasingly utilized as they provide greater tissue fixation/implant. New generation sutures

whose strength exceeds traditional braided suture material (but with handling capability similar to monofilament) are available both preloaded on anchors and as "free" sutures for use during side-to-side repairs. Alternative "knotless" devices for cuff repair are available as well.

4. **Suture Passing Devices.** A wide selection of devices are available for suture passage through tendon. The simplest type is that which "penetrates" the tendon at the desired site and grasps a single limb of the anchor's suture, retrieving it through the tendon as the instrument is withdrawn. These tools require only a single step but need precise targeting to successfully penetrate and grasp the suture in a single maneuver and can leave a fairly large (2–3 mm) defect in the tendon. Other suture passing instruments involve a two-step approach: the first step is penetrating the tendon and passing a "shuttle" suture. The second step is retrograde shuttling of the anchor (or side-to-side) suture back through the tendon. A knot pusher (the single loop-type is fairly easy to use) and a knot cutter (some newer suture materials require a proprietary cutting device) complete arthroscopic repair instrumentation.

2.4.3. Surgical Technique

Arthroscopic cuff repair begins with careful patient positioning to ensure adequate surgical exposure and appropriate surgeon viewing. Dual video monitors permit visualization while arthroscopically viewing from anterior, lateral, or posterior portals. The following discrete steps are carried out in systematic fashion; the surgeon can proceed to the mini-open repair at any time during the approach.

1. **Glenohumeral Arthroscopy.** Standard posterior arthroscopic and anterior portals are established for thorough diagnostic evaluation of the glenohumeral joint. Undersurface cuff debridement is frequently helpful in delineating cuff tear dimensions. A probe (or the shaver tip) can be helpful in ascertaining cuff tear size and the presence of intratendinous pathology. In cases of partial cuff tears, placement of a percutaneous "marking stitch" via a spinal needle will facilitate tear recognition on the bursal side, useful in both arthroscopic and mini-open repairs.

2. **Subacromial Arthroscopy.** The arthroscope is redirected into the subacromial space. A lateral working portal is established to perform a bursectomy, cuff tear assessment, and, when indicated, decompression. The lateral portal incision should be made in anticipation of possibly incorporating it (or avoiding it) when proceeding with the mini-open approach. A bursectomy may be necessary to adequately identify the torn cuff pattern, but care is taken to avoid inadvertent cutting of the marker suture. If a subacromial decompression is performed, it must be carried out in a timely manner to avoid swelling and soft tissue distension, which can compromise both arthroscopic and mini-open repairs.

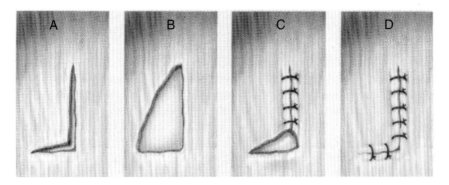

FIGURE 2.2. (A) An L-shaped tear with a vertical and longitudinal component. (B) The tissue has retracted causing a triangular tear pattern. (C) Closure of the vertical limb of the tear via side-to-side sutures. (D) The horizontal component has been repaired. This horizontal component typically requires use of bone anchors. (From Parten PM, Burkhart SS. Arthroscopic repair of full-thickness tears of the rotator cuff. In: Tibone JE, Savoie FH, Shaffer BS, (eds). Shoulder Arthroscopy. New York: Springer, 2003. Reprinted with permission.)

3. **Tendon Preparation.** Nonviable cuff tissue should be debrided. This may be accomplished using a basket and shaver for the cuff edge and an aggressive shaver blade or burr for the tuberosity. Only light decortication of the tuberosity is necessary.

4. **Tear Pattern Identification.** Tear pattern identification is probably the single most important step during arthroscopic or open cuff repair because it reveals how the repair is best achieved (Figure 2.2). For example, small tear patterns may be simple avulsions, requiring only tendon-to-bone reattachment. Conversely, larger tears typically have a longitudinal component as well, usually requiring a side-to-side repair first, followed by a tendon-to-bone repair. Tear pattern recognition is enhanced by viewing and grasping the torn tendon from multiple portals. Only in this way can one see how to best approximate the cuff. Switching sticks or cannulae whose diameter accommodates the scope sheath permit portal and instrument exchange.

5. **Mobilization/Interval Release.** Tears with poor mobility may require mobilization via an interval "slide" with release of the coracohumeral ligament, and/or along the base of the scapular spine between the supraspinatus and infraspinatus.[2,3] In general, these slides are more easily accomplished arthroscopically than open, particularly if releasing through a somewhat limiting "mini deltoid" split.

6. **Margin Convergence.** Larger U-shaped and L-shaped tears usually include a longitudinal component that can be re-approximated by side-to-side sutures. This "shifts" or converges the free margin of the cuff closer to the tuberosity (Figure 2.3).[4] Even large tears can be predominantly closed and converted to a simple tendon-to-bone configuration with only three or four side-to-side sutures. One of the distinct benefits of arthroscopic

suture passing instrumentation is the facility with which this margin convergence can be achieved, which is of great value during mini-open repairs as well.

7. **Tendon-to-Bone Repair.** Repair of the cuff to the lightly decorticated tuberosity is necessary in most cuff repairs, and can be accomplished using suture anchors, transosseous tunnels, or, if mini-open, a combination. Implants should be inserted at "deadman's angle," usually via a percutaneously portal just lateral to the acromial edge. Recent emphasis on a dual-row technique requires medial and lateral rows, with the exact number of anchors depending upon tear size.[5] Anchor seating should be confirmed by tensioning the suture(s) following placement. Use of double-loaded anchors (sutures/implant) increases the amount of tissue fixation per anchor, although it also doubles the number of tendon passes required. Performing suture anchor insertion and suture tendon passing techniques through a mini-open approach provides an ideal opportunity to visualize implant deployment, assess suture orientation relative to the anchor eyelet, and confirm repair security.

Suture management will be far easier if anchors are seated, and sutures are passed sequentially for each anchor prior to insertion of the next anchor. Knot tying can be done after each anchor's sutures are passed or can be delayed until passage of all anchors' sutures. These sutures should

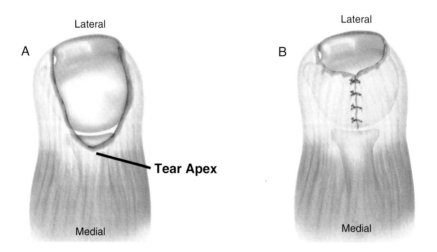

FIGURE 2.3. (A) An aerial view of a larger, U-shaped tear involving the supraspinatus and infraspinatus tendon with tear retraction such that the apex is just medial to the glenoid margin. Attempting to repair this through an open technique would likely be unsuccessful due to inability to translate the cuff laterally to the tuberosity. (B) By performing a side-to-side repair, margin convergence is achieved, rendering tendon-to-bone repair via suture anchors fairly straightforward. (From Parten PM, Burkhart SS. Arthroscopic repair of full-thickness tears of the rotator cuff. In: Tibone JE, Savoie FH, Shaffer BS, (eds). Shoulder Arthroscopy. New York: Springer, 2003. Reprinted with permission.)

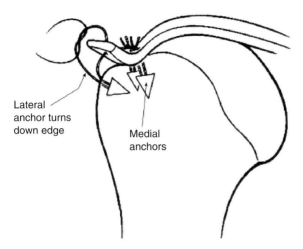

Lateral
anchor turns
down edge

Medial
anchors

FIGURE 2.4. The dual-row repair technique in which medial anchors secure the medial footprint using a horizontal mattress configuration, while lateral anchors ensure correction of any edge instability using simple vertical sutures. (From Parten PM, Burkhart SS. Arthroscopic management of massive rotator cuff tears. In: Tibone JE, Savoie FH, Shaffer BS, (eds). Shoulder Arthroscopy. New York: Springer, 2003. Reprinted with permission.)

be brought out through an accessory portal. The lateral anchors are next seated and their sutures passed in a simple vertical configuration. After all sutures have been passed, they are tied using the lateral sutures for traction as the medial row is secured, after which the lateral sutures are fixed. The order in which the sutures are secured may be modified based on experience and preference (Figure 2.4).

Suture management and knot tying are critical components of successful arthroscopic repair and require skill with sliding and nonsliding knots before reaching this step intraoperatively. The principles of knot security and loop security must be well understood to achieve satisfactory repairs. Confidence and skill can be developed by practicing arthroscopic knot tying during the mini-open approach.

8. **Assess Repair Integrity.** Regardless of the repair method, the cuff must be inspected for security through a passive range of motion. The arthroscope facilitates assessment by intra-articular placement, confirming restoration of the cuff's anatomical footprint.

2.5. Postoperative Management

The postoperative rehabilitation programs for the arthroscopic and mini-open rotator cuff repair are similar.[6] The postoperative protocol largely rests on the surgical technique employed and the surgeon's confidence in the repair. Because early motion can jeopardize healing,[7] a period of immobilization is generally preferred following cuff repair. My preferred approach following an arthroscopic repair, includes use of a sling for the first 4 weeks, with removal for daily hand, wrist, and elbow exercises, as well as for shower and dressing. The patient is not permitted to actively flex, elevate, or abduct the shoulder for the first 6 weeks, but allowed to use their hands for keyboard work, cutting food, and some simple hygiene. Passive exercises with a therapist are begun at week 4; active and assistive motion is begun at week 6; and resistance exercises are initiated at week 12.

This early immobilization protocol poses little risk. Risk of stiffness may prompt earlier sling discontinuation and initiation of therapy, though no active motion is permitted until the six week mark. It is important to convey to patients that, in comparison to the mini-open approach, arthroscopic repair does not heal more quickly, and will not permit earlier, more aggressive, or shorter rehabilitation.

2.6. Results and Complications

Both the mini-open[8–12] and arthroscopic[4,13–20] cuff repairs show consistently excellent results and high rates of patient satisfaction. A number of studies have shown comparable results between the two approaches.[21–24] Although no studies have yet conclusively demonstrated the superiority of either technique, stiffness is perceived to be less frequent following arthroscopic repair,[21,25] although repair integrity may be inferior, (at least based on early single row repair technique outcome reports). Further refinements in the arthroscopic technique, such as improved suture grasping suture configurations (i.e. locking rather than simple or mattress sutures) will ensure we will continue to pursue an ongoing evolving outcome landscape.[13,17,26–28] The rapid evolution of current advances in technology and techniques have outstripped our ability to keep pace with outcomes. We cannot yet prove the widespread impression that arthroscopic repairs will prove to be the standard. It is probably fair to say that the quality of the repair, however attained, is probably the most important factor in leading to a good outcome, and although learning arthroscopic cuff repair will likely enhance the results of even open repair techniques, surgeons must rely on their own judgment as to how this is best achieved.

2.6.1. Pearls in Your Transition

1. Stay behind your learning curve, not ahead of it. Transitioning to arthroscopic cuff repair need not be unidirectional. Even after mastering the arthroscopic repair "learning curve," the mini-open approach may have value in selected cases.

2. Recognize your own surgical skills and improve upon them through practice. Many teaching tools are available, including surgical technique models and cadaver workshops. A site visit to observe someone with

arthroscopic cuff repair expertise will further help avoid the pitfalls and appreciate the nuances of this demanding procedure.

3. Set an approximate time limit for reasonable progress and consider proceeding to open. Gary Gartsman, one of the technique's earliest pioneers, opened up his first 63 cases (G. Gartsman, personal communication, 1998). With advances in technique, we may no longer need to open this many cuffs before achieving a sense of proficiency and confidence, but doing so certainly provides a useful and proven transition strategy. With time and practice, arthroscopic cuff repair will become easier, but during your early experience, keep a low threshold for converting to a mini-open repair.

2.7. Conclusions

Arthroscopic cuff repair is promising, offering enhanced tear pattern recognition, margin convergence, and potentially improved clinical results. However, this technique can be technically imposing. By combining a stepwise progression of discrete arthroscopic maneuvers with the established mini-open repair, transition to an all-arthroscopic approach can be achieved.

References

1. Burkhart S. Point/counterpoint debate: cuff tears should be fixed arthroscopically. Paper presented at: Arthroscopy Association of North America Fall Meeting, December 2004.
2. Lo IK, Burkhart SS. The interval slide in continuity: a method of mobilizing the anterosuperior rotator cuff without disrupting the tear margins. Arthroscopy 2004;20:435–441.
3. Tauro JC. Arthroscopic repair of large rotator cuff tears using the interval slide technique. Arthroscopy 2004;20:13–21.
4. Burkhart SS, Danaceau SM, Pearce CE Jr. Arthroscopic rotator cuff repair: analysis of results by tear size and by repair technique-margin convergence versus direct tendon-to-bone repair. Arthroscopy 2001;17:905–912.
5. Lo IK, Burkhart SS. Double-row arthroscopic rotator cuff repair: re-establishing the footprint of the rotator cuff. Arthroscopy 2003;19:1035–1042.
6. Baker CL, Whaley AL, Baker M. Arthroscopic rotator cuff tear repair. J Surg Orthop Adv 2003;12:175–190.
7. Thomopoulos S, Williams GR, Soslowsky LJ. Tendon to bone healing: differences in biomechanical, structural, and compositional properties due to a range of activity levels. Biomech Eng 2003;125:106–113.
8. Baysal D, Balyk R, Otto D, Luciak-Corea C, Beaupre L. Functional outcome and health-related quality of life after surgical repair of full-thickness rotator cuff tear using a mini-open technique. Am J Sports Med 2005;33:1346–1355.
9. Shinners TJ, Noordsij PG, Orwin JF. Arthroscopically assisted mini-open rotator cuff repair. Arthroscopy 2002;18:21–26.
10. Hata Y, Saitoh S, Murakami N, Seki H, Nakatsuchi Y, Takaoka K. A less invasive surgery for rotator cuff tear: mini-open repair. J Shoulder Elbow Surg 2001;10:11–16.

11. Hersch JC, Sgaglione NA. Arthroscopically assisted mini-open rotator cuff repairs. Functional outcome at 2- to 7-year follow-up. Am J Sports Med 2000;28:301–311.
12. Fealy S, Kingham TP, Altchek DW. Mini-open rotator cuff repair using a two-row fixation technique: outcomes analysis in patients with small, moderate, and large rotator cuff tears. Arthroscopy 2002;18:665–670.
13. Boileau P, Brassart N, Watkinson DJ, Carles M, Hatzidakis AM, Krishnan SG. Arthroscopic repair of full-thickness tears of the supraspinatus: does the tendon really heal? J Bone Joint Surg Am 2005;87:1229–1240.
14. Gartsman GM, Khan M, Hammerman SM. Arthroscopic repair of full-thickness tears of the rotator cuff. J Bone Joint Surg Am 1998;80:832–840.
15. Murray TS, Lajtai G, Mileski RM, Snyder SJ. Arthroscopic repair of medium to large full-thickness rotator cuff tears (outcome at 2- to 6-year follow-up). J Shoulder Elbow Surg 2002;11:19–24.
16. Tauro JC. Arthroscopic rotator cuff repair (analysis of technique and results at 2- and 3-year follow-up). Arthroscopy 1998;14:45–51.
17. Wilson F, Hinov V, Adams G. Arthroscopic repair of full-thickness tears of the rotator cuff (2- to 14-year follow-up). Arthroscopy 2002;18:136–144.
18. Wolf EM, Pennington WT, Agrawal V. Arthroscopic rotator cuff repair: 4- to 10-year results. Arthroscopy 2004;20:5–12.
19. Park JY, Chung KT, Yoo MJ. A serial comparison of arthroscopic repairs for partial- and full-thickness rotator cuff tears. Arthroscopy 2004;20:705–711.
20. Jones CK, Savoie FH 3rd. Arthroscopic repair of large and massive rotator cuff tears. Arthroscopy 2003;19:564–571.
21. Buess E, Steuber KU, Waibl B. Open versus arthroscopic rotator cuff repair: a comparative view of 96 cases. Arthroscopy 2005;21:597–604.
22. Kim SH, Ha KI, Park JH, Kang JS, Oh SK, Oh I. Arthroscopic versus mini-open salvage repair of the rotator cuff tear: outcome analysis at 2 to 6 years' follow-up. Arthroscopy 2003;19:746–754.
23. Severud EL, Ruotolo C, Abbott DD, Nottage WM. All-arthroscopic versus mini-open rotator cuff repair: a long-term retrospective outcome comparison. Arthroscopy 2003;19:234–238.
24. Warner JJ, Tetreault P, Lehtinen J, Zurakowski D. Arthroscopic versus mini-open rotator cuff repair: a cohort comparison study. Arthroscopy 2005;21:328–332.
25. Norberg FB, Field LD, Savoie FH 3rd. Repair of the rotator cuff. Mini-open and arthroscopic repairs. Clin Sports Med 2000;19:77–99.
26. Gleyze P, Thomazeau H, Flurin PH, Lafosse L, Gazielly DF, Allard M. Arthroscopic rotator cuff repair: a multicentric retrospective study of 87 cases with anatomical assessment [in French]. Rev Chir Orthop Reparatrice Appar Mot 2000;86:566–574.
27. Wolf EM, Bayliss RW. Arthroscopic rotator cuff repair clinical and arthroscopic second-look assessment. In: Gazielly DF, Gleyze P, Thomas T, editors. The cuff. Paris: Elsevier; 1996:319.
28. Galatz LM, Ball CM, Teefey SA, Middleton WD, Yamaguchi K. The outcome and repair integrity of completely arthroscopically repaired large and massive rotator cuff tears. J Bone Joint Surg Am 2004;86:219–224.

3
Patient Positioning, Anesthesia Choices, and Portals

Richard L. Angelo

3.1. Patient Positioning

Both the lateral decubitus position and the beach chair position have their proponents. The choice is largely determined by the position used when the surgeon was learning shoulder arthroscopy, the ease and anticipated frequency of converting to a mini-open procedure, and the availability of surgical assistants and supportive devices for arm positioning. Benefits and compromises exist for each option.

3.1.1. Lateral Decubitus Orientation

The supine position is used during the induction of general anesthesia. The patient is then repositioned to the lateral decubitus orientation on a vacuum bag. Once a soft axillary roll is appropriately placed and the head supported in a neutral orientation, the patient is allowed to roll back approximately 15° and the bag is evacuated for support. The table is then rotated to place the anesthesiologist and necessary equipment near the middle of the operating table. The surgeon is thus provided unrestricted access to the involved shoulder. A monitor is located for easy viewing, usually across from the surgeon near the head of the table. The arm is supported in 30° to 40° abduction and 15° of forward flexion using 10#s to suspend rather than place significant traction on the shoulder (this shoulder position is varied during the case depending on the access necessary to specific locations). Numerous sterile sleeves and gauntlet devices are commercially available to support the arm. Cushions pad the dependent knee and ankle. A routine sterile prepration and drape are then performed. The lateral decubitus method eliminates the need for an assistant or mechanical device to support the arm. Internal and external rotation of the suspended arm affords acceptable access to the entire rotator cuff.

While the surgeon is working in the glenohumeral joint, the glenoid is typically oriented parallel with the floor. When working in the subacromial space, the surgeon may elect either to maintain this orientation (the acromion is vertical), or to rotate the camera head to view the acromion in a position parallel with the floor (as it would appear with the patient standing).

If the surgeon elects to convert to a mini-open approach, the unsterile portion of the suspension apparatus is removed and the patient's arm allowed to rest on the hip. Access to the supraspinatus and infraspinatus is readily obtained by extending the lateral subacromial portal proximally. An absorbable suture is introduced transversely through the deltoid at the inferior extent of the portal defect to prevent inadvertent distal extension and iatrogenic injury to the axillary nerve. The deltoid is then divided proximally along its fibers to the level of the acromion. If the surgeon converts to an open procedure for the subscapularis or biceps tendon through a standard deltopectoral approach, the vacuum bag is at least partially inflated (softened) and the patient is allowed to roll backward to a more supine position. The operating table is then adjusted to a gentle beach chair configuration, and acceptable position and support for the head and neck are verified.

3.1.2. Beach Chair Orientation

In the beach chair orientation, the patient's thorax is positioned to permit the involved shoulder to overhang the table. Alternatively, a specially designed table with a removable wing for exposure of the operative shoulder may be used. The operating table is then adjusted to create a beach chair configuration. Bony prominences are appropriately padded. A relatively more vertical orientation for the back will minimize the dependent position of the camera when in the posterior portal and avoid fogging of the lens. The anesthesiologist sets up near the patient's uninvolved shoulder and the viewing monitor is placed opposite the surgeon near the foot of the table. A surgical assistant or a sterile, maneuverable mechanical arm holder adjusts the position of the shoulder during the procedure, depending on the access necessary. The beach chair position allows greater mobility of the arm than does the lateral decubitus position, particularly with respect to internal and external rotation of the shoulder. The upright (anatomical) orientation for the arthroscope is maintained while working in both the glenohumeral and subacromial regions. Conversion to an open procedure for all regions of the cuff is relatively simple and usually requires only reducing the degree of thorax elevation.

3.2. Anesthesia Choices

3.2.1. General Anesthesia

Both endotracheal intubation (GET) and a laryngeal mask airway (LMA) provide safe, reliable options for the administration of general anesthesia. However, no durable analgesia is afforded once the patient awakens, and nausea and vomiting can sometimes be difficult to manage in the periop-erative period.

3.2.2. Interscalene Regional Block

Interscalene blocks (ISB) provide anesthesia, muscle relaxation, and postoperative analgesia, although supportive parenteral pain medication may be necessary during and in the immediate postoperative period.[1] At some institutions, ISB is used as the primary means of anesthesia and at others as an adjunct to general anesthesia. As with any invasive procedure, risk/benefit ratios determine its use. Proponents note its effectiveness, despite the frequent need for some additional narcotic support during the immediate postoperative period, and its relatively low risk of serious com-plications. Those in favor often practice in large or academic institutions where very dedicated anesthesia teams committed to regional anesthesia perform a large number of blocks, thus improving their expertise and minimizing complications.[2] Surgeons operating in smaller facilities, often in a community setting, relate a less favorable experience. They cite an increased frequency of potential serious complications including cardiac arrest, grand mal seizures, hematoma, and pneumothorax. Potential neu-rological injuries include damage to the recurrent laryngeal, vagal, and axillary nerves. Phrenic nerve dysfunction is common and can give rise to significant respiratory distress. Potential brachial plexus lesions include transient paresthesias (which have been reported to be as high as 9% at 24 h and 3% at 2 weeks postoperatively),[3] or a brachial plexus palsy which may be transient, require prolonged recovery, or be permanent in a small percentage of cases. Even with a successful block, the duration of pain relief averages only 9 to 10h, which may make pain management challenging in an outpatient setting.[1] Regardless of the surgical facility, a thorough disclosure of the potential risks should be discussed with the patient, preferably beforehand in an office setting during the preoperative visit.

3.2.3. Adjunctive Pain Management

The suprascapular nerve supplies 70% of the sensation to the shoulder joint. The efficacy of a local block of the suprascapular nerve has been debated, but it may result in up to a 30% reduction in postoperative nar-cotic usage and a fivefold reduction of nausea.[4] This block carries a low risk when performed with a blunt-ended needle and may be repeated as necessary, even in an office setting on the first postoperative day. In addi-tion, local infiltration of the portal sites with 1/2% bupivacaine is worth-while and pain pumps with indwelling catheters and cooling jackets using circulating ice water have also shown promise.

3.3. Portals

Properly located portals for arthroscopic rotator cuff repair are safe[5–7] and will provide the necessary field of view and instrument access to desired locations within the glenohumeral and acromioclavicular joints and subacromial space. Suture passage and management, in particular, require access to the subacromial region from multiple approaches.

3.3.1. General Technique

Bony landmarks are identified by careful palpation and mapped along with the anticipated portal locations using a surgical marker. (All anatomical references and diagrams are provided here with the patient in the lateral decubitus position.) Minor adjustments to the recommended distances from anatomical landmarks may be necessary for patients supported in the beach chair orientation or for particularly large or small patients. The posterior portal is typically established first. It is recommended that all subsequent portals be made from the outside working in under direct vision after first establishing the desired tract with a spinal needle.

A small skin incision is made at the chosen entry site, and a trocar and cannula are directed along the same path established by the spinal needle and into the joint or subacromial space. By avoiding the use of sharp trocars and excessive force to penetrate the capsule, articular cartilage damage is prevented. Consider using a screw-in or lock-in cannula, which are more secure and most easily introduced using a cannulated trocar delivered over a previously placed switching rod.

Primary portals are those used on a routine or frequent basis to perform an acromioplasty, mobilize and prepare the rotator cuff for repair, insert tuberosity anchors, and manage and tie sutures.

Primary Portals (Figure 3.1)

Posterior (P)
  Uses: Primary viewing portal; instrument approach to the articular surface of the infraspinatus and periglenoid capsule
  Field of View: Anterior capsule, glenohumeral ligaments, biceps, superior subscapularis, articular surface supraspinatus and infraspinatus tendons
  Entry Site: 1.5 cm inferior and 1.0 cm medial to the posterolateral corner of the acromion
  Path/Orientation: Cannula directed toward the coracoid tip
  Structures Transgressed: Posterior deltoid, infraspinatus

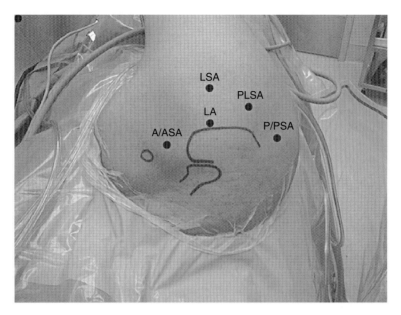

FIGURE 3.1. Abbreviations: P, posterior; PSA, posterior subacromial; A, anterior; ASA, anterior subacromial; LSA, lateral subacromial; PLSA, posterolateral subacromial; LA, lateral acromial.

Anterior (A)

Uses: View articular surface of the infraspinatus/posterior capsule; instrument approach to periglenoid capsule, supraspinatus, subscapularis, and biceps tendon/groove

Field of View: Infraspinatus tendon, posterior capsule

Entry Site: Lateral to the coracoid tip

Path/Orientation: Cannula directed toward the center of the glenohumeral joint

Structures Transgressed: Anterior deltoid, rotator interval

Posterior Subacromial (PSA)

Uses: View entire subacromial space, acromioclavicular joint and extra-articular biceps; instrument anterior acromion (i.e., cutting-block acromioplasty technique) and posterior bursa

Field of View: Subacromial bursa, bursal surface of rotator cuff, inferior acromial surface, coracoacromial ligament, acromioclavicular joint

Entry Site: Same as posterior glenohumeral (P) portal above

Path/Orientation: Trocar/cannula immediately inferior to the posterior margin of the acromion

Structures Transgressed: Posterior deltoid

Lateral Subacromial (LSA)

    Uses: View or instrument the subacromial space, acromioclavicular joint, and extra-articular biceps

    Field of View (Figure 3.2): Same as PSA portal with better view of the posterior bursal curtain and infraspinatus

    Entry Site: 2.5 to 3.0cm lateral to the lateral acromial margin [anterior–posterior (AP) location is determined with a spinal needle directed toward the center of the rotator cuff pathology]

    Path/Orientation: Direct spinal needle/cannula inferior to the lateral acromial margin and parallel to its inferior surface

    Structures Transgressed: Lateral deltoid

Posterolateral Subacromial (PLSA)

    Uses: Primary viewing portal for rotator cuff pathology

    Field of View (Figure 3.3): Same as LSA portal

    Entry Site: 1cm lateral and approximately 1cm anterior to the posterolateral corner of the acromion. (Exact AP location is again determined by a spinal needle directed toward the center of the rotator cuff pathology. Avoid placing this portal closer than 3cm from the LSA portal as it may interfere with instrument passage at that site.)

    Path/Orientation: Direct arthroscopic trocar and sheath toward the center of the cuff tear

    Structures Transgressed: Lateral deltoid

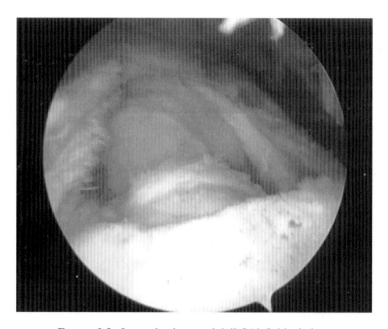

FIGURE 3.2. Lateral subacromial (LSA) field of view.

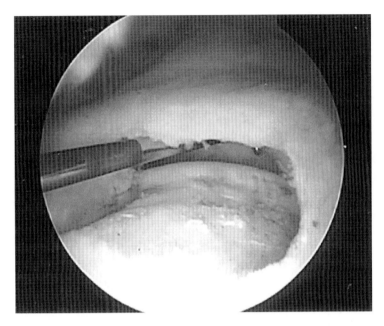

FIGURE 3.3. Posterolateral subacromial (PLSA) field of view.

Lateral Acromial (LA)
> **Uses:** Primary instrument approach to the greater tuberosity (i.e., drill, tap, anchor insertion)
> **Field of View:** Not applicable
> **Entry Site:** Immediately lateral to the lateral acromial boarder (exact AP location is determined by a spinal needle directed toward the center of the center of the prepared greater tuberosity)
> **Path/Orientation:** Instruments directed toward and at a 45° angle (in the frontal plane) to the tuberosity
> **Structures Transgressed:** Lateral deltoid

3.3.3. Accessory Portals

Accessory portals are employed selectively for subscapularis repair, biceps tenodesis, and partial distal claviculectomy (Figure 3.4).

Superomedial (SM): Neviaser
> **Uses:** Limited to direct instrumentation with small instruments, i.e., suture lasso; provides access to the medial cuff
> **Entry Site:** The soft triangle just medial to the junction of the posterior clavicle and the medial acromion

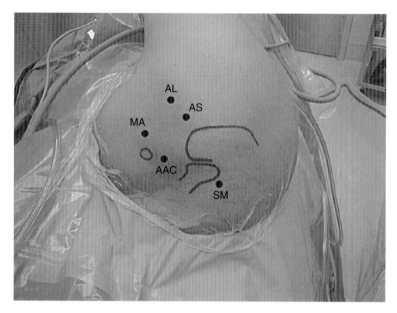

FIGURE 3.4. Abbreviations: SM, superomedial (Nevaiser); MA, midanterior; AL, anterolateral; AS, anterosuperior; AAC, anterior acromioclavicular.

Path/Orientation: Shoulder should be abducted <45°; while viewing from posterior or anterior, direct spinal needle 30° lateral and toward superior glenoid

Structures Transgressed: Trapezius

Anterosuperior (AS; also called superolateral)

Uses: Superior view of subscapularis insertion

Field of View: View of the subscapularis insertion onto the lesser tuberosity; biceps tendon

Entry Site: 1.0 cm directly lateral to the anterolateral corner of the acromion

Path/Orientation: Direct spinal needle/cannula through the most posterior aspect of the rotator interval adjacent to the anterior border of the supraspinatus toward the subscapularis insertion onto the lesser tuberosity

Structures Transgressed: Anterior deltoid, rotator interval

Anterolateral (AL)

Uses: View biceps groove, instrument subscapularis

Field of View: Subacromial bursa, bursal surface of subscapularis; biceps/groove

Entry Site: 3.0 cm lateral to the midanterior (MA) portal

Path/Orientation: Direct spinal needle/cannula toward biceps groove

Structures Transgressed: Anterior deltoid

Anterior Acromioclavicular (AAC)

Uses: Instrument the acromioclavicular joint

Field of View: Acromioclavicular joint (to assess adequacy of distal clavicular resection)

Entry Site: 3.0 cm anteroinferior and in line with the AC joint

Path/Orientation: Direct spinal needle/cannula toward the AC joint

Structures Transgressed: Anterior deltoid

3.4. Conclusions

With care and attention to detail, portals can be inserted to optimize the field of view and instrument access to the entire rotator cuff and associated pathology encountered. In addition, properly placed portals will immeasurably improve the ease and efficiency of repairing the rotator cuff arthroscopically.

References

1. Weber S, Jain R. Scalene regional anesthesia for shoulder surgery in a community setting: An assessment of risk. J Bone Joint Surg Am 2002;84;775–779.
2. Bishop J, Sprague M, Gelber J, et al. Interscalene regional anesthesia for shoulder surgery. J Bone Joint Surg Am 2005;87:974–979.
3. Urban M, Urquhart B. Evaluation of brachial plexus anesthesia for upper extremity surgery. Reg Anesth 1994;19:175–182.
4. Ritchie E, Tong D, Chung F, et al. Suprascapular nerve block for postoperative pain relief in arthroscopic shoulder surgery: a new modality? Anesth Analg 1997;84:1306–1312.
5. Nottage W. Arthroscopic portals: anatomy as risk. Orthop Clin North Am 1993;24:19–26.
6. Stanish W, Peterson D. Shoulder arthroscopy and nerve injury: pitfalls and prevention. Arthroscopy 1995;11:458–466.
7. Lo I, Lind C, Burkhart S. Glenohumeral arthroscopy portals established using and outside-in technique: neurovascular anatomy at risk. Arthroscopy 2004; 20:596–602.

4
Suture Anchor Options

F. Alan Barber

Suture anchors have played a significant role in the development of arthroscopic techniques to repair torn rotator cuff tendons.[1,2] As these arthroscopic techniques gained acceptance and became an achievable goal, our understanding and appreciation of suture anchor choices also expanded. Early anchor designs with metal wire barbs have given way to more effective methods of securing sutures in the osteoporotic bone of the humeral head.[3-7] An anchor that might be very acceptable to use with a straightforward, crescent-shaped single tendon tear may not be as helpful in a more complex tear or a more difficult-to-reach tear, such as one in the subscapularis tendon.

The challenge of rotator cuff repair is different from that of glenohumeral stabilization. The rotator cuff suture anchor is used in osteoporotic bone to attach sutures to this bone long enough to allow healing of a diseased tendon that is attached to a muscle that is likely to be atrophic and undergoing fatty infiltration. These biological factors often undermine the chance of clinical success.

Historically, rotator cuff tendons were attached to bone by placing sutures through bone tunnels in the humeral tuberosity.[8] Tunnels for sutures were either drilled or created by awls or punches, and then the suture was passed through them. Concerns about these sutures cutting through the tuberosity were sometimes addressed by placing reinforcing devices laterally and sometimes by locating the suture outlet more distally on the humerus. The inconsistency with this method of tendon fixation to bone has been demonstrated by load-to-failure testing of these suture tunnels.[9] A suture anchor repair is significantly stronger than the standard suture in bone technique irrespective of bone quality.[10] Also, the suture tunnel technique, though suitable for open procedures, is impractical for an arthroscopic repair.

To simplify attaching suture to bone, anchors were developed. The initial anchors were devised for glenohumeral surgery,[11,12] although numerous other applications have since been developed. The nature of the glenoid dictates that successful anchors should be relatively small and hold well in cortical bone. The contrast between the bone characteristics of the glenoid and of the humeral tuberosities is significant. Consequently, the characteristics for an ideal glenoid anchor are different from those of an ideal tuberosity anchor. As an example, because those patients undergoing arthroscopic rotator cuff repair are considerably older than the typical patient undergoing an arthroscopic Bankart or superior labral anterior and posterior (SLAP) repair, osteoporosis is a greater concern. The size and shape of the glenoid require an anchor that will not be as effective in the tuberosity, and the more osteoporotic bone of the humeral head requires a different holding mechanism to be maximally effective.

4.1. Anchor Evaluation

Surgeons have many anchors from which to choose.[3-7] These anchors vary in many ways. Size is one variable. For a push-in anchor, the overall size (drill size or outer diameter) is important to consider. For screw-in anchors, the difference between the major diameter and the minor (or core) diameter gives an indication of how large the flight of screw threads will be and how much bone they will grip to resist pullout.

The shape is another variable. The anchor shape determines how easily an anchor can be inserted and whether specialized techniques or instruments will be required. The composition of the anchor will influence its ease of insertion, its capacity for revision, and the load-to-failure strength, as well as whether it is absorbable and whether it requires a tap for insertion.

All anchors are attached to sutures. Because this is the main reason an anchor exists, the manner and configuration of this attachment is a key element. Recent advances and cost issues point to the improved efficacy of multiple sutures in a single anchor. The suture capacity of the eyelet, the type and location of the eyelet in the anchor, the presence of more than one eyelet, and the ability to reload the anchor with different sutures are all issues that should be considered by the surgeon. Other issues of concern include the method of anchor insertion, radiopacity, mode of anchor failure, and the holding strength of the anchor.

Many of the initial sutures anchors are no longer available[11] and have been replaced by newer, superior models. While not directly connected to anchor usage, creative new anchor designs and their associated instrument systems have also sought to simplify the challenge of arthroscopic knot tying, passing the suture through the tissue, and dealing with very osteoporotic bone.

What are the characteristics of a good anchor? An anchor must accomplish the following:

(1) fix the suture to the bone; (2) not pull out of that bone; (3) permit an easy surgical technique; and (4) not cause long-term problems.

Although anchors do have many advantages, they also have disadvantages: (1) anchors require special instruments that are specific for each anchor; (2) the use of anchors increases procedure cost; (3) there is a learning curve to master in using suture anchors; and (4) a foreign material is left behind that may complicate additional surgery.

4.2. Anchor Size

For the arthroscopic rotator cuff repair, anchor size is less of a concern because the humeral tuberosities provide a large area for insertion. Larger anchors have been shown to be stronger than smaller anchors,[3] although some of the newer, non-screw anchors are an exception to this trend.[6] With the increasing use of double row fixation and the possibility for revision surgery, larger anchors may not necessarily be better. When one considers the wide array of available anchors and the size of most surgical cannulas, my observation is that there is not really any need to use an anchor larger that 5mm in diameter. Increasing anchor diameter from 5.5mm to 6.5mm may actually be problematic. Larger anchors (e.g., 6.5mm and above) tend to cause crowding and limit the fixation points, and the increased holding strength provided by the larger size far exceeds the weakest link in the rotator cuff repair, which is the suture–tendon interface.[13] As a result, a larger anchor is often simply excessive.

Another important feature of a screw-in anchor is the surface area of the screw threads that bite into the bone and actually provide the holding power. Increasing the number of threads per centimeter, deepening those threads (increasing the difference between the major and minor diameters), and beveling the threads to improve compressive holding of osteoporotic bone make some screw anchors more effective and less likely to migrate than others of the same size.

Anchors can be too small as well. Most anchors that are well suited for a glenoid rim application are not recommended for use in the rotator cuff. The smaller size of these anchors (ranging from 2.0–3.5mm) fits into the confined space and dense bone of the glenoid rim but will not work as effectively (with the possible exception of subscapularis tendon repairs) in the less dense bone of the humeral tuberosity. Some of these smaller sutures cannot accommodate two #2 sutures commonly chosen for rotator cuff tendon repair, which is an additional limitation that makes them less desirable.

4.3. Anchor Shape

Anchors with different shapes are available. They can be classified as screw-in and non–screw-in anchors. The non-screw anchors may be further subdivided into toggle, push-in, and "morphing" anchors. The latter are a group of anchors that change their morphology after being placed into the bone. In addition, there are a group of anchors that act more like tacks and have a bar or disk attached that secures the tissue to the bone. While these devices eliminate the need to pass sutures and tie knots, the trade-off is less precise tendon fixation and a larger hole in the tendon, created from passing the device.

Screw anchors hold very effectively in the osteoporotic bone of the humeral head and tuberosities. They demonstrate excellent load-to-failure strengths. The use of the slipknot demands an open eyelet that allows the easy passage of the suture. This feature is common to both screw-in and non–screw-in anchors. With the advent of multiple sutures in an eyelet, anchors with large eyelets and multiple eyelets have appeared. In addition, most of the current anchors allow suture substitution should the surgeon wish to change the suture.

4.4. Anchor Eyelet

Another aspect of an anchor's shape is the eyelet. The eyelet can have a significant impact upon anchor performance in rotator cuff repair and is a potential site for suture failure.[14–16] Rotation of the suture eyelet relative to the line of force can affect suture fretting.[14] In addition, the line of suture load relative to the eyelet can affect the load-to-failure force.[16] Load-to-failure testing of anchors often applies a longitudinal pull in line with the axis of anchor insertion. However, this is not the manner in which anchors are used clinically. Inserting the suture anchor at an angle to the suture pull (the so-called "deadman" angle)[17] increases the load to failure. At the same time, this different angle places different loads on the eyelet and, with physiological cyclic loading, results in stresses that may abrade the eyelet and toggle the anchor in the bone.

The eyelet configuration varies as well. In order to accommodate two sutures, some anchors have one elongated vertically oriented eyelet while others have a wide horizontally oriented eyelet. The horizontal eyelet is less likely to result in binding sutures once one has been tied. This allows both sutures to be tied as slipknots. Some Arthrex (Naples, FL) anchors have eyelets made from a braided flexible suture (either polyester or FiberWire®). This flexible eyelet is very conducive to tying slipknots and can accommodate multiple sutures easily. Some anchors solve the problem of suture binding by having two independent suture channels. These channels may be at different angles to one another or on different sides of the anchor eyelet column.

The advantage of multiple sutures in a single anchor is to increase the number of fixation points without increasing the number of anchors. The decreased anchor congestion and the cost savings of this approach are appealing. In addition, distributing the loads over a greater number of tissue fixation points decreases the load per suture.[18] We recently investigated different suture combinations that might be used with multiple loaded anchors. In a study of the Super Revo® anchor (Linvatec, Largo, FL), three simple sutures were compared to two simple sutures, two simple sutures with a mattress suture sharing the simple suture holes, and two simple sutures with a mattress suture placed more medially. Interestingly, with a cyclic load applied at a deadman angle to anchor insertion direction, the three simple sutures demonstrated a superior performance in cyclic load testing to the other knot patterns.

4.5. Suture Material

Each anchor comes with one or more sutures. The trend among the newer anchors is to hold two sutures (recently, anchors with three sutures have been developed). The conventional braided polyester sutures are being replaced with stronger materials that use ultra-high molecular weight (UHMW) polyethylene.[7] The first of these was FiberWire® introduced by Arthrex, which has a core consisting of multiple strands for small polyethylene fibers. This significantly increases the suture strength. In fact, #2 FiberWire® is as strong as #5 braided polyester suture.[7] In response to the widespread acceptance of FiberWire®, a suture based upon a weave of UHWM polyethylene (Dynema) was introduced. This material is provided by various companies under different brand names (Force Fiber®, Herculine™, Maxbraid™, and Ultrabraid®). It is stronger than FiberWire®, and without the central core of polyethylene strands is more elastic. However, despite this increased strength, knots tied with this material can still slip. In a study comparing these sutures, 28% of FiberWire® knots slipped at less than 150N and 13% slipped with forces less than 75N.[19]

Both FiberWire® and the Dynema sutures may be more abrasive to the eyelet of a biodegradable suture anchor than braided polyester sutures. Another source of eyelet failure may be introduced by "running" these sutures through an eyelet (as with tying a sliding knot) and with cyclic loads during shoulder motion.

4.6. Anchor Material and Anchor Removal

A significant trend in the development of new suture anchors is a move toward biodegradable materials. The vast majority of suture anchors released in the initial years of anchor development were made of metal; recent anchors are predominately biodegradable. The material selected is primarily poly L-lactic acid (PLLA). However, some anchors are now made out of a copolymer of dextro (D) and levo (L) stereoisomers (PDLLA) in various combinations. It should be remembered that PLLA takes about 5 years to biodegrade and adding D-lactide to the polymer speeds this process.

One clear advantage of biodegradable anchors is that they create less of a problem with revision surgery than do metal anchors. If another anchor must be inserted into the area of a biodegradable anchor, a drill can simply clear the insertion track and the new anchor placed. There are very few metal anchors that have associated instruments that permit the surgeon to unscrew and remove the anchor. None of the metal non-screw anchors offer a means to easily remove them.

4.7. Anchor Placement

Placement of the suture anchor has been the subject of recent debate. The normal rotator cuff attachment site is known as its *footprint*. In the past, little attention has been paid to how well this footprint was recreated by the tendon repair. Until the recent appreciation of margin convergence[20] and interval slide techniques[21,22] allowed surgeons to achieve an easier reattachment of the cuff tendon edge to the greater tuberosity, most surgeons were quite satisfied to get the tendon somewhere near the bone attachment point without too much tension.

The different options for anchor placement include: (1) locating the anchors at the edge of the articular humeral cartilage to reduce the tension on the tendon; (2) locating the anchors more laterally but on top of the tuberosity; (3) locating the anchors on the side of the humeral shaft (over the edge) in the cortical bone and using a tension band suture to compress the tendon down to the prepared site on the greater tuberosity;[23] and (4) using a double row of anchors[24] (one to fix the tendon near the articular cartilage and the second more laterally to fix the rest of the rotator cuff tendon across the full extent of the normal cuff footprint).

Snyder supports an anchor position adjacent to the articular margin.[25] He has serial magnetic resonance imaging (MRI) evidence of "margin extension" of the proximally attached tendon distally to cover the normal cuff footprint during the healing process.[26] The footprint is seen to "fill in" starting from the attached cuff tendon edge and moving laterally until a normal-appearing cuff footprint develops. Double row fixation techniques increase surgical costs, can result in anchor crowding, and potentially complicate any subsequent revision procedure. However, when a single row repaired rotator cuff is viewed from the glenohumeral joint, tendon gaping is often seen with arm motion. This lifting up of the repaired tendon suggests that joint fluid can bathe the footprint area and raises concerns as to how robust the tendon-to-bone healing response will be.

The bone density of the greater tuberosity is another variable.[27] The anterior area of the greater tuberosity is denser than the posterior, and the more distal areas hold an anchor differently than more proximal. Anchor load-to-failure strength will vary according to the position of the anchor in the greater tuberosity, its position (depth) relative to the cortical surface, and how far it is inserted from the articular cartilage margin (the insertional footprint of the tendon).

4.8. Anchor Failure

There are many potential sources of failure in a tendon–suture–anchor–bone construct. The tissue (osteoporotic bone, degenerating tendon, or atrophic muscles with fatty infiltration)[28] may significantly compromise the long-term success of a repair. Any single step in the surgical technique (angle of anchor insertion, depth of anchor insertion, orientation of the eyelet, abrasion or damage to the suture, or knot security) may be a source of failure. The suture size, material, resistance to abrasion, type of knot used, and number of sutures in a single anchor may present problems. The rehabilitation protocol prescribed (and whether it is actually followed) may lead to poor results. Finally, the issues previously covered concerning the suture anchors (size, shape, material, and eyelet design) may be a source of failure. The surgeon must give each of these areas careful consideration and attention to achieve an ultimately successful outcome.

Probably the most common source of rotator cuff tendon repair failure is the tendon itself. Several authors feel that this is the most common mechanism.[13,29] There may be little that can be done to overcome this, but using knots that grasp the tendon more effectively and using multiple sutures that will distribute the holding forces across a larger area may be effective strategies to deal with this limitation. In addition, biodegradable anchors have the potential to fail at the eyelet, and different suture types may have a tendency to show less secure knot fixation.

The depth of anchor insertion has an effect on the mode of failure. It has been demonstrated that anchors with a deep placement failed from the suture cutting through the bone. These anchors are also likely to rotate and translate toward the cortex.[30,31] In contrast, anchors whose eyelet was slightly above the bone level (proud) failed by the suture breaking at the eyelet.[30]

4.9. Rehabilitation

The purpose of rehabilitation after a rotator cuff repair is to maintain motion and regain muscle strength while protecting the repair. The healing footprint of the tendon-to-bone repair requires several months to mature.

In reality, many patients do not follow the prescribed protocols and subject their repair to higher loads than is desirable. The fact that an arthroscopic rotator cuff repair causes very little postoperative pain contributes to this problem. Sometimes the patient returns to the clinic and proudly displays a considerable range of active shoulder motion far sooner than is desirable. In order to attempt to mitigate these events, the fixation system should be strong enough to tolerate functional loads even in the early postoperative course.

4.10. Current Anchor Developments

Consolidations in the industry and the introduction of newer, more effective designs have led to a decrease in the number of suture anchor models available. A review of recently released anchors reveals some trends. Most of the new anchors provide two sutures. The suture material options include both the conventional braided polyester and the newer, high-strength sutures. The addition of two sutures to the anchor is accomplished by either enlarging the existing eyelet or providing two suture eyelets. Both screw-in anchors and push-in anchors are still being developed, but the most commonly chosen material is biodegradable. PLLA suture anchors predominate.

The following list (in alphabetical order by manufacturer name) is by no means comprehensive and is not meant to serve as a recommendation of one anchor over another. Instead, these suture anchors are cataloged in an effort to offer the reader a better understanding of some of the newer anchors available that may be suitable for rotator cuff repair.

4.10.1. Arthrex (Naples FL)

Bio-Corkscrew™ (Figure 4.1): This is one of the anchors made from a copolymer of lactic acid (dextro and levo forms). This PDLLA material has a more rapid degradation than the standard PLLA. The eyelet is not made from a polymer but from a #4 braided polyester suture loop that is molded into the core body to create a unique suture eyelet that results in less suture–eyelet abrasion when tying the attached sutures. The load-to-failure strength of the anchor in cancellous bone is good. The Bio-Corkscrew™ is available with two braided polyester #2 sutures (1 green and 1 white), with two solid color #2 FiberWire® sutures, or with two #2 TigerTail® (FiberWire® with stripes) sutures. The anchor comes in two sizes: 5.0 and 6.5 mm.

Bio-Corkscrew™ FT (Figure 4.2): The Bio-Corkscrew™ FT (which stands for "fully threaded") is a 5.5-mm diameter bioabsorbable (PLLA)

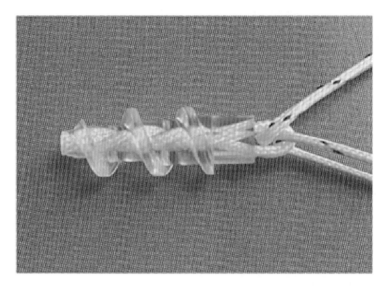

FIGURE 4.1. The Bio-Corkscrew™ is made from PDLLA and has a braided suture eyelet.

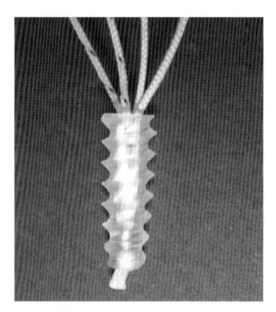

FIGURE 4.2. The Bio-Corkscrew™ FT is a PLLA, fully threaded anchor with a braided eyelet holding two FiberWire® sutures.

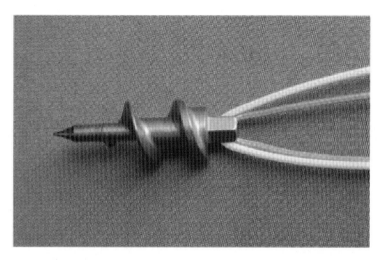

FIGURE 4.3. The Corkscrew™ II anchor is made of titanium and has two sutures.

suture anchor designed to be inserted flush with the cortical bone surface to maximize fixation strength and anchor stability. The Bio-Corkscrew™ FT has a FiberWire® eyelet recessed into the body of the anchor to reduce suture abrasion at the eyelet during knot tying. It comes preloaded with two #2 FiberWire®® sutures (one solid blue; one white with black Tiger-Tail suture).

Corkscrew II™ (Figure 4.3): This is the original titanium anchor revised to have two individual suture eyelets and is suitable for rotator cuff repair. It carries two sutures (either #2 FiberWire® or braided polyester). The anchor threads are widely spaced to work in cancellous bone, and the anchor is 5 mm in diameter. The anchor insertion shaft has a vertical laser mark on the distal part to indicate the suture eyelet orientation.

4.10.2. Arthrocare (Sunnyvale, CA)

Magnum™ knotless fixation implant: This is a metal anchor with a single #2 braided polyester suture. It is inserted into the bone in a closed configuration [Figure 4.4(A)], and, when deployed, the toggle opens to fix the anchor in the bone [Figure 4.4(B)]. It has a very high load-to-failure strength. The anchor's internal mechanism provides cinchable and reversible tension to allow adjustments to the single suture.

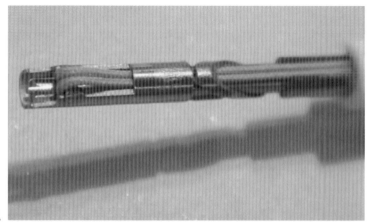

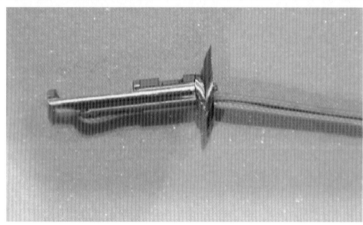

FIGURE 4.4. The MagnumBio-Corkscrew™ anchor (A) has a single suture, and toggles open (B) when deployed.

4.10.3. Depuy Mitek (Westwood, MA)

SpiraLok™ (Figure 4.5): This is a screw anchor with dual eyelets and two sutures. There are two separate suture eyelets on an eyelet shaft that are oriented at 90° to each other. The anchor is made from PLLA and has a blue color. The sutures available include braided polyester, Orthocord™ (composed of polydioxanone (PDS) and UHMW polyester), and Panacryl (an absorbable suture). It is available in 5.0 and 6.5 mm sizes.

Fastin RC (Figure 4.6): This is a metal screw-in anchor that holds two sutures through dual eyelets. This anchor is 5.0 mm in diameter and, because of the strength provided by its metal composition, has a small central core with deep screw threads that allow a very good load-to-failure strength and good fixation in the bone of the humeral head. The sutures

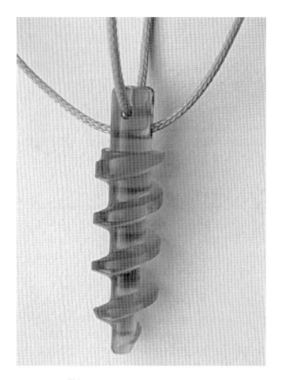

FIGURE 4.5. The SpiraLok™ anchor is made from PLLA and has two sutures in two separate eyelets.

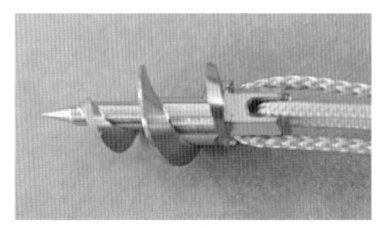

FIGURE 4.6. The Fastin RC is a metal anchor with two separate eyelets and two sutures.

available include #2 braided polyester, Orthocord™ (partially biodegradable), and Panacryl (a fully biodegradable suture).

4.10.4. Linvatec (Largo, FL)

Impact™ (Figure 4.7): This is an impaction, non-screw anchor that is white and made from SR-PDLLA (self-reinforced poly dextro (4%) levo (96%) lactide acid). It has two separate eyelets placed parallel to one another in the shaft of the anchor which maintain the ability to tie sliding knots. The proximal suture (white) must be tied first. It is 3.5mm in diameter and 10.5mm long. The sutures available are #2 braided polyester and #2 Herculine™ (the Linvatec version of Dynema).

Duet™: In contrast to the Impact™ anchor, the Duet™ (Figure 4.8) is a screw-in anchor made from the same SR-PDLLA as the Impact™ anchor. It holds two #2 Herculine™ or #2 braided polyester sutures through two separate eyelets that are in an eyelet shaft located above the screw threads. It is 6.0mm in diameter.

Super Revo®: This is a conventional titanium screw-in anchor that has been modified with a widened eyelet to hold two #2 Herculine™ or two #2 braided polyester sutures (Figure 4.9). These sutures share the same eyelet. If sliding knots are desired, careful attention should be given to eyelet position when anchor insertion is complete so one suture does not bind the other during knot tying. The anchor is 5.0mm in diameter. A three-suture version called the ThRevo™ anchor is also available.

4.10.5. Smith & Nephew Endoscopy (Andover, MA)

BioRaptor™ (Figure 4.10): This is a non-screw push-in anchor with a ribbed design. It is white and biodegradable (made of PLLA) and holds

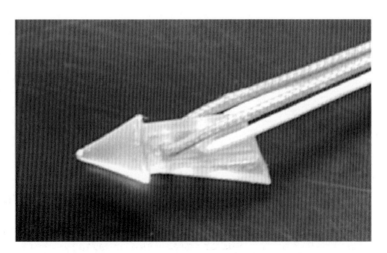

FIGURE 4.7. The Impact™ anchor is self-reinforced PDLLA [SR-PD(4)L(96)LA] and has two sutures that pass through separate eyelets in the anchor shaft.

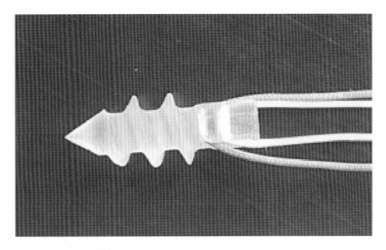

FIGURE 4.8. The Duet™ anchor is made from SR-PD(4)L(96)LA and holds two sutures in separate eyelets on a shaft above the screw threads.

two #2 braided polyester sutures. It also comes with either one or two #2 Ultrabraid® (Dynema–UHMW polyethylene) sutures. These sutures pass through a single eyelet that is positioned in the mid portion of the anchor, thus avoiding a superior stump above the ribs. It is narrower (3.7 mm) in diameter; this may limit its suitability for rotator cuff repair.

Twinfix™ AB (Figure 4.11): This screw-in anchor is white and made of PLLA. It accommodates two sutures through dual eyelets located toward

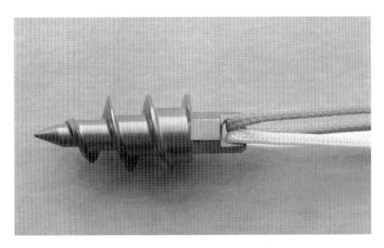

FIGURE 4.9. The Super Revo® anchor is titanium and comes with two sutures (TwoVo configuration) or three sutures (ThreeVo configuration) in an oversized eyelet.

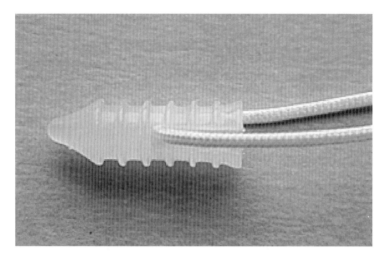

FIGURE 4.10. The BioRaptor™ is a PLLA anchor with two sutures in a single eyelet placed in the middle of the shaft of this push-in anchor.

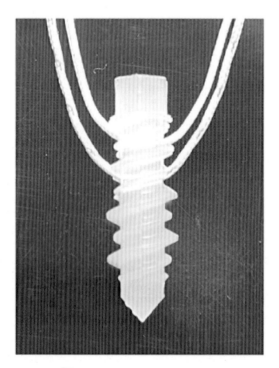

FIGURE 4.11. The Twinfix™ AB is made of PLLA and holds two sutures in dual eyelets that are located toward the upper portion of the screw.

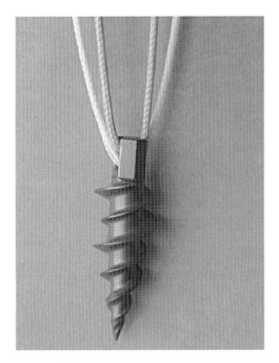

FIGURE 4.12. The Twinfix™ Ti is a titanium anchor that holds two sutures in a large eyelet at the top of the anchor.

the upper portion of the screw and not in a post at the top of the anchor. The sutures are made of #2 braided polyester. The anchor comes in 5.0- and 6.5-mm diameters.

Twinfix™ Ti (Figure 4.12): This titanium screw-in anchor comes pre-loaded with two #2 braided polyester sutures, or two #2 Ultrabraid® sutures (one white and one striped, called Cobraid). Ultrabraid® is the Smith & Nephew version of Dynema suture. The anchor is available in 5.0 and 6.5 mm diameters.

Twinfix™ Quick T (Figure 4.13): This anchor provides a single-step, transtendon tissue repair method that uses a pretied knot behind a T bar made of nonabsorbable polymer (plastic). The screw portion of the anchor is the Twinfix™ Ti titanium screw and is available with both 3.5- and 5.0-mm diameters. The T portion measures 10 mm×1.5 mm and has 4 spikes that are 0.1 mm in length. A single #2 braided polyester suture is attached to the anchor, and the second eyelet is empty. The pretied knot is advanced by a single lumen knot pusher to hold the tissue against the bone.

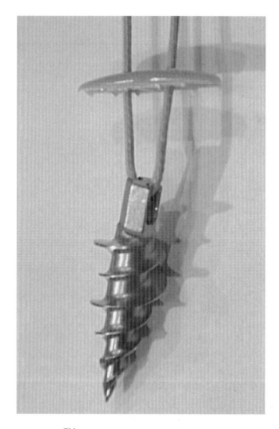

FIGURE 4.13. The Twinfix™ Quick T has a pretied knot behind a T bar made of nonabsorbable polymer (plastic) that is advanced by a knot pusher to hold the tissue against the bone.

4.10.6. Stryker Endoscopy (San Jose, CA)

BioZip™: This suture anchor is a white screw-in anchor that accommodates two #2 braided polyester or two #2 ForceFiber® (Stryker version of Dynema) sutures through two separate suture channels [Figure 4.14(A,B)]. These channels are located on opposite sides of the central shaft of the suture anchor. The anchor is made of PLLA and comes in 5.0 and 6.5mm sizes.

Our understanding of anchor mechanics is now focusing attention on eyelet friction during suture passing and knot tying. This has causes some surgeons to prefer nonsliding knots to slipknots. Winged anchor designs seem to be less effective.

While the concept of the deadman angle is clearly valid, its direct application to the humeral head does not provide the best insertion angle. When the anatomy of the older osteoporotic humeral head is considered,[32] placing

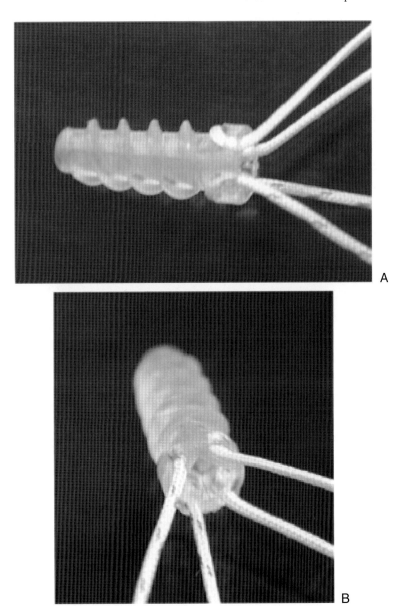

A

B

FIGURE 4.14. The BioZip™ is a PLLA anchor with sutures in two eyelets (A and B) on opposite sides of the anchor head.

the anchor at a 45° angle will plunge it into the central cavity, which has few trabeculae (Figure 4.15). A more acute angle is preferable (see arrow). Suture anchors that are inserted on the greater tuberosity should enter at an oblique angle to catch the dense subcortical bone.

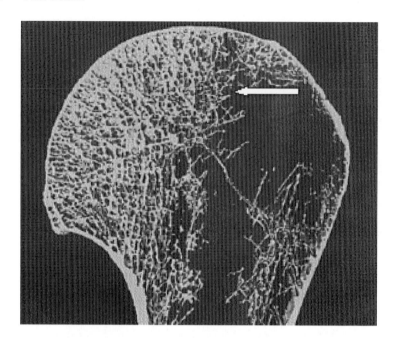

FIGURE 4.15. The insertion angle should place the anchor into the denser subchondral bone rather than into the more osteoporotic center of the humeral head. (Reprinted from DC Meyer et al., Association of osteopenia of the humeral head with full-thickness rotator cuff tears, J Shoulder Elbow Surg 2004;13:333–337 with permission from the Journal of Shoulder and Elbow Surgery Board of Trustees.)

References

1. Gerber C, Schneeberger AG, Beck M, Schlegel U. Mechanical strength of repairs of the rotator cuff. J Bone Joint Surg Br 1994;76:371–380.
2. Snyder SJ. Technique of arthroscopic rotator cuff repair using implantable 4-mm Revo suture anchors, suture Shuttle Relays, and no. 2 nonabsorbable mattress sutures. Orthop Clin North Am 1997;28:267–275.
3. Barber FA, Herbert MA, Click JN. The ultimate strength of suture anchors. Arthroscopy 1995;11:21–28.
4. Barber FA, Herbert MA, Click JN. Suture anchor strength revisited. Arthroscopy 1996;12:32–38.
5. Barber FA, Herbert MA, Click JN. Internal fixation strength of suture anchors — update 1997. Arthroscopy 1997;13:355–362.
6. Barber FA, Herbert MA. Suture anchors — update 1999. Arthroscopy 1999; 15:719–725.
7. Barber FA, Herbert MA, Richards DP. Sutures and suture anchors: update 2003. Arthroscopy 2003;19:985–990.
8. Harryman DT 2nd, Mack LA, Wang KY, Jackins SE, Richardson ML, Matsen FA 3rd. Repairs of the rotator cuff. Correlation of functional results with integrity of the cuff. J Bone Joint Surg Am 1991;73:982–989.

9. Burkhart SS, Johnson TC, Wirth MA, Athanasiou KA. Cyclic loading of transosseous rotator cuff repairs: tension overload as a possible cause of failure. Arthroscopy 1997;13:172–176.
10. Reed SC, Glossop N, Ogilvie-Harris DJ. Full-thickness rotator cuff tears. A biomechanical comparison of suture versus bone anchor techniques. Am J Sports Med 1996;24:46–48.
11. Richmond JC, Donaldson WR, Fu F, Harner CD. Modification of the Bankart reconstruction with a suture anchor. Report of a new technique. Am J Sports Med 1991;19:343–346.
12. Wolf EM. Arthroscopic capsulolabral repair using suture anchors. Orthop Clin North Am 1993;24:59–69.
13. Burkhart SS, Diaz Pagan JL, Wirth MA, Athanasiou KA. Cyclic loading of anchor-based rotator cuff repairs: confirmation of the tension overload phenomenon and comparison of suture anchor fixation with transosseous fixation. Arthroscopy 1997;13:720–724.
14. Meyer DC, Nyffeler RW, Fucentese SF, Gerber C. Failure of suture material at suture anchor eyelets. Arthroscopy 2002;18:1013–1019.
15. Rupp S, Georg T, Gauss C, Kohn D, Seil R. Fatigue testing of suture anchors. Am J Sports Med 2002;30:239–247.
16. Bardana DD, Burks RT, West JR, Greis PE. The effect of suture anchor design and orientation on suture abrasion: an in vitro study. Arthroscopy 2003;19: 274–281.
17. Burkhart SS. The deadman theory of suture anchors: observations along a south Texas fence line. Arthroscopy 1995;11:119–123.
18. Burkhart SS, Wirth MA, Simonich M, Salem D, Lanctot D, Athanasiou K. Knot security in simple sliding knots and its relationship to rotator cuff repair: how secure must the knot be? Arthroscopy 2000;16:202–207.
19. Pedowitz RA, Espinosa L, Abbi G, Odell R, Mahar A. Very strong sutures can still slip: evaluation of five knot types and two suture materials for shoulder arthroscopy. Arthroscopy 2004;20(suppl):E 21.
20. Burkhart SS, Danaceau SM, Pearce CE Jr. Arthroscopic rotator cuff repair: analysis of results by tear size and by repair technique-margin convergence versus direct tendon-to-bone repair. Arthroscopy 2001;17:905–912.
21. Tauro JC. Arthroscopic "interval slide" in the repair of large rotator cuff tears. Arthroscopy 1999;15:527–530.
22. Lo IK, Burkhart SS. Arthroscopic repair of massive, contracted, immobile rotator cuff tears using single and double interval slides: technique and preliminary results. Arthroscopy 2004;20:22–33.
23. Boileau P, Brassart N, Watkinson DJ, Carles M, Hatzidakis AM, Krishnan SG. Arthroscopic repair of full-thickness tears of the supraspinatus: does the tendon really heal? J Bone Joint Surg Am 2005;87:1229–1240.
24. Apreleva M, Ozbaydar M, Fitzgibbons PG, Warner JJ. Rotator cuff tears: the effect of the reconstruction method on three-dimensional repair site area. Arthroscopy 2002;18:519–526.
25. Millstein ES, Snyder SJ. Arthroscopic management of partial, full-thickness, and complex rotator cuff tears: indications, techniques, and complications. Arthroscopy 2003;19(suppl 1):189–199.
26. Snyder SJ. Arthroscopic cuff repair with suture shuttle. Paper presented at: 22nd Annual San Diego Shoulder meeting, La Jolla, CA, 2005.

27. Tingart MJ, Apreleva M, Lehtinen J, Zurakowski D, Warner JJ. Anchor design and bone mineral density affect the pull-out strength of suture anchors in rotator cuff repair: which anchors are best to use in patients with low bone quality? Am J Sports Med 2004;32:1466–1473.
28. Goutallier D, Postel JM, Bernageau J, Lavau L, Voisin MC. Fatty muscle degeneration in cuff ruptures. Pre- and postoperative evaluation by CT scan. Clin Orthop 1994;304:78–83.
29. Cummins CA, Strickland S, Appleyard RC, Szomor ZL, Marshall J, Murrell GA. Rotator cuff repair with bioabsorbable screws: an in vivo and ex vivo investigation. Arthroscopy 2003;19:239–248.
30. Bynum CK, Lee S, Mahar A, Tasto J, Pedowitz R. Failure mode of suture anchors as a function of insertion depth. Am J Sports Med 2005;33: 1030–1034.
31. Mahar A, Tucker B, Upasani V, Oka R, Pedowitz R. Failure mode of suture anchors as a function of insertion depth in human cadaver humeri. Arthroscopy 2004;20(suppl):E 22.
32. Meyer DC, Fucentese SF, Koller B, Gerber C. Association of osteopenia of the humeral head with full-thickness rotator cuff tears. J Shoulder Elbow Surg 2004;13:333–337.

5
Suture Management and Passage

Richard K.N. Ryu

As arthroscopic rotator cuff repair techniques become ubiquitous, mastering basic surgical steps is of paramount importance if satisfactory results are to be achieved on a consistent basis. We have learned that the critical steps in an arthroscopic rotator cuff repair consist of (1) appropriate portal placement for optimal viewing and for manipulation of tissue and equipment;[1,2] (2) tear pattern recognition, such that appropriate mobilization techniques are utilized to complete an anatomical repair without undue tension;[2] (3) rotator cuff mobilization, including supraglenoid release, subacromial space release, possible anterior interval release, or double interval release, to include the infraspinatus and supraspinatus junction;[3–5] (4) greater tuberosity preparation, in which the subchondral bone is not violated, accompanied by anchor insertion oriented at 45° to the long axis of the humerus, to maximize pullout strength;[6] (5) suture management and passage, either retrograde or antegrade, through the free edge of the tear or in a side-to-side pattern, in which tissue is captured and coapted without sacrificing pullout strength;[7,8] (6) deft knot tying such that loop and knot security are achieved while re-attaching the edge of the cuff tear to the anatomical footprint.[6]

This chapter deals specifically with suture passage and management encountered in the routine arthroscopic rotator cuff repair. After the first four steps listed above have been accomplished, the next challenge is to effectively pass suture through the rotator cuff in an effort to produce an effective and biomechanically favorable construct, permitting early passive range of motion during the biological healing process.

Two basic techniques are available when contemplating re-approximation of the free edge of the tear to the footprint on the greater tuberosity: the retrograde and the antegrade techniques. Each will be described in detail, including pertinent variations of the two techniques.

5.1. Retrograde Suturing

The retrograde approach can be achieved with a two-step suture hook-and-shuttle technique or with a retrograde penetrating device that is used to pierce the rotator cuff and grasp the appropriate suture limb, all in a single step.

The advantages of the retrograde approach are (1) the instruments are re-usable, thereby cutting costs significantly; (2) passage of the suture hook or penetrator/retriever does not require a separate cannula and, furthermore, can be accomplished percutaneously through a 3-mm mini-puncture wound from a variety of angles, as dictated by the tear pattern; (3) for delaminated tears with retraction of either the inferior or superior leaf, the retrograde technique permits a more proximal suture passage thereby capturing both leaves of a chronic delaminated tear that might otherwise be too medial for a "jawed" device.

The disadvantages include (1) an extra step is required to retrieve the suture shuttle before the limb can be passed through the tissue if the shuttle technique is employed; (2) grasping the suture limb by the penetrator–retriever can sometimes be difficult if an awkward angle is required. This can be solved with the extra step of "handing-off" the suture limb with a grasper through a separate portal in order to complete the sequence.

The sequence for a suture hook retrograde shuttle technique is simple. Utilizing percutaneous starting positions dictated by the tear pattern, the hollow suture hook (Spectrum[TM] Tissue Repair, Linvatec, Largo, FL), the tip of which can be changed to alter the angle of the instrument, is passed through the bursal surface of the tear, exiting the inferior free edge of the rotator cuff. A #1 polydioxanone (PDS) (Ethicon, Somerville, NJ) suture is threaded through the hollow portion of the suture hook and retrieved through a lateral cannula. Prior to passage of the suture hook, the sutures to be retrograded through the rotator cuff are segregated and kept separated within this same cannula. The #1 PDS suture is retrieved and a simple loop tied within the #1 PDS. One limb of the suture is then loaded into the loop; by simply retrograding the #1 PDS suture, the limb of the suture is pulled through the rotator cuff (Figure 5.1). Care should be taken to avoid tangling the suture tails, as crossed sutures between the anchor and the undersurface of the rotator cuff can compromise knot tying, especially sliding knots. If a vertical mattress suture configuration is desired, such as that used in double row fixation (Figure 5.2), the suture shuttle can be used to pass both suture limbs. If a simple stitch is required, only a single pass is necessary before tying is accomplished. With the retrograde suture shuttle technique, the sutures can be tied after each passage. This does not compromise the ability to retrograde the suture hook through the free edge of the rotator cuff tear. In actuality, anchoring of the rotator cuff facilitates subsequent suturing, as resistance to the passage of the suture hook allows greater precision. This is in contradistinction to the antegrade technique, in which tying of the sutures in serial fashion can compromise accessibility for the suturing device to the free edge of the rotator cuff tear.

As an example of a retrograde piercing/retriever-type device, an angled or straight Penetrator[TM] (Arthrex, Naples, FL) can be passed from an appropriate portal through the substance of the rotator cuff, exiting the free edge. At this time, if the suture limb is easily retrieved, the jaws of the

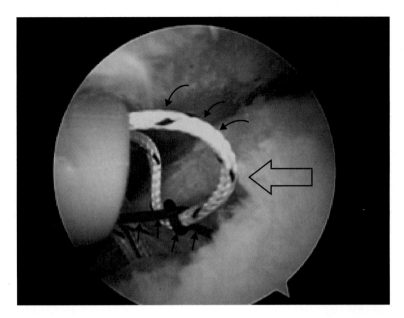

FIGURE 5.1. Suture limb retrograded through the cuff edge with #1 PDS shuttle. PDS shuttle (*small straight arrows*), suture limb (*curved arrows*), and cuff edge (*large arrow*).

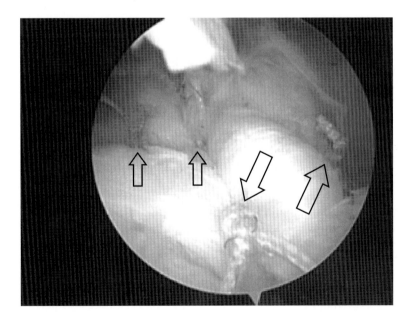

FIGURE 5.2. Proximal row of double row fixation requiring vertical mattress configuration and passage of both limbs of the suture. Vertical mattress suturing (*small arrows*) and simple stitch at the lateral end of double row fixation (*large arrows*).

Penetrator™ are opened, and the suture limb grasped and retrograded. If the angle of penetration is acute and if it is difficult to manipulate the Penetrator™ so that the suture limb can be easily captured, a grasping tool is introduced through a separate portal, delivering the suture to the Penetrator™. This maneuver can make the retrieval and subsequent retrograde passage much easier to accomplish without placing undue stress on the tissue and on any knots that may have already been tied.

5.2. Antegrade Suturing

Antegrade suturing, like the retrograde technique, can be accomplished with suture hooks and PDS suture shuttles passing the instruments lateral to medial and inferior to superior. Additionally, numerous ingenious antegrade suturing devices have been developed that permit suturing in a fashion similar to what a surgeon would do in a mini-open technique, namely passing a needle with suture attached through the bottom or top of the free edge of the tear.

The advantages of the antegrade technique include (1) it is ergonomically desirable as the suturing action mimics the open approach, passing suture from lateral to medial; (2) it is possible to create an oblique mattress suture with a single pass using a dual parallel long-needle instrument (OPUS ArthroCare, Austin, TX) and improving suture pullout strength; and (3) current instrumentation is designed for a single pass, obviating the need for a suture shuttle, and streamlining the process by eliminating a step.

The disadvantages of the antegrade technique are (1) if a long-needle instrument is utilized, opening the jaw of the instrument can be difficult if the tear is lateral, and the cannula must be withdrawn. Soft tissue interposition can occur making suture management difficult. (2) For complex tears with delamination, the jaws of the instrument may limit the medial reach of the suture, necessitating a separate step to stabilize the delaminated portions of the tear.

Several commercially available devices use the so-called long-needle technique. Some of these devices are preloaded; others allow you to load the suture limb onto the tip of the device, e.g., the Scorpion™ (Arthrex), after the suture anchors have been inserted. The jaws of the Scorpion™ and similar devices usually measure between 15 and 20mm in depth, and are opened once past the edge of the lateral cannula. The inferior portion of the jaw is then placed under the free edge of the tear (Figure 5.3). The Scorpion™ is manipulated so that an appropriate bite is created; by squeezing the handle, the long needle is passed through the tip of the instrument, piercing the suture material and pulling it through the superior surface of the rotator cuff tear proximal to the torn edge (Figure 5.4). The use of FiberWire® (Arthrex) or its equivalent is of critical importance with this technique because the suture must withstand the tip of the long needle without completely severing. The instrument can then be withdrawn and used to grasp

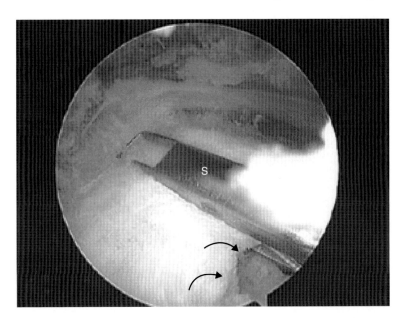

FIGURE 5.3. Scorpion™ (Arthrex) antegrade instrument taking "bite" of rotator cuff tear prior to long needle deployment. Cuff edge (*curved arrows*), Scorpion™ (S).

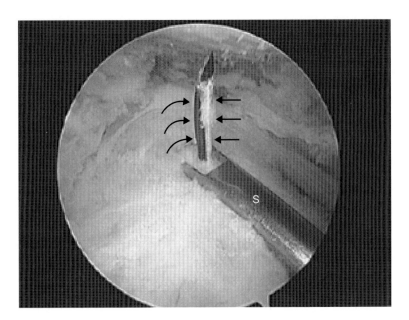

FIGURE 5.4. Long needle deployed through the rotator cuff. FiberWire® (Arthrex) suture (*small straight arrows*), long-needle tip (*curved arrows*), and Scorpion™ (Arthrex) (S).

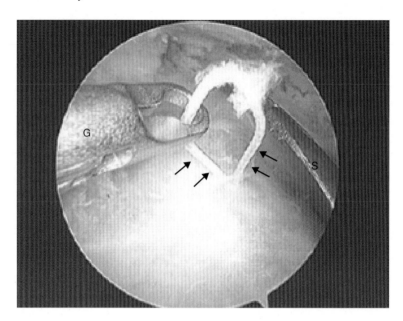

FIGURE 5.5. Frayed suture limb retrieved with grasping tool from separate portal. Suture limb (*small arrows*), grasping tool (G), and Scorpion™ (Arthrex) (S).

the passed suture, delivering the suture through the same cannula. Alternatively, through a separate cannula, the suture can be retrieved (Figure 5.5) and in a second step, re-introduced into the appropriate cannula for tying knots. If all of the anchors are placed, and the suture pairs segregated in a separate cannula, use of the Scorpion™ provides for a simple and efficient means of passing sutures quickly and reliably through the substance of the rotator cuff. Because the mobility of the free edge of the tear can be compromised by the early tying of sutures, it is recommended that once the sutures have been delivered through the cuff that the matched pairs are not tied but rather placed in a separate cannula and then tied in sequence once all of the suturing has been completed. The benefit of using sutures that are color coded or identified via a different pattern is clear when determining the order of knot tying.

As noted above, the drawbacks to these antegrade instruments include the necessity of using a separate cannula and of ensuring that the cannula conforms to the shape and design of the Scorpion™ or like devices so that the instrument can be opened without soft tissue entanglement. Often the cannula must be withdrawn far laterally for the jaws to open maximally, and concern for entrapping soft tissue during suture passage is present. Another potential liability is the inability to handle retracted delaminated rotator cuff tears. Although it is possible to place a stitch in advance through the retracted leaf and to utilize this traction stitch when the antegrade long-needle passage is being accomplished, this additional step can be cumbersome. The retrograde suture shuttle technique permits simultaneous passage and treatment of the retracted leaf.

The antegrade technique can also be performed with a suture hook and PDS suture beginning at the free end of the tear and piercing lateral to medial. Use of a separate portal through which a grasper is applied to the free edge of the tear is often necessary in order to generate enough tissue tension so that the suture hook can be passed through the cuff edge without the tissue moving away from the pressure (Figure 5.6). The steps remain essentially the same as PDS suture is used as a shuttle to pull the suture through the substance of the cuff. The proximal end of the PDS suture, as it exits the more medial portion of the rotator cuff, is retrieved through any free portal and is simply pulled to draw the appropriate loaded suture limb through the cuff in an antegrade fashion.

In this age of increasing cost awareness combined with the desire to optimize patient care and outcome, the cost of the various implants, as well as those instruments specifically designed for suture passage, must be considered. The retrograde technique, which uses hollow suture hooks or nondisposable penetrator–retrievers, offers the greatest cost containment in that the instruments are reusable, requiring only occasional sharpening.

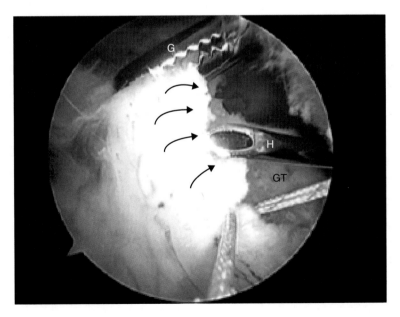

FIGURE 5.6. Antegrade suturing with suture hook. Grasper stabilizes cuff edge to permit efficient tissue piercing. Cuff edge (*curved arrows*), grasping tool (G), suture hook (H), and greater tuberosity (GT).

The antegrade long-needle devices do have a fixed cost per usage and are intended as disposable items. These considerations may be a factor in selecting the technique with which you are most comfortable and which gives you the greatest likelihood of a satisfactory surgical outcome. Clearly, clinical and practical judgment will determine the technique used and the associated costs.

5.3. Side–Side Suturing

When faced with a side-to-side repair in a retracted L-shaped tear, repairing the tendon to bone before addressing the side-to-side suturing pattern can provide tear stability and permit a more anatomical approximation of the side-to-side repair. In some situations, such as a large retracted U-shaped tear, an initial side-to-side margin convergence repair is mandatory in order to converge the free edge of the tear to the greater tuberosity for bony fixation [Figure 5.7(A–C)]. There are two basic techniques available for side-to-side cuff suturing. In some tears, the use of a simple crescent-shaped suture hook (Spectrum™, Linvatec) is sufficient. Working through a cannula, the suture hook is simply passed either anterior to posterior or posterior to anterior, capturing tissue on both sides of the defect beginning proximally and working towards the greater tuberosity. Even in large, retracted tears, in which single suture hook passage seems unlikely, side-to-side suturing with a single pass of the suture hook, facilitated by placing a grasping instrument through a pre-existing portal and stabilizing one side of the side-to-side tear, can be readily accomplished [Figure 5.8(A,B)]. The sutures are tied in sequence, and the additional stability provided by early knot tying allows for expedited side-to-side suturing as the tear pattern becomes more stable. Once the margin is converged to the greater tuberosity, anchoring of the cuff to bone is easily accomplished without undue tension on the repair [Figure 5.9(A,B)].

Another technique which can be employed when the side-to-side gap is too great and a single device cannot bridge the gap effectively, consists of a suture "hand-off." A loaded piercing device is passed through one side of the tear, and the suture is delivered into the gap. Through a portal on the opposite side, a Penetrator™ (Arthrex) is passed and the suture is captured and retrograded, completing the suture passage through the far side of the tear [Figure 5.10(A,B)].

FIGURE 5.7. (A) Large, retracted U-shaped tear viewing from lateral portal. Retracted cuff edge (*arrows*), glenoid (G), and greater tuberosity (GT). (B) Side-to-side suturing with suture hook viewed from lateral portal. Cuff edge (*arrows*), suture hook (H), and acromion (A). (C) Margin convergence accomplished as cuff edge is converged to the greater tuberosity with side-to-side sutures. Converging cuff edge (*dotted line*) and greater tuberosity (GT).

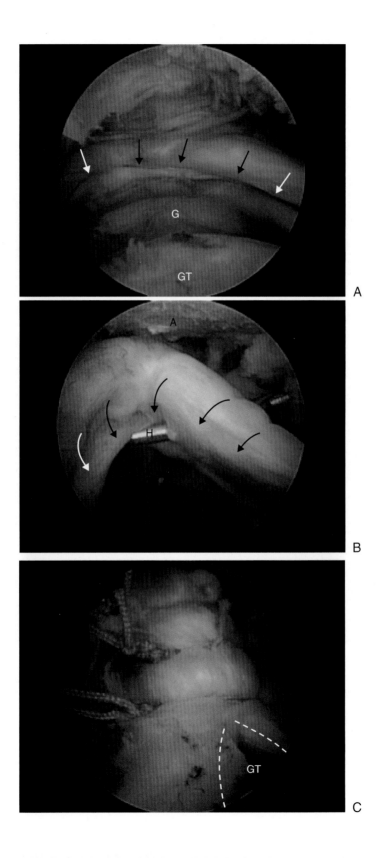

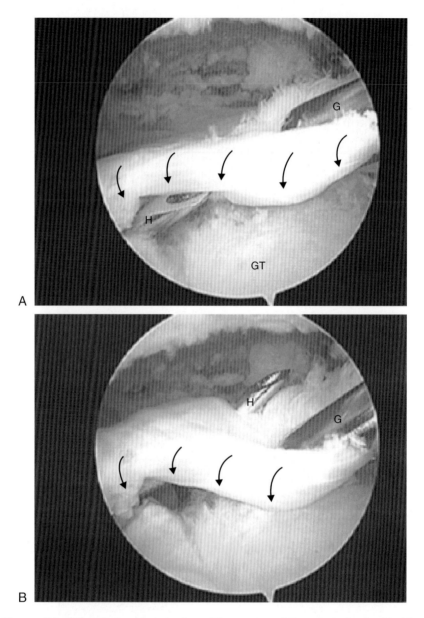

FIGURE 5.8. (A) Side-to-side suturing with passage of the suture hook aided by grasper stabilizing far side of the gapping tear. Cuff edge (*arrows*), grasping tool (G), suture hook (H), and greater tuberosity (GT). (B) Suture hook piercing far side of tear; the suture hook is delivered by the grasper. Cuff edge (*arrows*), grasping tool (G), and suture hook (H).

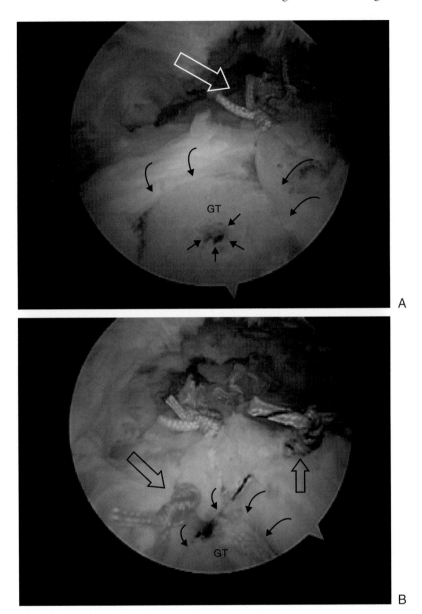

FIGURE 5.9. (A) Margin of the cuff tear converged to the greater tuberosity. Side–side sutures (*large arrow*), converged cuff edge (*curved arrows*), anchor target hole (*straight arrows*), and greater tuberosity (GT). (B) Tear repair completed with cuff-edge-to-bone fixation. Suture limbs from the anchor (*large arrows*), cuff edge (*curved arrows*), and greater tuberosity (GT).

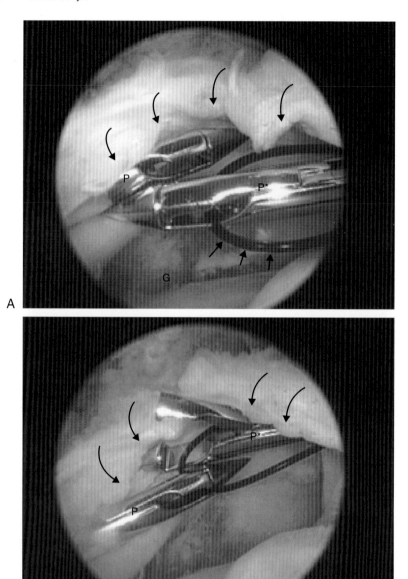

FIGURE 5.10. (A) Loaded Penetrator™ (Arthrex; P*) set to hand-off PDS suture (*straight arrows*) to second Penetrator™ (P). Cuff edge (*curved arrows*) and glenoid (G). (B) Hand-off completed as suture transferred from Penetrator™ (P*) to Penetrator™ (P). Cuff edge (*curved arrows*).

5.4. Conclusions

Once sutures have been effectively retrograded or antegraded through the free edge of the tear, all side-to-side elements of the tear addressed, and all remaining knots securely tied, an anatomical repair should be present. As the shoulder is taken through a range of motion, no undue tension at the repair site should be present. If a decompression accompanied the rotator cuff repair, visual confirmation of satisfactory clearance as the shoulder is taken through a range of motion should also be verified. Meticulous attention to surgical detail combined with practicing the suture management and passage techniques described should lead to consistently satisfying results with arthroscopic rotator cuff repair.

References

1. Bennett W. Arthroscopic repair of full-thickness supraspinatus tears (small to medium): a prospective study with 2 to 4 year follow-up. Arthroscopy 2003; 19:249–256.
2. Gartsman GM, Khan M, Hammerman SM. Arthroscopic repair of full thickness tears of the rotator cuff. J Bone Joint Surg 1998;80:832–840.
3. Jones C, Savoie F. Arthroscopic repair of large and massive rotator cuff tears. Arthroscopy 2003;19:564–571.
4. Tauro J.C. Arthroscopic rotator cuff repair: analysis of technique and results at 2 and 3 year follow-up. Arthroscopy 1998;14:45–51.
5. Lo IK, Burkhart SS. Arthroscopic repair of massive, contracted, immobile rotator cuff tears using single and double interval slides: technique and preliminary results. Arthroscopy 2004;20:22–33.
6. Lo IK, Burkhart SS. Current concepts in arthroscopic rotator cuff repair. Am J Sports Med 2003;31:308–324.
7. Murray TF, Lajtai G, Mileski RM, et al. Arthroscopic repair of medium to large full-thickness tears: outcome at 2-to-6 year follow-up. J Shoulder Elbow Surg 2002;11:19–24.
8. Burkhart SS, Athanasiou KA, Wirth MA. Margin convergence: a method of reducing strain in massive rotator cuff tears. Arthroscopy 1996;12:335–338.

6
Arthroscopic Knot Tying

Ian K.Y. Lo

Routine and reproducible arthroscopic knot tying remains one of the most difficult skills for the novice arthroscopist to master when creating a stable rotator cuff repair construct. Despite recent advances in both suture welding and knotless anchor technology, arthroscopic knot tying still remains the most popular method of fixation when performing suture anchor–based shoulder reconstructions. Unlike open shoulder surgery techniques, arthroscopic knots are generally formed outside the joint with the suture already passed through the anchoring device and tissue to be repaired. Unfortunately, an endless number of combinations of knots (sliding vs. static, simple vs. complex, etc.) can accomplish this task. This further complicates an already confusing topic.

6.1. Knot Definitions

When tying an arthroscopic knot there are two limbs of the suture: the *post limb* and the *wrapping limb*. The post limb is the straight portion of the suture; this limb is purely defined as the suture limb that is under the most tension. Because arthroscopic knots are tied outside the body, they are generally slid along the long straight post limb. The wrapping limb is the free portion of the suture that wraps around the post limb, creating the knot.

For a knot to be effective, it must possess both knot security and loop security. Knot security is defined as the effectiveness of the knot at resisting slippage when load is applied and depends on three factors: friction, internal interference, and slack between throws.

Friction is greater for a knot tied with braided multifilament suture than for comparable knots tied with monofilament suture. Internal interference refers to the complex weave of the two suture limbs relative to one another and can be increased by increasing the complexity of the weave and increasing the length of contact between the suture limbs. Slack between throws decreases knot security. Slack between throws can be decreased by remov-

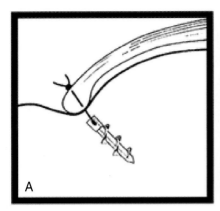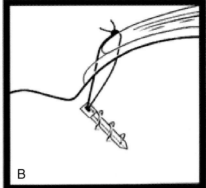

FIGURE 6.1. Loop security. (A) A tight suture loop holds the soft tissue tightly apposed to the prepared bone bed. (B) A loose loop allows the soft tissue to pull away from the prepared bone bed, regardless of how securely the knot may be tied. (Reprinted from Burkhart SS, et al., Loop security as a determinant of tissue fixation security, Arthroscopy 1998;14:773–776, with permission from The Arthroscopy Association of North America.)

ing any twists between the two suture limbs prior to seating a half hitch and by past pointing. Loop security is the ability to maintain a tight suture loop as a knot is tied.[1,2] Thus, it is possible for any tied knot to have good knot security but poor loop security (e.g., a loose suture loop) and therefore be ineffective in approximating the tissue edges to be repaired, creating an unstable construct (Figure 6.1).

6.2. Knots To Know

There are two general situations the arthroscopist may encounter when tying an arthroscopic knot, based on whether the suture can or cannot freely slide through the anchoring device and tissue. When the suture can freely slide, a sliding knot may be used. Sliding knots are advantageous because the complete knot is tied extracorporeally, and the knot can be slid down the post limb without unraveling or jamming prematurely. Commonly used sliding knots include the Duncan loop, Tennessee slider, Nicky's knot, Roeder knot, SMC knot, and the Weston knot (Figure 6.2).

When the suture does not slide through the tissue and anchoring device, only a static (or nonsliding knot) may be used. Nonsliding knots are generally formed from a stack of half hitches. The most commonly used nonsliding knots are the Revo knot, as popularized by Snyder, and the surgeon's knot (Figure 6.3).[3]

Although a multitude of arthroscopic knots are described, the arthroscopist needs to know only two knots: one static and one sliding knot. In

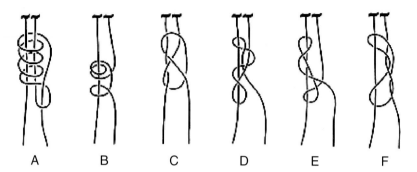

FIGURE 6.2. Commonly used sliding knots. (A) Duncan loop. (B) Nicky's knot. (C) Tennessee slider. (D) Roeder knot. (E) SMC knot. (F) Weston knot. (Reprinted from Lo IK, et al., Arthroscopic knots: determining the optimal balance of loop security and knot security, Arthroscopy 2004;20:478–502, by permission of The Arthroscopy Association of North America.)

fact, if preferred, a surgeon's knot may be tied in both situations (meaning only one knot is necessary to master) because tying a static knot is as effective in both situations (when using a double diameter knot pusher, see below) and avoids the theoretical disadvantages of suture abrasion, anchor abrasion, or damaging the soft tissue. However, when tying a sliding knot I prefer the Roeder knot because it provides the maximum loop security and knot security compared to other commonly used arthroscopic knots.[3]

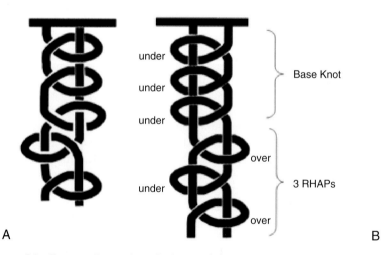

FIGURE 6.3. Commonly used static knots. (A) Revo knot. (B) Surgeon's knot. RHAPs, reversing half hitches on alternating posts. (From Lo IKY. Essential principle of tying secure arthroscopic knots. In: The Handbook of the 23rd Fall Course of The Arthroscopy Association of North America. Reprinted with permission.)

6.3. Tying a Surgeon's Knot (Static Knot)

The surgeon's knot consists of a base knot of three half hitches in the same direction and on the same post followed by three reversing half hitches on alternating posts [Figure 6.3(B)]. There are two basic types of half hitches (i.e., under/over, over/under) which are named according to the position of the wrapping limb relative to the post limb as viewed by the surgeon during knot tying (Figure 6.4). When tying a surgeon's knot, the first three half hitches can be either three over/under or three under/over half hitches. Because the first three half hitches are in the same direction, they will not lock; this actually acts similar to a sliding knot.

However, for the next three throws (i.e., half hitches four, five, and six) the direction of the half hitch is changed (called *reversing the half-hitch*, e.g., over/under to under/over), and the post is changed (called *alternating the post*, i.e., tying the half hitch on the opposite post) for each successive throw. This creates the most convoluted suture weave possible, maximizing internal interference and, therefore, knot security.

One method of reversing the half hitch and alternating the post is to rethread the knot pusher after each throw and reverse the half hitch. However, this can be a time-consuming process. A much quicker way to perform this exercise is to reverse the half hitch and alternate the post by tensioning the wrapping limb.[4] To perform this, after placing a base knot (either a sliding knot or a series of half hitches), the next half hitch is advanced down the post limb [Figure 6.5(A)]. As the half hitch approaches the knot, the post limb is relaxed and the wrapping limb is pulled, flipping the knot [Figure 6.5(B)]. This alternates the post and reverses the half hitch. The half hitch is then past pointed to tighten the knot [Figure 6.5(C)]. Practically speaking, when tying a static surgeon's knot, six half hitches are thrown extracorporeally all in the same direction (i.e., all under/over or all over/under). However, when advancing the half hitch down into the joint, half hitch four and six are flipped to create the reversing half hitches and alternating post sequence.

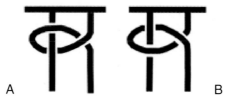

A   B

FIGURE   6.4. Half   hitch   configurations.   (A)   Under/over.   (B)   Over/under. (From Lo IKY. Essential Principle of Tying Secure Arthroscopic Knots. In: The Handbook of the 23rd Fall Course of The Arthroscopy Association of North America. Reprinted with permission.)

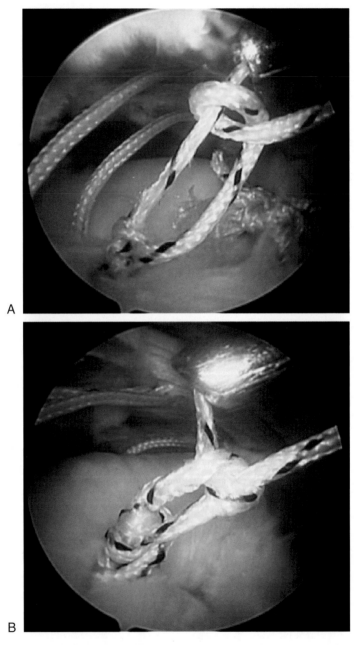

FIGURE 6.5. Arthroscopic photograph through a posterior portal demonstrating reversing the half hitch and alternating the post by tensioning the wrapping limb. (A) The half hitch is advanced down the post limb, approaching the base knot. (B) The wrapping limb is then tensioned, which reverses the half hitch and alternates the post. (C) The half hitch is then tightened by past pointing.

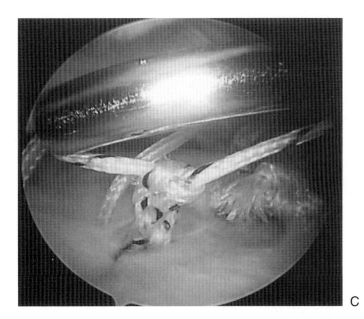

C

FIGURE 6.5. *Continued*

6.3.1. Tying a Surgeon's Knot with a Double Diameter Knot Pusher

The difficulty when tying a surgeon's knot or stacked half hitches is that when using a standard single diameter knot pusher the first half hitch has a tendency to unravel while the second half hitch is being thrown [Figure 6.6(A)]. This can be particularly concerning if the second half hitch is on the opposite post because the knot may lock prematurely, resulting in a loose loop and loss of loop security [Figure 6.6(B)].

To eliminate this potential problem, tying stacked half hitches may be performed using a double diameter knot pusher (Surgeon's Sixth Finger™, Arthrex, Naples, FL). This instrument is composed of an inner metal knot pusher and an outer plastic sleeve (Figure 6.7). When using this instrument to tie half hitches, the suture (usually the suture limb on the tissue side) is fed through the cannulated inner metal knot pusher and out the proximal portion of the instrument. Any excess suture is wrapped around the fingers of one hand to apply alternating tension when tying the knot [Figure 6.8(A)]. The free hand is used to place successive half hitches around the knot pusher. With this knot pusher, the outer plastic sleeve is used to push the half hitch into the joint. However, after the initial half hitch has been placed, the inner metal knot pusher is used to hold the first half hitch in place as subsequent half

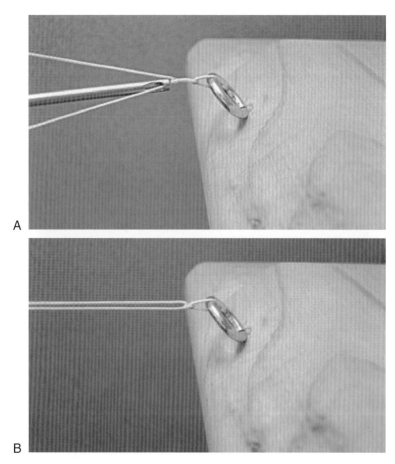

A

B

FIGURE 6.6. Clinical photograph demonstrating a series half hitches tied with a single diameter knot pusher. (A) As the second half hitch is being thrown, the first half hitch has a tendency to unravel and back off. (B) A second locking half hitch may prematurely lock the knot, resulting in a loose loop and loss of loop security.

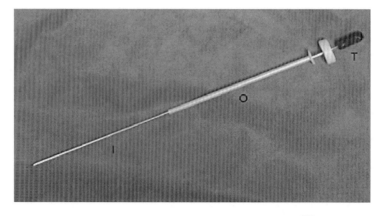

FIGURE 6.7. Clinical photograph of the Surgeon's Sixth Finger™ double diameter knot pusher. Note the inner metal knot pusher (I) with an outer plastic sleeve (O). The suture threader (T) is used to pass the suture limb through the cannulated inner metallic tube.

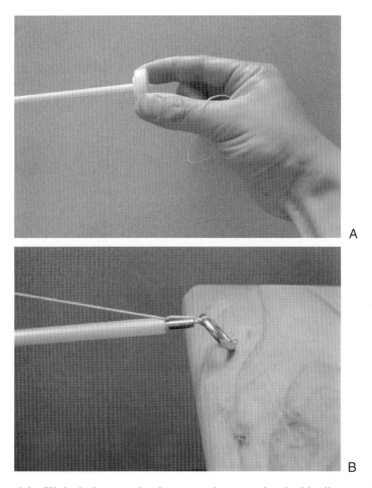

FIGURE 6.8. Clinical photographs demonstrating use of a double diameter knot pusher. (A) The suture is fed through the cannulated inner metal cannula and out the proximal portion of the knot pusher. Excess suture is wrapped around the fingers of one hand to apply and release tension. (B) As the plastic sleeve is used to push successive half hitches down the inner metal knot pusher, the inner metal knot pusher is used to hold the initial half hitches securely. This ensures a tight loop and maximizes loop security.

hitches are thrown and pushed into the joint using the outer plastic sleeve [Figure 6.8(B)]. In addition, to remove twists using the Surgeon's Sixth Finger™, the outer plastic sleeve is rotated so that the knot will lie flat (Figure 6.9). Thus, the use of the Surgeon's Sixth Finger™ maximizes loop security and knot security when tying a surgeon's knot or stacked half hitches.

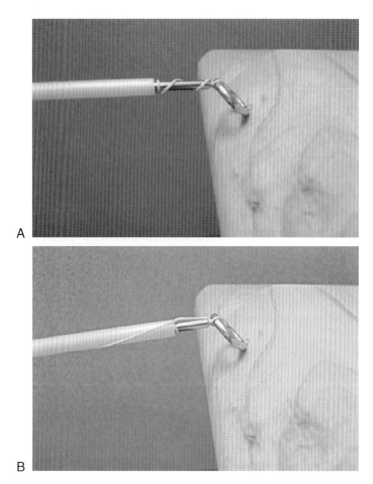

A

B

FIGURE 6.9. Clinical photograph demonstrating untwisting of the half hitch using the outer plastic sleeve of a double diameter knot pusher. (A) Twisted. (B) Untwisted.

6.4. Tying the Roeder Knot (Sliding Knot)

The Roeder knot is a complex, locking sliding knot. The Roeder knot is formed by throwing the first loop around the post strand only, the second loop around both limbs, and the third loop around only the post limb [Figure 6.10(A)]. The tail of the wrapping limb is then passed between the two parallel strands between the second and third loops [Figure 6.10(B)]. The knot is seated and then slid into the joint by simultaneously pushing on the knot and pulling on the post limb [Figure 6.10(C)]. Once seated, the knot is then locked.

Locking is performed by pulling on the wrapping limb, which kinks the post and prevents it from backing off back with subsequent loss of loop

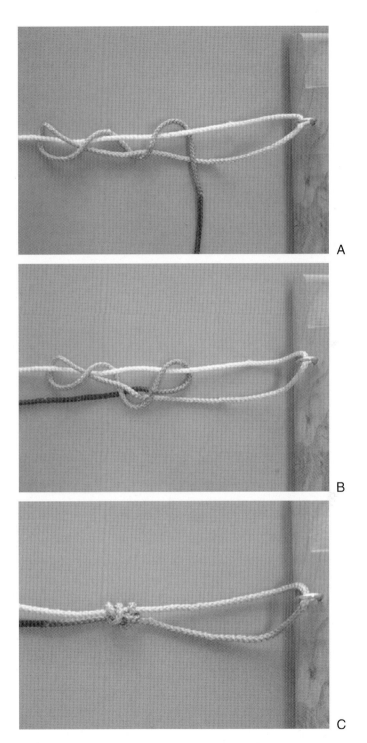

FIGURE 6.10. Roeder knot. (A) The Roeder knot is formed by throwing the first loop around the post strand only, the second loop around both limbs, and the third loop around the post limb only. (B) The tail of the wrapping limb is then passed between the two parallel strands and between the second and third loops. (C) The knot is then slid down the post limb and seated.

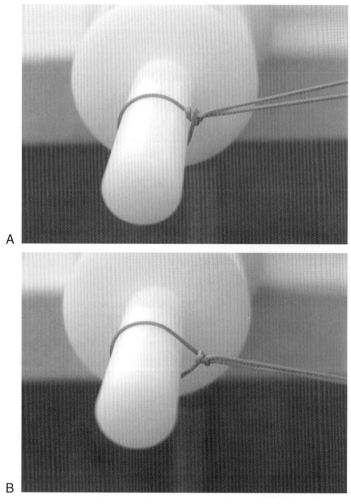

A

B

FIGURE 6.11. Expansion of the suture loop with locking of the sliding knot. (A) A Nicky's knot has been tied to a 30-mm circumferential post and close apposition of the suture to the post is demonstrated. (B) Locking the knot by tensioning the wrapping limb flips the knot and prevents the knot from slipping backwards, but also enlarges the suture loop. Note how the suture loop is pulled away from the 30-mm circumferential post. (Reprinted from Lo, IK. Arthroscopic knots: determining the optimal balance of loop security and knot security, Arthroscopy 2004;20: 489–502, with permission from The Arthroscopy Association of North America.)

security. However, when performing this maneuver one must be careful to not cause expansion of the suture loop (Figure 6.11). This effect can be seen in almost all the sliding knots, which require a flipping maneuver to lock. To minimize this effect, a knot pusher can be used to apply counter pressure to prevent the knot from backing off when locking the knot [Figure 6.12(A)]. After placing the Roeder knot, all knots are backed up

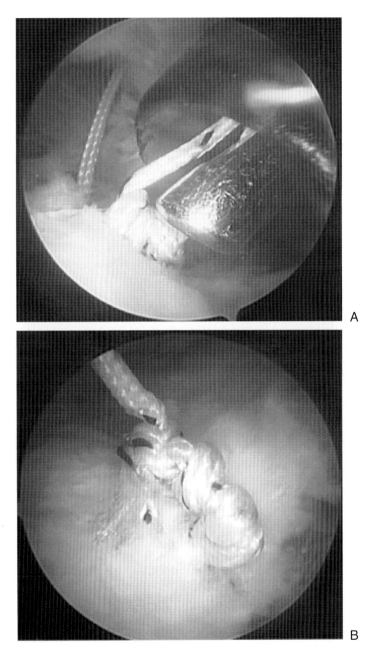

FIGURE 6.12. (A) Arthroscopic view through a posterior subacromial portal demonstrating locking of the Roeder knot. The wrapping limb is pulled while applying counter pressure with the knot pusher. (B) Arthroscopic view through a lateral subacromial portal demonstrating a Roeder knot secured with three reversing half hitches on alternating posts.

by three reversing half hitches and alternating posts, which maximizes knot security and loop security [Figure 6.12(B)].

When tying a sliding knot, the post should be kept short and the wrapping limb seen extracorporeally should be kept approximately half the total length of the suture. This is so that the two limbs will be of approximately equal length when the sliding knot is delivered into the joint. This occurs because, as the knot slides into the joint, the knot takes the wrapping limb into the joint with it, shortening it, while the post limb lengthens.

6.5. Practical Tips When Tying an Arthroscopic Knot

1. **Dry Land Training.** It is important to become completely facile with arthroscopic knot tying in the laboratory prior to attempting arthroscopic knot tying. Tying an arthroscopic knot should become the easiest and quickest part of any arthroscopic reconstruction and not a source of anxiety.

2. **Visualization.** Visualization is a key component for successful arthroscopic knot tying. This is particularly important to maximize knot security and loop security during arthroscopic knot tying by untwisting loops and ensuring there is no inadvertent soft tissue interposition.

3. **Cannula Use.** Arthroscopic knots should be tied through a cannula and should be placed directly over or close to the area to be tied. An assistant should stabilize the cannula in line with the sutures to ensure there is no inadvertent soft tissue interposition or abrasion of the suture against the cannula. Clear cannulas are very helpful during knot tying, particularly when swelling is extreme. In these cases, knot tying can be completely performed within the cannula itself. Only one pair of sutures should be in the cannula at a time during knot tying. Other suture pairs should be held separately in a temporary holding portal.

4. **Retrieving Sutures.** When retrieving sutures, many of the suture limbs may be overlapped and twisted upon one another. However, one can untangle the limb and retrieve the suture all in one simple step. The key is to retrieve the suture as close to its exit as possible. To minimize entanglement or entrapment of other sutures, you must perform the retrieval by retrieving both suture limbs simultaneously and grabbing the suture limbs as close to their exit point as possible. During rotator cuff repair, one limb should be grabbed as close to the anchor as possible and then other suture limb should be grabbed as it exits the rotator cuff without crossing over any other sutures. When the suture is then retrieved

through a cannula, this creates an unobstructed pathway for subsequent knot tying.

5. **Finding the Lost Suture.** Occasionally, when there is a "jungle" of sutures in the glenohumeral or subacromial space, it can be difficult to determine which suture limbs match each other. The easiest way to match sutures is to first retrieve one limb. There is usually one limb that is always easily seen (usually the suture limb on the anchor side) and can be retrieved safely. To identify the matching suture limb, the retrieved suture is then pulled, allowing a small amount of the suture to run through the anchor eyelet. However, this will also pull on the matching limb and one can then identify and retrieve the suture limb that has moved.

Furthermore, when swelling becomes significant particularly in the subacromial space, the bursa may completely obstruct the visualization of suture limbs. In this situation, one can use a single diameter knot pusher to push the suture into the subacromial space into an area where it is visible and can be retrieved. When performing this maneuver, it is important to attempt to reproduce the same angle of approach and to use the same soft tissue tunnel. If the same angle of approach or the same soft tissue tunnel is not used, then a bridge of tissue may become trapped within the suture loop. This will bind the deltoid/deltoid fascia against the rotator cuff. If this occurs, it is important to recognize and debride the intervening soft tissue bridge.

6. **Determining Suture Sliding.** Once the suture pair has been retrieved, it is important to determine if the suture slides freely through the anchor and tissue. If the suture does not slide freely through the anchor and tissue, then a static knot (e.g., surgeon's knot) should be tied. If the suture slides freely through the anchor, then a sliding knot (e.g., Roeder knot) or, alternatively, a static knot can be tied.

7. **Unraveling the Twists.** Prior to tying the knot, the suture limbs must not be crossed inside the cannula. This can lead to loss of both knot security and loop security. To remove the twists between the suture limbs, a single diameter knot pusher is advanced down either limb of the suture into the joint and the twists are removed. The suture limbs are then separated as they exit the cannula, and a finger is used to separate the limbs during tying of a complex sliding knot (Figure 6.13). A hemostat may then be clamped on the post limb, which is usually chosen as the limb that is on the tissue side of the repair construct.

When using a double diameter knot pusher, untwisting the suture limbs prior to tying the surgeon's knot is usually not necessary because the twists may be removed during tying by rotating the outer plastic sleeve (Figure 6.9).

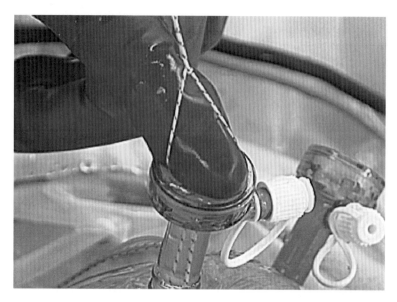

FIGURE 6.13. Clinical photograph demonstrating separation of the suture limbs using a finger during tying of a complex sliding knot.

6.6. Conclusions

Tying an effective arthroscopic knot remains a necessary and fundamental skill to master for performing arthroscopic rotator cuff repair. Adherence to the principles outlined in this chapter will aid the arthroscopist in mastering this skill expeditiously and transforming a seemly demanding process into a routine and rapid step in obtaining a stable repair construct.

References

1. Burkhart SS, Wirth MA, Simonich M, Salem D, Lanctot D, Athanasiou K. Knot security in simple sliding knots and its relationship to rotator cuff repair: how secure must the knot be? Arthroscopy 2000;16:202–207.
2. Burkhart SS, Wirth MA, Simonich M, Salem D, Lanctot D, Athanasiou K. Loop security as a determinant of tissue fixation security. Arthroscopy 1998;14:773–776.
3. Lo IK, Burkhart SS, Chan KC, Athanasiou K. Arthroscopic knots: determining the optimal balance of loop security and knot security. Arthroscopy 2004;20: 489–502.
4. Chan KC, Burkhart SS. How to switch posts without rethreading when tying half-hitches. Arthroscopy 1999;15:444–450.

7
Role of Arthroscopic Decompression and Partial Clavicle Resection

John S. Rogerson

Arthroscopic subacromial decompression (ASAD) and arthroscopic distal clavicle resection have become two of the most commonly performed surgical procedures of the shoulder. The arthroscopic technique has evolved significantly from the open anterior acromioplasty as described by Neer and others[1,2] and the open distal clavicle excision described by Mumford and Gurd.[3,4]

Even though these procedures have become commonplace, the indications remain controversial and the learning curve should not be underestimated. This chapter focuses on the technical aspects of the procedures, the indications and contraindications, and the avoidance of complications.

7.1. Historical Perspective

The arthroscopic technique for subacromial decompression was first described by Johnson in 1986.[5] Ellman presented the first series with follow-up and a detailed description of the operative technique.[6] Esch and colleagues evaluated their results with ASAD and related them to the severity of associated rotator cuff tears.[7] Paulos and Franklin presented one of the largest early series (80 patients) and introduced the use of the midlateral subacromial portal.[8]

All of these authors originally described the procedure with the scope viewing from the posterior portal and the instruments entering from a lateral approach. Sampson and colleagues first described the "cutting block" technique for precision acromioplasty in 1991.[9] This technique places the scope laterally and introduces shaving and burring instruments from a posterior portal, using the posterior half of the acromion as a guide for resection. The authors also emphasized the importance of the supraspinatus outlet X ray in both preoperative planning and postoperative evaluation and the benefits of evaluating the flatness of the cut from both the lateral and the posterior portals.

7.2. Etiology and Type of Impingement

The indications for arthroscopic subacromial decompression remain controversial. The necessity of performing an associated ASAD with rotator cuff repair is being questioned.[10] The extent of subacromial decompression, if one chooses to perform one, and the advisability of "co-planing" versus resection of the distal clavicle is also debated.[11]

Much of the controversy regarding ASAD focuses on the etiology and type of impingement. Patients complaining of pain with overhead activities can generally be differentiated into one of the following categories: (1) secondary impingement; (2) posterior superior "internal" impingement; (3) chronic secondary impingement with pathological subacromial changes; (4) primary "extrinsic" impingement; and (5) anterior subcoracoid impingement.

The location and character of associated rotator cuff tears often correlates with the specific type of impingement.

7.2.1. Secondary Impingement

The concept of secondary impingement originates with Codman who proposed an intrinsic tendinous degeneration as the essential lesion in rotator cuff disease.[12] The microvascular studies by Rathbun and McNab,[13] Moseley and Goldie,[14] and Rothman and Parke[15] support this concept. This vascular compromise results in tissue devitalization characterized as "angiofibroblastic hyperplasia" by Nirschl.[16] The subsequent pain and weakness of the supraspinatus compromises its function as a humeral head depressor and allows the superior vector forces of the deltoid to dominate, producing a "secondary" impingement of the cuff into the acromion.

F. Jobe and colleagues enlarged this concept to include patients with underlying anterior glenohumeral ligament instability.[17] As the humeral head subluxes anteriorly, the cuff is secondarily compressed against the coracoacromial arch. Morgan points out that posterior inferior capsular contracture produces an obligate anterior superior humeral head translation with elevation and subsequent superior impingement.[18]

Secondary impingement is more prevalent in a younger patient population actively involved in sports activities that entail overhead arm motion and should be suspected when the bony architecture is unremarkable. The subluxation–relocation test, as described by Jobe and colleagues, is helpful in differentiating secondary causes of impingement.[17]

With the arm abducted 90° degrees and externally rotated, an anterior force is applied by the examiner's hand on the posterior aspect of the humeral head. This accentuates the impingement pain in an unstable shoulder as the head and overlying cuff drive into the anterior edge of the acromial arch (subluxation). Conversely, posterior pressure on the head alleviates the impingement discomfort (relocation).

Cuff tears associated with secondary impingement from tendinosis degeneration are most commonly articular sided or intratendinous.

7.2.2. Posterior Superior "Internal" Impingement

Walsch and colleagues[19] and C. Jobe[20] have described a variety of secondary impingement noted in overhead athletes that occur when the arm is maximally externally rotated while abducted and extended (such as in the cocking phase of throwing). In this position, the posterior–superior articular surface fibers of the supraspinatus are placed under tension and sheer but are also compressed between the humeral head and adjacent glenoid rim, resulting in posterior superior synovitis and partial undersurface tears.

Morgan describes a subset of throwers with "glenohumeral internal rotation deficit" (GIRD).[18] This posterior–inferior capsular contracture produces a posterior–superior humeral head translation where the arm is cocked with "internal" impingement. Whether any underlying anterior instability is a factor in this compression is still unresolved.

While easily confused with primary or secondary anterior impingement, careful examination usually demonstrates pain more at the posterior–superior aspect of the rotator cuff with the arm abducted and externally rotated and extended. In this subgroup, rotator cuff tears are articular sided and are frequently associated with "peel-back" superior labral anterior to posterior (SLAP) lesions.

7.2.3. Chronic Secondary Impingement with Pathological Subacromial Changes

If the underlying cause of the secondary impingement is not rectified with a diligent rehabilitation program (i.e., scapular alignment, posterior capsule stretching), the cuff and humeral head elevate. The decreased acromial–humeral head distance results in inflammation and anterior mechanical irritation in the subacromial space with the development of a traction spur in the coracoacromial (CA) ligament. This anterior acromial osteophyte can lead to "awning" impingement and subsequent extrinsic bursa side cuff wear and tear. One observes articular and bursal partial tears in the same patient, with progression to full-thickness tears and anterior acromial undersurface fraying and osteophytes.

7.2.4. Primary "Extrinsic" Impingement

Neer introduced the concept of extrinsic impingement of the anterior acromion, coracoacromial arch, and the acromioclavicular joint on the underlying rotator cuff and biceps tendon.[1] He also emphasized that forward flexion of the arm is the dominant functional position and that anterior decompression, not lateral acromionectomy, is the appropriate operative approach for significant cuff degeneration. His impingement sign is performed with the patient seated in front of the examiner, who stabilizes the scapula as the arm is elevated slightly lateral to the midline to impinge the tuberosity against the acromion. Pain thus produced is eliminated by injecting 10 cc of 1% xylocaine into the subacromial bursa beneath the anterior acromion (impingement injection test) to confirm the diagnosis. Hawkins and Kennedy described a second impingement sign in which the arm is flexed forward 90° and then forcibly internally rotated, jamming the supraspinatus tendon against the anterior edge of the coracoacromial ligament to produce pain.[21]

Patients with primary extrinsic impingement frequently have a bony architecture with an anterior acromial hook or spur that presses directly on the cuff and biceps with forward elevation of the arm and is associated with bursal-sided rotator cuff tears.

7.2.5. Anterior Subcoracoid Impingement

Gerber and colleagues have described this type of anterior impingement between the humeral head and the coracoid process.[22] The coracoid tip may be enlarged, fractured, or iatrogenically altered, such as occurs with a laterally positioned Bristow transfer of the coracoid tip onto the anterior glenoid rim. Fractures of the coracoid from the recoil of a rifle in hunters may heal with lateral displacement. These changes are best noted on axillary view X rays or a computed axial tomography (CAT) scan with the arm flexed 90° and internally rotated.

Whatever the underlying etiology, the tip of the coracoid is positioned more lateral than normal, and as the arm is brought into forward flexion there is a compression of the rotator cuff between the humeral head and the tip of the coracoid. This produces pain with Neer's forward flexion test, but it occurs usually between 80° and 130° of flexion rather than at full flexion. Hawkin's flexion and internal rotation test is consistently positive, but the pain is lower and more anterior than with superior impingement. The patient also demonstrates decreased horizontal adduction with pain similar to that found with acromioclavicular disease, but the pain is again more at the tip of the coracoid and not at the acromioclavicular (A-C) joint.

Subscapularis tendon degeneration and partial tearing are associated with this type of impingement, and treatment needs to be directed at the coracoid process with a partial lateral resection.

7.3. Athroscopic Subacromial Decompression Controversies and Indications

There are basically two schools of thought regarding ASAD. There are those (Matsen,[10] Nirschl[16]) who contend that all impingement is "secondary" and decompression is almost never indicated, and others (Neer[1,2] and Rockwood[23]) who believe that most impingement is "extrinsic" and almost always needs subacromial decompression, especially if associated with full-thickness rotator cuff tears. Review of the literature, common sense, and arthroscopic experience would argue against both of these extremes.

First, however, one must define a contemporary arthroscopic subacromial decompression. It is not just an arthroscopic replication of the open procedure described by Neer[1,2] and Rockwood.[23] One should avoid taking full-thickness bone off the anterior acromion, which risks detachment of the deltoid insertion or fully resecting the CA ligament. Rather, the goal is to convert a pathological coracoacromial arch to a physiological arch, maintaining the superior deltoid fascial attachments and releasing, but not resecting, the CA ligament.

The most commonly cited concern with subacromial decompression is iatrogenic harm to the coracoacromial arch and destabilization of the glenohumeral joint with anterior–superior subluxation of the head. Although not uncommonly seen in open decompression surgery when the anterior deltoid is detached and fails to heal, it has only rarely been reported with the arthroscopic technique, again when the deltoid fascia was inadvertently released with electrocautery.[24] In fact, this superior migration is not routinely reported even with large os acromial resections. Some decrease in acromio–humeral distance after ASAD has been reported, however, when associated cuff tears are left unrepaired.[25]

When decompression is performed arthroscopically with a cutting block technique, a type I flat surface, which is a normal variant of acromial shape, is produced. One is not truly losing the "arch," but instead removing the excess congenital hook or protruding CA ligament calcification blocking flexion. Because the deltoid is not detached, immediate motion can be instituted postoperatively, so adhesions and stiffness are not a significant clinical problem.

Another argument against ASAD is that the results of minimal debridement and osteophyte resection are equivalent to decompression.[26] A review of the literature, however, reveals an absence of double-blind studies and little or no correlation of results in regard to bursal- versus articularsided tears.

One needs to treat all varieties of impingement with a diligent conservative treatment program, including scapular and rotator cuff retraining, range-of-motion (ROM) exercises to regain full internal and external rotation, nonsteriodal anti-inflammatory drugs (NSAIDs), differential subacromial/A-C joint injection, and activity modification for 3 to 6 months in an effort to avoid operative intervention.[27] If, however, full-thickness rotator cuff tears are associated with impingement, one may need to pursue earlier surgical management, as long-term conservative care with progressive resistance exercises can lead to gradual enlargement and further retraction of the tear.

If conservative care proves unsuccessful, one then needs to try to differentiate primary extrinsic versus secondary impingement versus secondary impingement with pathological adaptive subacromial changes and determine a preoperative plan. This distinction is based on the clinical picture, physical examination, imaging studies, and differential injections, and is confirmed by arthroscopic findings.

The following general guidelines apply at the time of arthroscopy:

- Partial articular-sided tears with no subacromial pathology (anterior CA spur or fraying) are treated with either debridement, partial articular-sided tendon avulsion (PASTA) repair, or conversion to full-thickness tear and repair (based on the extent of the tear) and do not require ASAD.
- Partial bursal-sided tears with evidence of extrinsic subacromial impingement (anterior CA spur or fraying) are treated with either tear debridement, flap repair, or conversion to full-thickness tear and repair (based on the extent of the tear) and are combined with an ASAD.
- Full-thickness tears are repaired completely or partially, and the need for ASAD is determined based on chronicity (acute less likely), bony morphology (type II and III more likely), and evidence of extrinsic impingement (spur or fraying).
- A perfectly smooth undersurface anterior acromion indicates no significant extrinsic impingement and does not need a decompression.
- Internal impingement, isolated A-C osteolysis, anterior subcoracoid impingement, and irreparable cuff tears with associated glenohumeral arthritis likely to later require arthroplasty should not be decompressed.

7.4. Acromioclavicular Controversies and Indications

The A-C joint is a common but sometimes overlooked source of shoulder pain. Degenerative disease of the A-C joint frequently accompanies extrinsic impingement and cuff deterioration. Osteophytic overgrowth on the undersurface of the distal clavicle and medial acromion can impinge on the underlying rotator cuff tendon and muscle. The pain of an arthritic or osteolytic joint can also mimic that of anterior impingement.

Conversely, A-C disease may also be isolated (osteolysis) and must be distinguished from and treated apart from the rest of the uninvolved shoulder. One must decide preoperatively utilizing physical findings, X rays, magnetic resonance imaging (MRI), bone scan, and differential injections as necessary if the A-C joint is a pain generator in the clinical syndrome.

Patients with bursal cuff disease and symptomatic A-C disease warrant an A-C resection at the time of ASAD. The controversy involves co-planing of the inferior tip of the distal clavicle where the A-C joint is asymptomatic at the time of ASAD. Gross reported a significant number (approximately 30%) of patients that later became symptomatic at the A-C joint after co-planing.[11] Tasto and colleagues have shown that resection of the inferior A-C capsule destabilizes the A-C joint.[28] In contrast, Snyder,[29] Weber,[30] and Barber[31] looked at their series of ASAD with co-planing and noted a very low incidence of late A-C disease.

In my practice, I am careful not to violate the capsule or A-C joint at the time of ASAD if the A-C X ray is normal and the joint asymptomatic.

If the joint is asymptomatic but has small osteophytes inferiorly, I perform a minimal osteophyte resection, leaving the capsule largely intact. However, if there is considerable X ray evidence of A-C degeneration and large inferior osteophytes off the clavicle and/or acromion, I proceed without hesitation to a complete A-C resection at the same time with the ASAD.

7.5. Anatomy

Knowledge of the coracoacromial anatomy is crucial for diagnostic accuracy, operative facility, and the avoidance of complications. The bony architecture is composed of the acromion, the A-C joint, the coracoid process, and the greater humeral tuberosity. The shape of the acromion and contour of its undersurface are best evaluated with Neer's supraspinatus outlet view. Bigliani and colleagues described three distinct acromial shapes: type I, flat; type II, curved; and type III, hooked.[32] They found an increased correlation between the type III hooked acromion and underlying full-thickness rotator cuff tears (69.5% for type III and 3% for type I). This radiographic view is also valuable in determining the overall slope and thickness of the acromion and in predetermining those cases where the cutting block technique of acromioplasty would be inappropriate.

The greater tuberosity of the humerus forms the floor of the coracoacromial space. It is important to note its size and shape and any osteophytic overgrowth, sclerosis, erosion, or cysts. It is best evaluated radiographically with an anterior–posterior view with the arm in external rotation.

It is important to remember that the subacromial bursa is an anterior structure. It extends from the anterior one half to one third of the acromion to just medial to the A-C joint to 1 to 2 cm anterior to the acromion and 2 to 3 cm laterally. The bursal wall is frequently thickened and troublesome posteriorly and has been named the *posterior bursal curtain*. This curtain frequently "closes" as one backs the scope posteriorly to get a larger field of view of the subacromial bursa. It is frequently necessary to resect a portion of this structure when performing subacromial surgery.

The anatomy of the coracoacromial ligament is pertinent to the technique of acromioplasty. It attaches to the front and undersurface of the acromion as a thick band and continues around the anterolateral corner to attach to the lateral ridge for a variable distance. Anteriorly, the coracoacromial ligament attaches to the anterior inferior edge of the acromion, while the deltoid fascia attaches more superiorly (Figure 7.1).

As the coracoacromial ligament is detached, it falls away easily from the overlying anterior deltoid muscle and fascia. Laterally, however, the coracoacromial ligament blends intimately with the deltoid muscle fascia along the lateral acromion.[33] Care must be taken not to aggressively detach the fascia or resect too much bone laterally, as this may result in a deltoid detachment.

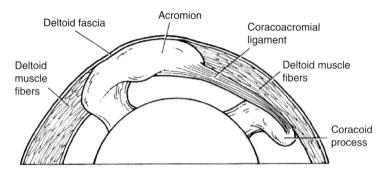

FIGURE 7.1. Lateral view of coracoacromial ligament and deltoid fascia attachment on anterior acromion. (a) Deltoid fascia, (b) deltoid muscle fiber, (c) coracoacromial ligament insertion on undersurface and lateral edge of acromion. (Reprinted from James C.Y. Chow, Advanced Arthroscopy, copyright 2001 with permission from Springer.)

Edelson and Luchs and others have noted various degrees of transformation of the coracoacromial ligament into bone at its acromial insertion.[34] Gartsman labeled this phenomenon *anterior acromial protruberance.*[35] Rockwood in his open technique recommends resecting 8 to 10 mm of full-thickness anterior bone and then reattaching the deltoid fascia.[36] This technique of full-thickness anterior bone resection back to the level of the A-C joint has insinuated itself into some authors' early description of arthroscopic subacromial decompression.[33]

For the most part, the anterior acromial protruberance is really an inferior extension of calcification into the coracoacromial ligament insertion. One does not need to vertically resect full-thickness acromial bone anteriorly to remove it; in fact, great care should be taken not to resect too much superior anterior bone, as this may detach the anterior deltoid fascia, producing an operative disaster.

The best radiographic views for determining the amount of anterior acromial protruberance are the axillary view and the supraspinatus outlet view. The axillary X ray is also an excellent view for evaluation of the A-C joint, particularly for picking up posterior A-C arthritis that may be missed on a routine anterior–posterior view.

7.6. Diagnosis

The history is important. Pain with the cocking and acceleration phase of throwing is most likely secondary to an underlying instability or posterior superior impingement. Nocturnal and rest pain is often indicative of a rotator cuff tear, whereas patients with cuff tendinitis develop pain with progressive activity.[37] Other causes of shoulder pain, such as scapular thoracic bursitis, suprascapular nerve syndrome, cervical radiculopathy, and referred pain from the gallbladder, liver, lung, or heart also need to be differentiated.

The clinical signs and X rays noted previously are most valuable in making a diagnosis of impingement. Concomitant rotator cuff disease or A-C joint disease can be evaluated with an arthrogram, MRI, or combined magnetic resonance arthrogram (MRA). The arthrogram may be more accurate in determining full-thickness rotator cuff tears but less sensitive in picking up partial-thickness lesions or intratendinous pathology. An MRA with abduction external rotation view is more sensitive in demonstrating partial articular-sided cuff tearing and delamination.[38] Isolated A-C joint injection and/or bone scan may be helpful in differentiating A-C joint versus subacromial disease. It is important to know the status of the A-C joint prior to arthroscopic decompression so that residual pathology in this location is not left unattended.

7.7. Preoperative Planning

Careful preoperative evaluation is necessary to determine the appropriate operative approach and to avoid complications. Anterior–posterior, outlet, and axillary views are the key to evaluating the acromion. The anterior–posterior view demonstrates the orientation of the A-C joint and the lateral slope of the acromion. The outlet view is utilized to determine the shape of the acromion (type II or type III) and the overall thickness.[39,40] On the outlet view, lines are drawn on the undersurface of the acromion: one from the front tip of the acromion to the posterior edge and a second line along the posterior half of the undersurface of the acromion extending out anteriorly. The distance between these two lines at the anterior margin approximates the amount of undersurface anterior bone that will be resected if one utilizes the cutting block technique (Figure 7.2).

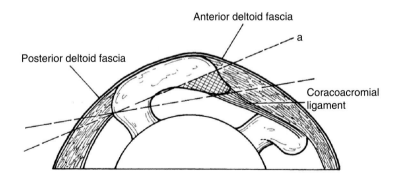

FIGURE 7.2. Preoperative planning for ASAD. (A) Cutting-block line. (Reprinted from James C.Y. Chow, Advanced Arthroscopy, copyright 2001 with permission from Springer.)

The axillary view is used to determine the shape of the acromion (cobra vs. square tipped) and whether there is any anterior acromial protruberance or subtle A-C arthritis.

If on the outlet view one notes a very thin or curved acromion, the cutting block line on the undersurface of the posterior half of the acromion may actually exit the superior aspect of the acromion, taking off too much anterior bone. In these cases, the cutting block technique, as described by Sampson and colleagues,[11] would be inappropriate. Instead, the lateral approach would be more applicable, removing just a small anterior hook and not producing a type I flat acromion.

Preoperatively, one should determine (1) the technique to be utilized for ASAD (cutting block vs. limited anterior resection) and (2) the need for an A-C resection.

7.8. Surgical Procedure

7.8.1. Positioning and Setup

The procedure may be performed utilizing either beach chair or lateral decubitus positions. When utilizing lateral decubitus, the table is turned approximately 100° to 110° from the anesthesiologist, who is then situated at the patient's abdomen. Long anesthesia tubing is required. The TV monitor tower with contained video equipment is positioned directly anterior to the patient's head and chest. The shoulder holder is attached to the operating table on the anterior side of the body near the foot. The inflow pump is positioned so that it can be observed by the surgeon during the procedure.

The lateral decubitus position is modified, as described by Gross and Fitzgibbons.[41] This position rolls the patient back 25° to 30°, placing the glenoid orientation parallel to the floor (Figure 7.3).

The patient is placed in the beanbag with the U position toward the head and the tails extending to the superior–anterior and posterior chest cephad to the axilla for support. The shoulder is isolated with large plastic U drapes facing inferiorly to block fluid extravasation toward the neck with either position. Traction is applied to the patient's arm, and appropriate head support is then utilized so that the head is in exact neutral. The arm is positioned at approximately 30° of abduction and 10° of flexion with 7 to 15 pounds of traction applied, depending on the patient's size and muscularity. A second dual-traction apparatus may be applied if a stabilization procedure needs to be performed.

7.8.2. Surgical Technique

7.8.2.1. Glenohumeral Diagnostic Arthroscopy

The anatomy of the shoulder is outlined with a marking pen prior to the operative procedure and the portals marked. The glenohumeral joint is

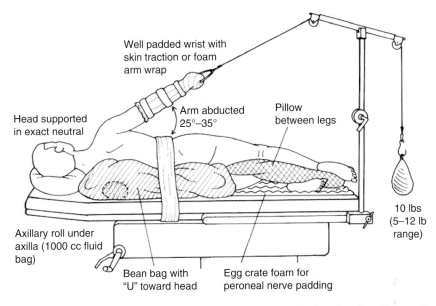

Well padded wrist with
skin traction or foam
arm wrap

Arm abducted
25°–35°

Pillow
between legs

Head supported
in exact neutral

Axillary roll under
axilla (1000 cc fluid
bag)

Bean bag with
"U" toward head

Egg crate foam for
peroneal nerve padding

10 lbs
(5–12 lb
range)

FIGURE 7.3. Patient position with appropriate support for head and axillary roll. (Reprinted from James C.Y. Chow, Advanced Arthroscopy, copyright 2001 with permission from Springer.)

then examined completely from both a posterior and a high anterior portal, established at the superior aspect of the rotator interval. This will later be the anterior portal for the subacromial bursoscopy. Any pathology within the glenohumeral joint is appropriately addressed.

Partial undersurface or small complete rotator cuff tears are frequently marked with a tag suture placed through an 18-gauge needle introduced superiorly into the joint and retrieved out the anterior portal. This suture marker is beneficial later when subacromial bursoscopy is performed, as it provides a quick reference to the questionable cuff area from the superior view. The scope is then removed from the glenohumeral joint and through the same posterior skin portal, redirected at a 10° caudad angle to the acromion into the subacromial bursa and far enough anteriorly to enter the bursal chamber. If the bursa is easily entered and distended, then the inflow is brought in at the scope with a pump and a lateral portal is then made on the basis of an accurately placed 18-gauge needle.

If the bursa is significantly inflamed or not easily distended, with poor visualization, then the scope trocar and sheath is brought directly out anteriorly just lateral to the coracoacromial ligament to exit from the previously made high anterior skin portal. The outflow cannula is then placed on the tip of the trocar and pushed back into the subacromial space so that it lies under the anterior half of the acromion. The sheath is separated slightly, the scope is inserted into the posterior cannula, and flow and visualization are established. A lateral portal is then directed with an 18-gauge needle.

The bursa is then viewed from posteriorly and debrided from the lateral portal until good visualization is established. Any suspicious areas of the rotator cuff that may have been previously identified with a suture marker are debrided and examined from both the posterior portal and the lateral portal.

7.8.2.2. Lateral Approach "Limited Anterior Resection" Technique

Preoperatively, I will have decided whether I am going to use a lateral approach "limited anterior resection" or a "cutting-block" approach for the decompression. If the patient has a thin curved acromion and a lateral approach is appropriate, I place my lateral portal 3.5 to 4 cm lateral to the acromion and about midway between the midportion of the acromion and the anterolateral corner. I make sure with an 18-gauge needle that I can get the shaver along the anterior–inferior edge of the acromion and a short distance down the anterolateral side and that it can be directed slightly upward at the acromion for ease in burring and shaving.

The undersurface of the anterior half of the acromion is then debrided with an aggressive shaver and/or a cautery ablation system (Figure 7.4).

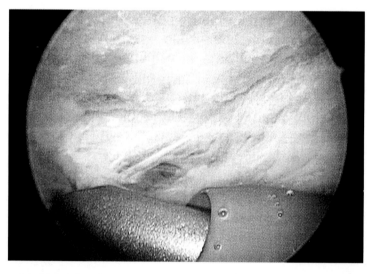

FIGURE 7.4. Debridement of anterior half of acromion and bursa (anterolateral corner of acromion to right.) (Reprinted from Rogerson J. Avoiding complications associated with arthroscopic subacromial decompression, distal clavical resection, and rotator cuff repair. In: J Serge Parisien, Current Techniques in Arthroscopy, copyright 1998 with permission from Thieme.)

Care should be taken with either instrument to stay on the undersurface of the bone and not pop off anteriorly or laterally into the deltoid fibers, which are very vascular. The anterolateral corner of the acromion is identified with an 18-gauge needle directed from superiorly, and the debridement is started at this point and progresses medially toward the A-C joint and also posteriorly.

From the preoperative planning, the amount of bone to be resected is known, as is the diameter of the burr. Starting at the anterolateral corner, the appropriate amount of anterior hook is resected from anterior to medial. Care is taken not to remove full-thickness bone anteriorly and thereby detach the anterior deltoid fascia. This cannot be subsequently repaired as in open operative procedures. After the anterior bone is resected from lateral to medial, tapering of the remaining posterior bone is then accomplished from anterior to posterior to the mid portion of the clavicle, or the scope can be placed laterally and the shaver introduced posteriorly to taper from posterior to anterior. Because of the thin and curved nature of the acromion, the goal is not to produce a completely flat undersurface but to perform a smooth and even taper. Whether one tapers from anterior to posterior or posterior to anterior, the scope is always placed laterally to evaluate the decompression in two planes.

7.8.2.3. The "Two Portal Cutting Block" Technique

If on the basis of the preoperative planning, it is determined that the patient has a thick acromion and a prominent hook anteriorly, I routinely utilize the cutting block technique as described by Sampson.[9] After the anterior one half of the acromion is debrided and the anterior lateral bony edges outlined with minimal resection, the scope is placed in the lateral portal to view the arch of the acromion.

The burr is introduced though the posterior portal on the undersurface of the posterior one half of the acromion. Using this as a cutting block the burr is advanced anteriorly with a sweeping motion medially to laterally (Figure 7.5).

The anterior hook of the acromion is resected and the undersurface flattened in the sagittal plane (Figure 7.6). Take care not to advance the burr anteriorly into deltoid fibers or fascia.

If the A-C joint is to be resected, the burr is then swept more medially to remove the inferior A-C capsule and expose the A-C joint. The lateral 10 to 15 mm of the inferior tip of the clavicle is resected from posterior to anterior. Manual pressure from above can usually deliver much of the remaining clavicle for resection.

The scope is then placed posteriorly and rotated upward, visualizing the line of orientation of the A-C joint and remaining superior clavicular bone.

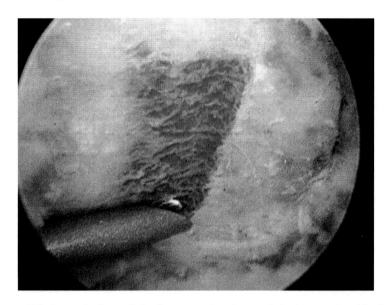

FIGURE 7.5. Lateral view of the burr starting forward during cutting block resection. (Reprinted from Rogerson J. Avoiding complications associated with Arthroscopic subacromial decompression, distal clavical resection, and rotator cuff repair. In: J. Serge Parisien, Current Techniques in Arthroscopy, copyright 1998 with permission from Thieme.)

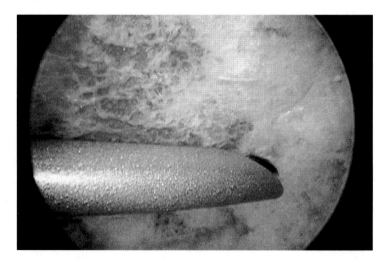

FIGURE 7.6. Completed resection with flat acromial undersurface from posterior to anterior and intact deltoid fascia. (Reprinted from Rogerson J. Avoiding complications associated with arthroscopic subacromial decompression, distal clavical resection, and rotator cuff repair. In: J. Serge Parisien, Current Techniques in Arthroscopy, copyright 1998 with permission from Thieme.)

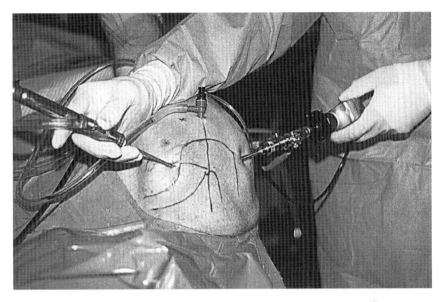

FIGURE 7.7. Scope placed posteriorly with burr introduced from anterior–inferior A-C portal. (Reprinted from James C.Y. Chow, Advanced Arthroscopy, copyright 2001 with permission from Springer.)

The burr (with the aid of an 18-gauge needle) is then introduced through an anterior and slightly inferior A-C portal and directed from anterior to posterior and lateral to medial to remove the remaining superior cortical shell of distal clavicle (Figure 7.7).

Rotation of the scope from superior to medial exposes the posterior cortex and posterior–superior capsule to view [Figure 7.8(A,B)]. If bursal tissue compromises visualization, either it can be debrided or the scope can be inserted through the lateral portal. If superior visualization is poor, a 70° scope can be utilized.

If there is no evidence of degenerative disease of the A-C joint and no inferior osteophytes, I do not take the decompression into the joint or bevel it. If inferior osteophytes are present, minimal resection is performed. If manual pressure from above demonstrates significant A-C instability or exposes bare bone, a complete A-C resection is performed.

In patients with isolated A-C disease, decompression is not performed. The scope is then redirected into the subacromial bursa from the posterior portal. I still place a lateral portal and introduce a bipolar cautery/ablation tip or a shaver to debride the fat pad and inferior capsule of the A-C joint.

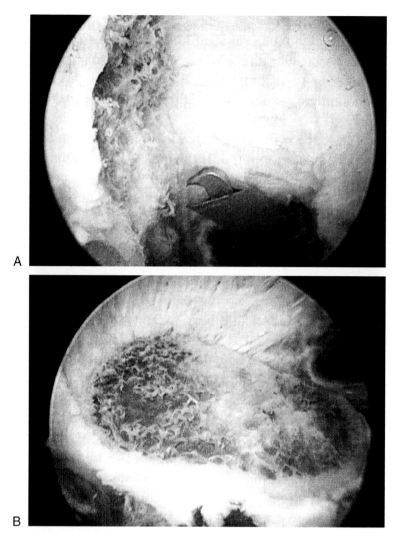

FIGURE 7.8. (A) Superior clavicle resected exposing superior capsule. (B) Scope rotated medially to view completed clavicle resection. Posterior superior capsule intact. (Reprinted from James C.Y. Chow, Advanced Arthroscopy, copyright 2001 with permission from Springer.)

Once the A-C joint has been exposed, a burr is introduced from an anterior–inferior A-C portal and directed from anterior to posterior and inferior to superior, resecting approximately 1.0 to 1.5 cm of the clavicle (and the medial acromial facet if the joint is inclined medially). The scope can be inserted through the lateral portal for visualization of the posterior clavicle if needed.

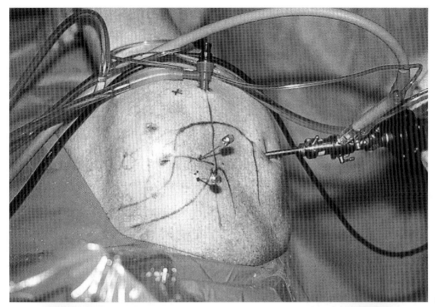

A

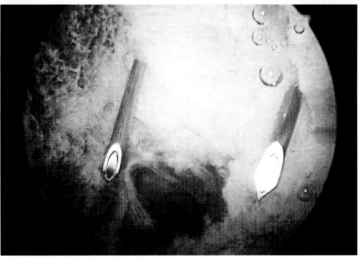

B

FIGURE 7.9. (A) Needles placed percutaneously in a parallel fashion to measure the amount of distal clavicle resection. (B) Arthroscopic view of gap with needles. (Reprinted from James C.Y. Chow, Advanced Arthroscopy, copyright 2001 with permission from Springer.)

The gap is then examined to make sure all cortical bone superiorly is removed and resection is even from anterior to posterior. It is measured with two parallel percutaneous 18-gauge needles from above; 10 to 15 mm of bone is resected with more bone removed in patients with any previous A-C instability [Figure 7.9(A,B)].

The pump pressure is then reduced and hemostasis of larger vessels is obtained with the electrocautery device; 10 cc of 0.25% bupivacaine with epinephrine are instilled into the subacromial space and the incisions are closed with simple 4-0 nylon sutures and a sterile dressing applied. No immobilization is utilized for ASAD or A-C resection unless associated rotator cuff repair is performed.

7.9. Postoperative Management

Passive support and motion of the affected shoulder is provided by the opposite arm if needed. Pendulum exercises are started the next day. Home ROM exercises are utilized the first week. Physical therapy may or may not be utilized depending on the patient's progress with the home program. Closed chain scapular stabilizing exercises are initiated immediately. Open chain exercises are initiated based on the rotator cuff status and quality of repair. Light-duty work is instituted early (1/2 to 2 weeks), but heavy labor usually begins at 6 to 12 weeks postoperatively after decompression and/or A-C resection and 4 to 6 months for rotator cuff repair; sports activities are individualized and variable.

7.10. Complications

The most common complications associated with arthroscopic ASAD and distal clavicle excision are (1) inadequate, uneven, or over-resection; (2) heterotopic bone formation; (3) muscle injury, either deltoid or rotator cuff; and (4) excessive bleeding.

Inaccurate bone resection is best avoided by thorough preoperative planning. Utilization of the cutting block technique, when appropriate, leads to more consistent results with less likelihood of deltoid detachment. Care should be taken to avoid soft tissue interposition between the burr and the posterior acromion, resulting in excess superior angulation.

The amount of bone to be resected arthroscopically from the tip of the clavicle is still unresolved. If the posterior–superior A-C ligaments are well preserved, the length of the clavicle to removed can be reduced.[42] Bigliani found a 91% success rate in A-C resection with just 5 to 6 mm of resection in patients with arthritis or osteolysis and stable joints.[43] If the posterior and superior ligaments are violated or previously injured, then the remaining tip of the clavicle becomes more unstable and more resection is needed.[44,45] Bigliani had only 37% satisfactory results in patients with painful A-C joints after second-degree A-C separations. However, he continued to perform minimal (5–6 mm) resections in this subgroup. Other investigators have had much improved results with second-degree and even third-degree separations with either open or arthroscopic technique when 1.5 to 2 cm of clavicle was resected.[46,47]

My present practice is as follows:

1. In A-C joint disease with or without decompression with intact A-C and coracoclavicular ligaments: 10 to 12 mm of resection.
2. In A-C joint disease with or without decompression with previous A-C ligament injury but generally intact coracoclavicular ligament (second-degree separation or mild third-degree separation): 15 to 17 mm of resection.
3. Chronic symptomatic, unstable, third- or fourth-degree A-C separation with both A-C and coracoclavicular compromise: open modified Weaver–Dunn reconstruction and deltotrapezial fascial repair.

Care should be taken to measure the distance between the clavicle and the acromion with two 18-gauge needles from above; if needed, this should be performed at both the anterior and posterior aspect of the clavicle. It is easy to obtain an uneven gap in resection with more bone removed anteriorly than posteriorly.

Incomplete resection of the superior cortical bone during distal clavicle resection is not uncommon. Clear visualization of this area using either a 30° or 70° arthroscope is necessary to remove all the superior bone. If a cortical egg shell of bone is left behind, elevation and cross-chest maneuvers will remain painful and the bone will also serve as a nidus of heterotopic bone formation.

Caution should be exercised when using burrs for resecting the tip of the clavicle. It is easy to wrap up the soft underlying cuff musculature in the instrument. I prefer to use a well-hooded burr with the open side always facing up or in toward the cancellous middle of the clavicle. Suction should be just enough to clear debris. Care also should be utilized at the anterior acromion during ASAD. Avoid full-thickness anterior bone resection and deltoid detachment by gingerly advancing the burr anteriorly on the undersurface of the acromion. Take care not to plunge into the deltoid fascia or muscle fibers.

The vascularity around the tip of the clavicle and A-C joint is plentiful. Cauterization of the fat pad underneath the A-C joint before the debridement is helpful. It is also beneficial to outline the tip of the clavicle frequently with a cautery device as the clavicle is being resected medially because the periosteal vessels are numerous.

7.11. Conclusions

Arthroscopic subacromial decompression should only be performed when indicated by preoperative and, more important, by arthroscopic evaluation indicating extrinsic bursal-side wear. The appropriate technique of ASAD is dictated by the bony anatomy. The approach to the A-C joint should be determined preoperatively based on clinical, X-ray, and MRI findings.

102   J.S. Rogerson

Finally, intraoperative attention to potential complications will generally lead to positive surgical outcomes.

References

1. Neer C. Anterior acromioplasty for chronic impingement syndrome in the shoulder: a preliminary report. J Bone Joint Surg Am 1972;54:41–50.
2. Neer C. Impingement lesions. Clin Orthop 1983;173:70–77.
3. Mumford E. Acromioclavicular dislocation. A new operative treatment. J Bone Joint Surg 1941;23:799–802.
4. Gurd F. The treatment of complete dislocation of the outer end of the clavicle. Ann Surg 1941;113:1094–1098.
5. Johnson L. Shoulder arthroscopy. In: Johnson LL, editor. Arthroscopic surgery: principles and practice. St. Louis: CV Mosby; 1986:1371–1379.
6. Ellman H. Arthroscopic subacromial decompression: analysis of one to three year results. Arthroscopy 1987;3:173–181.
7. Esch J, Ozerkis LR, Helgager JA, et al. Arthroscopic subacromial decompression: results according to the degree of rotator cuff rear. Arthroscopy 1988;4:241–249.
8. Paulos LE, Franklin JL. Arthroscopic shoulder decompression development and application — five year experience. Am J Sports Med 1990;18:235–244.
9. Sampson TG, Nisbet JK, Glick JM. Precision acromioplasty in arthroscopic subacromial decompression of the shoulder. Arthroscopy 1991;7:301–307.
10. Matsen F. Rotator cuff. The shoulder Rockwood and Matsen. New York: WB Saunders; 1998:755–839.
11. Gross R, Fischer B, McCarthy J, Arrogo J. Arthroscopy 1999;15:241–248.
12. Codman E. Rupture of the supraspinatus tendon and other lesions in or about the subacromial bursa. In: Todd T, editor. The shoulder. Boston: 1934:73–75.
13. Rathbun J, McNab I. The microvascular pattern of the rotator cuff. J Bone Joint Surg Br 1970;52:540–553.
14. Moseley H, Goldie I. The arterial pattern of the rotator cuff on the shoulder. J Bone Joint Surg Br 1963;45:780–789.
15. Rothman R, Parke W. The vascular anatomy of the rotator cuff. Clin Orthop 1965;41:176–186.
16. Nirschl R. Rotator cuff tendinitis: basic concepts of pathoetiology. Instr Course Lect 1989;38:439–445.
17. Jobe F, Kvitne R, Giangarra C. Shoulder pain in the overhand or throwing athlete: the relationship of anterior instability and rotator cuff impingement. Orthop Rev 1989;18:963–975.
18. Morgan C, Rajan S. Posterior Inferior capsulotomy for glenohumeral internal rotation deficit in baseball pitchers. Arthroscopy 2004;20(suppl 1):9.
19. Walsch G, Boylau P, Noel E, et al. Impingement of the deep surface of the supraspinatus tendon on the posterior superior glenoid rim: an arthroscopic study. J Shoulder Elbow Surg 1992;1:238–245.
20. Jobe C. Posterior superior glenoid impingement: expanded spectrum. Arthroscopy 1995;11:530–536.

21. Hawkins R, Kennedy J. Impingement syndrome in athletes. Am J Spans Med 1980;8:151–158.
22. Gerber C, Terier F, Ganz R. The role of the coracoid process in chronic impingement syndrome. J Bone Joint Surg 1985;678:703–708.
23. Rockwood C Jr, Lyons F. Shoulder impingement syndrome: diagnosis, radiographic evaluation and treatment with a modified Neer acromioplasty. J Bone Joint Surg Am 1993;75,409–424.
24. Bonsel S. Detached deltoid during arthroscopic subacromial decompression. Arthroscopy 2000;16:745–748.
25. Kempf JF, Gleyze P, Bonnomet F. A multicenter study of 210 rotator cuff tears treated by arthroscopic acromioplasty. Arthroscopy 1999;16:56–66.
26. Nirsch R. Rotator cuff tendinitis: basic concepts of pathoetiology. Instr Course Lecture 1989;38:439–445.
27. Rubin B, Kibler W. Fundamental principles of shoulder rehabilitation: conservative to postoperative management. Arthroscopy 2002;18(suppl 2):29–39.
28. Roberts R, Tasto J, Hazel R. Acromioclavicular joint stability after arthroscopic coplaning. Arthroscopy 1998;14:419–420.
29. Snyder S, Buford D. Coplaning the AC joint at the time of acromioplasty. Paper presented at: American Shoulder and Elbow Surgeons Opening Meeting, Miami, FL, March 2000.
30. Weber S. Coplaning the acromioclavicular joint at the time of acromioplasty: a long-term study. J Arthroscopy 1999;15;555.
31. Barber F. To coplane or not coplane: how does the remaining AC joint respond? Paper presented at: 19th Annual Meeting AANA, Miami Beach, FL, April 2000.
32. Bigliani LU, Morrison DS, April EW. The morphology of the acromion and its relationship to rotator cuff tears. Orthop Trans 1986;10:216.
33. Gallino M, Vatiston B, Annaratone G, et al. Coracoacromiol ligament: a comparative arthroscopic and anatomic study. Arthroscopy 1995;11:564–567.
34. Edelson JG, Luchs J. Aspects of coracoacrornial ligament anatomy of interest to the arthroscopic surgeon. Arthroscopy 1995;11:715–719.
35. Gartsman GM. Arthroscopic acromioplasty for lesions of the rotator cuff. J Bone Joint Surg 1990;72A:169–180.
36. Rockwood CA Jr. Surgical treatment of the shoulder impingement syndrome: a modification of the Neer anterior acromioplasty in 71 shoulders. Orthop Trans 1990;14:251.
37. Esch JC, Baker CL. Rotator cuff disease and impingement. In: Whipple TL, editor. Arthroscopic surgery — the shoulder and elbow. Philadelphia: Lippincott; 1993:161–163.
38. Nottage WM. Evaluation and treatment of partial thickness articular and bursal cuff tears 2005. Paper presented at: 22nd San Diego Shoulder meeting, San Diego, CA, June 2005.
39. Gartsman GM. Arthroscopic acromioplasty for lesions of the rotator cuff. J Bone Joint Surg Am 1990;72:169–180.
40. Wuh HCK, Snyder SJ. Modified classification of the supraspinatus outlet view based on the configuration and the anatomical thickness of the acromion. Paper presented at: the Fifty-Ninth Annual Meeting of the American Academy of Orthopedic Surgeons, Washington, DC, February 1992.

41. Gross RM, Fitzgibbons TC. Shoulder arthroscopy: a modified approach. Arthroscopy 1985;1:156–159.
42. Flatow EL, Bigliani L. Arhtroscopic acromioclavicular joint debridement and distal clavicle resection. Oper Tech Orthop 1999;1;240–247.
43. Bigliani LU, Nicholson GP, Flatow EL. Arthroscopic resection of the distal clavicle. Orthop Clin North Am 1993;24:133–141.
44. Klimkiewicz J, Sher J, et al. Biomechanical function of acromioclavicular ligaments in limiting anterior posterior translation of the acromioclavicular joint. Paper presented at: the open meeting of the American Shoulder and Elbow Surgeons, San Francisco, CA, 1997.
45. Fukuda K, Craig EV, An K, et al. Biomechanical study of the ligamentous system of the acromioclavicular joint. J Bone Joint Surg Am 1986;68:434–440.
46. Smith MJ, Stewart MJ. Acute acromioclavicular separations: a 20 year study. Am J Sports Med 1979;7:62–71.
47. Jacobs B, Wade PA. Acromioclavicular joint injury — an end result study. J Bone Joint Surg Am 1966;48A:475–486.

8
Tendon-to-Tuberosity Repair: Medial Footprint Fixation

Stephen J. Snyder, Aaron A. Bare, and Mark J. Albritton

Arthroscopic fixation of the torn rotator cuff tendon to the humeral tuberosity includes bone and tendon preparation, anchor placement, suture passing, and knot tying. Currently, a wide range of techniques and products are available to perform a rotator cuff repair. Included in this list is an extensive array of anchors, suture passing tools, and arthroscopic knots. In spite of all the new equipment available ostensibly to facilitate the task of arthroscopic cuff repair, we prefer the long-established method of using screw-in suture anchors and braided permanent sutures.

Once the suture anchor is well seated into the subchondral bone on the medial edge of the rotator cuff footprint, stitching the suture to the rotator cuff and securing the strands with a sliding locking knot will stabilize the repair. Our choices of stitching techniques include simple, mattress, or a combination of the two.

An arthroscopic shoulder surgeon must have a complete understanding of suture anchors, knots, and suturing techniques to ensure a successful outcome. He or she must possess all of the skills for arthroscopic rotator cuff repair prior to attempting operation on a patient. We recommend that interested surgeons practice and perfect all the requisite steps on an ALEX® shoulder model in an arthroscopic laboratory and attend arthroscopic shoulder courses to develop the skills required properly to perform the procedure.

8.1. Indications and Contraindications

Indications for arthroscopic rotator cuff repair hinge on both the patient and the surgeon. All rotator cuff tears that have a repairable tendon and adequate bone stock to allow secure anchor purchase into the subchondral bone are indications for arthroscopic repair. In our estimation, this encompasses virtually all repairable rotator cuff tears.[1,2]

The quality of the rotator cuff tendon tissue and amount of retraction are important factors in the decision-making process. Our experience has shown that a full- thickness tear that includes two or three cuff tendons and is retracted medial to the level of the glenoid, especially when coupled with significant muscle atrophy, is often untreatable by direct surgical repair. However, a partial rotator cuff repair may be helpful in some of these patients if they qualify for surgery.

Revision rotator cuff surgery may also be amenable to arthroscopic rotator cuff repair with suture anchor fixation. Removal of retained metal or bioabsorbable hardware can leave bony defects that are too large to assure anchor purchase. Bioabsorbable anchors may also leave large bone cavities as they degrade. In these cases, larger anchors, such as a 6.5 mm anchor, may be needed to ensure adequate bone purchase for secure fixation.

Contraindications for suture anchor arthroscopic rotator cuff repair are very few. Inadequate bone stock or large subchondral cysts may prevent adequate bone purchase and holding strength of the suture anchor. Also, similar to other elective surgeries, patients with significant medical conditions should be thoroughly evaluated and treated before any surgical intervention is undertaken.

8.2. Preoperative Planning

Preoperative planning includes a complete evaluation of the patient's shoulder, paying particular attention to the patient's strength, range of motion, location of pain, and the presence of atrophy. Pathology of the cervical spine, acromioclavicular joint, and biceps tendon, as well as the presence of subacromial impingement, are evaluated. Performing a neurological examination is also important, as cervical radiculopathy and suprascapular nerve dysfunction can mimic rotator cuff disease. Evaluating a patient with the shoulders exposed lessens the chance of missing subtle findings such as muscle atrophy, scapular winging, or bursal swelling. Both shoulders should be visualized to assess asymmetry. Other important factors to consider during preoperative planning are the age of the patient, the size of the tear, amount of retraction, the presence of muscle atrophy, and the presence of additional intra-articular pathology.

Active range of motion with the patient standing, as well as passive range of motion with the patient supine, should be documented to rule out adhesive capsulitis. The presence of adhesive capsulitis should be treated with physical therapy prior to surgical treatment of the rotator cuff.

Imaging studies complement the physical examination and aid in making a correct diagnosis. We recommend four views of the shoulder: an anterior–posterior (AP) view, outlet or arch view, acromioclavicular (AC) or Zanca view, and an axillary view. The acromial arch is classified according

TABLE 8.1. Modified Bigliani Morrison Acromial Classification.

Type 1: Flat acromial undersurface that extends away from the humeral head
Type 2: Gentle, curved undersurface parallels the contour of the humeral head
Type 3: Inferior-pointing or prominent anterior osteophyte that narrows the outlet of the
   supraspinatus tendon
Type A: Thin acromion, less than 8 mm
Type B: Average thickness, between 8–12 mm
Type C: Thick acromion, more than 12 mm

to a modified Bigliani and Morrison classification and is based on the contour of the anterior–inferior surface along with the acromial thickness (Table 8.1). Each acromion is designated with both a letter and number (i.e., 2B, 1C, or 3A). This classification system assigns importance to both the thickness and morphology of the acromion, helping to determine the exact amount of bone to resect, thus avoiding persistent postoperative impingement or acromial fractures.

A good quality magnetic resonance imaging (MRI) scan provides an estimation of the cuff tear size and the quality of the remaining tissue. The complete MRI scan includes T1 and T2 images in the coronal, sagittal, and axial planes. Fat saturation images amplify fluid collections in the bursa and help to differentiate fluid from fat. The sagittal cuts permit evaluation of muscle atrophy medial to the tendon origins. Normal muscle will encompass approximately 90% of the supraspinatus outlet. The amount of muscle atrophy gives an estimation of the patient's tissue quality and may influence the surgeon's decision on whether to proceed with surgery.

We recommend that all shoulder surgeons review and interpret their patient's MRI scan prior to viewing the MRI report. Any discrepancy in the readings should be discussed with the radiologist for mutual edification. We always recommend that the scan be performed on a 1.5 Tesla closed MRI with dedicated shoulder coils. Closed scanners provide imaging quality superior to open scanners.

Massive rotator cuff tears can be a challenge to repair arthroscopically. Some may be repaired using standard technique, albeit with more suture anchors, while others can be only partially repaired. Certain select patients, especially younger ones with massive, retracted nonrepairable rotator cuff tears, may be candidates for rotator cuff allograft supplementation, such as a Graft Jacket Allograft® (Wright Medical, Arlington, TN).

A gadolinium-enhanced MRI is useful to evaluate the undersurface contour of the rotator cuff in some cases. The contrast allows better visualization of the failed cuff or sometimes of a small partial tear. In addition, this scan allows valuable information regarding the labrum and articular surfaces.

8.3. Surgical Procedure

8.3.1. Positioning and Setup

We prefer to perform all shoulder arthroscopy with the patient under general anesthesia and in the lateral decubitus position, supported by a beanbag. As the patient is turned from the supine to lateral position, an axillary pad is placed under the dependent thorax to avoid injury to the underside neurovascular structures. It is also important to carefully pad both legs, paying particular attention to the common peroneal nerve at the knee and the malleoli.

The room setup for arthroscopic rotator cuff surgery includes a table located in the center of the operating room, angled approximately 45° posterior from the anesthesiologist to allow adequate working space. A video tower containing the electrical equipment, such as the video monitor, light source, camera box, and a motorized shaver box, is positioned in front of the patient at the level of the shoulder and angled to afford an unobstructed view for the surgeon. The arthroscopic pump is located adjacent to the portable video cart at a location that can be seen by the surgeons throughout the surgical procedure.

We find it convenient to utilize three locations to store all equipment required to perform the procedure. The instrument back table is located at the foot of the operating table. This table keeps the accessory equipment such as extra cannulas, punches, and scopes, as well as instrument trays. The scrub technician can utilize this table to load suture anchors during the procedure.

The first Mayo stand is located on the front side of the operating room table, at the level of the patient's chest. The table is located across the patient's body from the surgeon and is within easy reach. This stand holds instruments and equipment most commonly utilized by the surgeon. The remote controls for the pump, mechanical shaver, and electrocautery, as well as the arthroscope with the corresponding sheath, are stored on this stand. The surgical technician can add or remove equipment as needed during the procedure.

A second Mayo stand is positioned behind the surgeon. This tray holds all the instruments necessary to begin the procedure. This includes a skin marking pen, the arthroscopic sheaths, obturators, and cannulas. A separate metal basin is kept on this stand for sharp instruments such as scalpels and spinal needles. This avoids passing sharp instruments from technician to surgeon and minimizes the risk of injury.

Finally, a STaR Quiver® (Arthrex, Naples, FL) is attached to the upper arm after the STaR® (Arthrex, Naples, FL) Sleeve is applied. This is a handy device that conveniently holds the switching sticks, grasper forceps, and other small hand tools currently being used so that they are readily available for the surgeon's use (Figure 8.1).

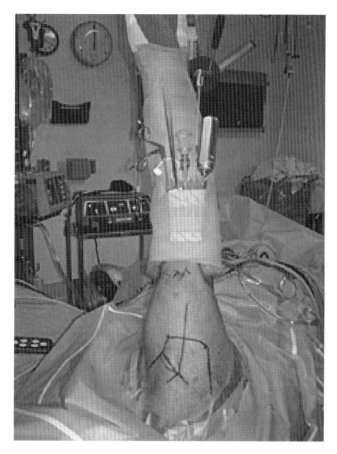

FIGURE 8.1. A STaR Quiver® holds switching sticks, cannulas, and grasper forceps.

8.4. Surgical Technique

8.4.1. Instrumentation

After a thorough, 15-point diagnostic arthroscopy, the undersurface of the rotator cuff is inspected, tears involving the articular surface are debrided, and the footprint is prepared to the edge of the articular cartilage. With the patient's arm in the bursal position, the undersurface of the acromion and acromioclavicular joint are smoothed and the rotator cuff and tuberosity are prepared. Direct visualization of the footprint area through the lateral portal (the so-called 50-yard line) gives the surgeon the best balanced view of the torn tendon. It allows him or her to assess the tear pattern for the repair and decide the appropriate number of suture anchors necessary for optimal rotator cuff fixation.

Current choices for tendon fixation include a vast assortment of metal and bioabsorbable anchors. We prefer to use metal anchors. The new Super ThRevo® (Linvatec, Largo, FL) anchors are preloaded with three sutures, either polyester or polyethylene, affording the option of performing simple, mattress, or a combination of stitches all using a single anchor. The additional versatility of the ThRevo® anchor allows the surgeon to perform the best possible suture combination while avoiding the need for "double row" type of fixation that adds cost and time to the repair.

Currently, we prefer metal rather than bioabsorbable anchors for rotator cuff repair for several reasons. Not only are they typically 30% less costly, they are also less brittle and very unlikely to break during insertion. Also, the location of the anchor can easily be followed by postoperative radiographs so that necessary action can be taken if an anchor is dislodged. Metal anchors will not biodegrade and can often be removed if necessary for revision situations. On rare occasions, bioabsorbable anchors can produce large osteolytic bone defects. This situation can make revision fixation in the ideal position along the footprint impossible.

8.4.2. Steps for Arthroscopic Rotator Cuff Repair

The first step in suture repair of the rotator cuff is to perform any necessary side-to-side repairs. The technique includes direct side-to-side stitching for vertical tears and two-step repair for oblique tears. After the side-to-side repairs are completed, a spinal needle is used to locate the angle for optimal screw insertion. This location is usually just off the lateral border of the acromion. The needle helps choose a spot on the prepared tuberosity 2 mm lateral from the articular cartilage. The angle of the needle (and anchor insertion) should be directed medially into the strong subchondral bone at 45°, the so-called tent peg angle. A small incision is made in the skin, and a 1-mm punch is used to create a starting hole for the anchor (Figure 8.2). The goal is to obtain excellent screw purchase beneath subchondral bone without penetrating the articular surface. An easy mistake is to insert the anchor too vertically along the margin into weaker cancellous bone in the lateral tuberosity. Also, the anchor should be buried in bone so that the suture eyelet is just below the surface and does not sit proud. Parenthetically, if the anchor is placed too deeply, the sutures exiting the eyelet will drape around the edge of the bone and be at risk for early failure. The surgeon should know how the anchor was loaded within its insertion device (i.e., screwdriver). The anchor must be loaded so that the eyelet is aligned with the orientation line on the end of the screwdriver. The braided suture ends will then exit the eyelet and face the rotator cuff when the anchor is properly seated.

The size of the anchor (i.e., ThRevo® 5 mm) should be taken into consideration, especially when using more than one anchor. If additional anchors are needed, they should be spaced far enough apart and angled

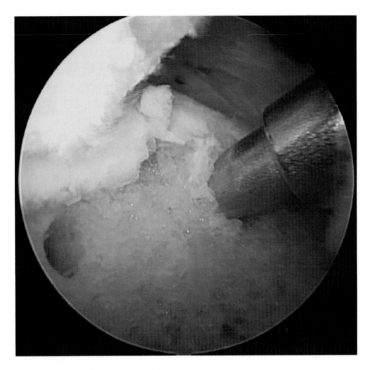

FIGURE 8.2. The punch is inserted 2 mm off the articular surface at a 45° angle to the footprint.

away from other anchors to avoid weakening the bone bridge between the two anchors. After the initial anchor is in place, begin stitching the rotator cuff from posterior to anterior, utilizing either simple or mattress suture patterns. The development of the Spectrum II suture hook system and Suture Savers® facilitate suture passing and management. Suture Savers® (Linvatec, Largo, FL) are used for each simple or mattress stitch. The Savers® prevent confusion with suture management and keep sutures organized prior to tying. After inserting the first anchor, all three sutures should be passed and stored in Suture Savers® prior to inserting additional anchors.

If the sutures have been managed correctly and there are no twists, sliding/locking knots, such as the SMC knot, are used to secure the rotator cuff to the tuberosity. Nonsliding knots, such as the modified-Revo® knot, are utilized in situations where the sutures do not slide through the suture eyelet. The sutures are tied in a sequential fashion, from anterior to posterior, removing the Suture Savers® one at a time to expose the sutures for retrieval.

The following 22 steps outline our technique for rotator cuff fixation to the tuberosity:

1. Begin the repair by closing any side-to-side cuff tears. Use a direct pass with a Spectrum® Crescent (Linvatec, Largo, FL) needle across the tear when possible. Pass a Suture Shuttle® and carry it out the opposite cannula.

2. Load the braided #2 suture into the Shuttle® eyelet and carry it across the tear by pulling back on the Suture Shuttle Relay®.

3. Tie the two sutures together using a sliding/locking knot finished with three half hitches, changing the post between each one.

4. If the side-to-side tear is oblique, it is often necessary to use a two-step technique. Pass the 45° suture hook through the stump of tendon remaining on the bone and pass a Shuttle®, retrieving it into the anterior cannula with a grasping forceps.

5. Pull the first limb of the suture through the stump of tendon on the tuberosity with the Shuttle Relay®.

6. Pass the next 45° Spectrum® suture hook through the cuff just anterior to the side-to-side split and carry the Shuttle® out the anterior cannula.

7. Pull the second limb of the suture back through the anterior side of the cuff to finish the two-step side-to-side stitch. Tie the sutures.

8. Insert the first ThRevo® anchor into a small pilot hole a few millimeters lateral to the articular cartilage at the end of the side-to-side tear. Angle the anchor approximately 45° below the subchondral bone (Figure 8.3).

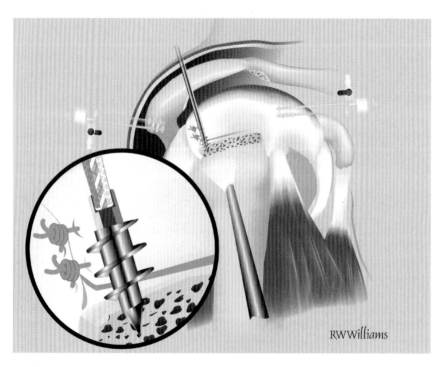

RWWilliams

FIGURE 8.3. A screw-in suture anchor is inserted along the medial aspect of the footprint adjacent to the articular margin. (Courtesy of Conmed Linvatec.)

9. Ensure that the eyelet of the anchor is oriented toward the cuff and the horizontal seating line on the driver is just below the cortical surface.

10. Retrieve the posterior–medial suture (exiting the anchor nearest the cuff) and carry it into the anterior cannula. Be certain to keep from crossing the sutures.

11. Pass the Spectrum 2® needle through the cuff posterior to the side-to-side tear and carry the Shuttle® out the anterior cannula. Again, be careful to retrieve the Shuttle® on the cuff side of the other sutures to avoid twists.

12. Load the suture into the eyelet outside the anterior cannula and pull it through the cuff and out into the posterior cannula (Figure 8.4).

13. Retrieve the partner of the first suture into the posterior cannula. Be sure not to cross it with the other sutures.

14. Store both of the sutures together in a green Suture Saver® outside the posterior cannula. Place a clamp on the Saver® to secure the sutures in place. Retrieve the medial (cuff side) limb of the middle suture into the anterior cannula.

15. Pass the Spectrum2® needle through the cuff on the posterior side of the side-to-side tear and send and retrieve the Shuttle® into the anterior cannula.

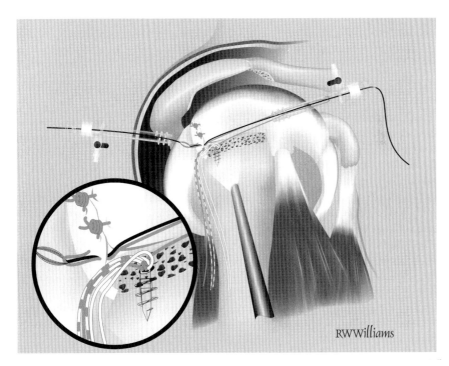

FIGURE 8.4. Sutures are shuttled through the edges of the margin convergent repair. (Courtesy of Conmed Linvatec.)

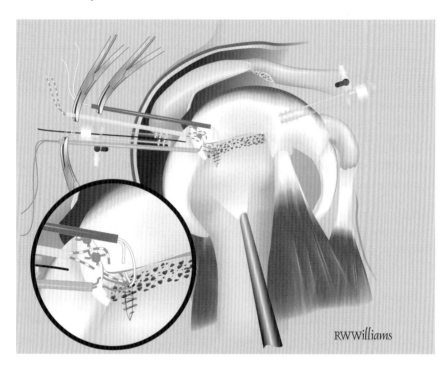

FIGURE 8.5. Suture savers are used to keep the sutures from entanglements and for easy retrieval. (Courtesy of Conmed Linvatec.)

16. Load the first limb of the mattress suture into the Shuttle® eyelet and carry it back through the tissue.

17. Retrieve the second limb of the middle suture (the one exiting the anchor away from the cuff) and store it in the anterior cannula. (Be sure to retrieve it on the cuff side of the other two sutures to avoid twisting.)

18. Pull the second limb of the mattress suture through the cuff into the posterior cannula.

19. Store both limbs of the mattress suture in a yellow Suture Saver® outside the posterior cannula. Retrieve the medial (cuff side) limb of the third suture into the anterior cannula.

20. Pass the third suture as a simple stitch just anterior to the side-to-side tear and store it in a red Suture Saver® (Figure 8.5).

21. Tie the first set of sutures by releasing the clamp on the Saver®, pulling both sutures into the cannula with a crochet hook, and tie using a sliding/locking knot (Figure 8.6). Alternatively, it may be more convenient to leave the Suture Savers® in place, insert the remaining ThRevo® anchors, pass the sutures and store them in additional Savers®.

22. At the completion of suture placement, the camera is moved into either the anterior or posterior cannula and the sutures are tied from the lateral cannula. Once all knots are tied, the final view of the repair is visualized through the lateral cannula (Figure 8.7).

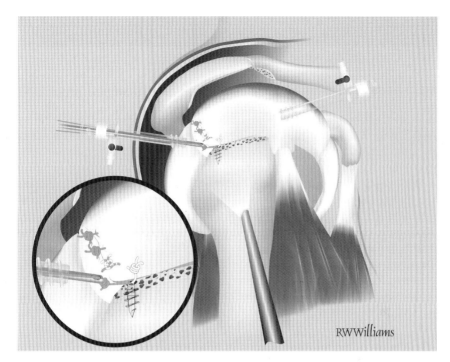

FIGURE 8.6. Knot tying begins posteriorly to assist visualization. (Courtesy of Conmed Linvatec.)

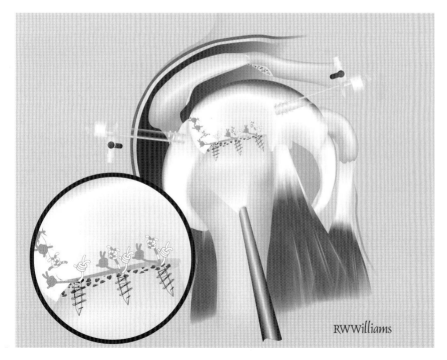

FIGURE 8.7. Rotator cuff repair to the tuberosity is completed. (Courtesy of Conmed Linvatec.)

8.5. Postoperative Management

As every rotator cuff tear is unique, so is the rehabiltation process. The rehabilitation regimen depends on the severity of the tear, the quality of the soft tissue, the bone purchase achieved by the anchor, and the security of the knot fixation at the tuberosity. In general, most patients with full-thickness rotator cuff repairs are protected in a neutral UltraSling® rotation brace for 4 weeks after the surgery.

We encourge patients to begin active elbow, wrist, and hand exercises the day of surgery, as well as to work on squeezing a rubber ball that is attached to the sling. Shoulder shrugs and scapular adduction exercises are also begun on the first postoperative day. Pendulum exercises are initiated at the first postoperative visit at approximately 1 week. Gentle isometric exercises in internal and external rotation are added at this time if the posterior cuff and subscapularis are intact.

At approximately 3 to 4 weeks, we encourage pool therapy for passive mobilization. Formal physical therapy with active assisted elevation exercises are begun at 6 weeks. Resisted rotator cuff exercises are gradually added to the therapy regimen based on the cuff specific factors mentioned above. By 3 months, most patients are allowed to resume normal daily activities. Strenuous sports, heavy lifting, and quick, aggressive movements are gradually phased in during months 4 through 6. Patients should be counseled that it will likely take 1 year to regain substantial strength, especially for large and massive rotator cuff tears.

8.6. Results and Complications

Avoidance of complications during arthroscopic rotator cuff repair requires attention to detail throughout the procedure. Anchor placement, stitching technique, and knot tying all present avenues for mistakes. Suboptimal surgical technique invites errors that may affect outcomes. However, excellent technique will result in optimal tendon-to-bone fixation and lead to excellent surgical results.[3]

Complications of rotator cuff repairs have been reported by various authors.[3-5] Overall, reported complications are limited and include hardware failure as well as postoperative infections and stiffness. For over 1400 rotator cuff repairs performed by the senior author, three infections have been encountered. In two cases, anchors have become prominent and required removal. In these early cases, the anchors were placed too vertical in the footprint. Three patients required manipulation to restore motion caused by postoperative stiffness.

References

1. Snyder SJ. Repair of full-thickness rotator cuff tendon and bursal flap tears. In: Shoulder arthroscopy, 2nd ed. Philadelphia: Lippincott Williams and Wilkins; 2003:230–250.
2. Snyder SJ. Arthroscopic Treatment Of Massive Rotator Cuff Tears. In: Shoulder arthroscopy, 2nd ed. Philadelphia: Lippincott Williams and Wilkins; 2003:251–262.
3. Murray TF, Lajtai G, Mileski RM, et al. Arthroscopic repair of medium to large full-thickness rotator cuff tears: outcome at 2 to 6 year follow-up. J Shoulder Elbow Surg 2002:11:19–24.
4. Millstein ES, Snyder SJ. Arthroscopic management of partial, full-thickness, and complex rotator cuff tears: indications, techniques, and complications. Arthroscopy 2003;19(suppl 1):189–199.
5. Park JY, Chung KT, Yoo MJ. A serial comparison of arthroscopic repairs for partial and full thickness rotator cuff tears. Arthroscopy 2003;20:705–711.

9
Tendon-to-Tuberosity Repair: Lateral Footprint Fixation

Gary M. Gartsman

Presently, there is no one technique for tendon-to-tuberosity repair that has been proven superior in any prospective, randomized clinical study.[1,2] At this point, the orthopedic surgeon must decide on a surgical technique based on another surgeon's personal preference and on a small number of relatively short-term clinical studies. As this textbook aims to capture not only the variations in technique but also the intellectual reasoning behind them, some background is necessary.

My training was in open shoulder surgery. Before the introduction of suture anchors, I repaired the torn supraspinatus over a decorticated area of bone with nonabsorbable braided sutures placed through bone tunnels. Various techniques allowed orthopedic surgeons to create the bone tunnels that were positioned so that one end of the suture exited the bone in the area of the rotator cuff footprint and the other exited the proximal humerus 1 to 2 cm distal to the greater tuberosity. It was not always simple to create the bone tunnels, and on occasion the fixation was less than robust. Therefore, when suture anchors were introduced in the mid- to late 1980s, many surgeons embraced them. I attempted with suture anchors to recreate the appearance of my repair with bone tunnels. The technical issue, of course, was where to put the anchors: in the footprint, distal to the tuberosity, or in both locations. I tried all three methods. When I placed the anchors only in the footprint, I created a lateral flap of tendon distal to the mattress sutures. When I added lateral anchors, the repair looked better, but the cost and radiographic appearance of all these anchors gave me pause. When I placed the anchors laterally, the bone was less osteoporotic, the cortex was intact, the tendon was lateralized and repaired anatomically, and there was no lateral flap. The tendon appeared to lie on the footprint. I also noted that the line of pull of the tendon was not in line with the angle of anchor insertion, and I believed that anchor pullout would be more difficult. I subjected none of these concepts to any rigorous theoretical or laboratory analysis.

During the period from 1982 to 1993, I began and then improved upon my shoulder arthroscopic techniques. When I practiced this technique in the laboratory, I simply inserted the anchor in the same location that I had used successfully with my open repairs, distal to the tuberosity. It seemed so straightforward. I could introduce the anchor through the lateral cannula and avoid the percutaneous entry required of a medial insertion. When I finished tying the knots, the repair looked just like my open repairs, and for me that was the goal. I was not trying to create an arthroscopic operation. I was just trying to replicate arthroscopically the technique that I had used successfully with open repair, as had others. I have been generally pleased with my results and have used the following technique, with minor changes in over 1600 consecutive arthroscopic repairs of full-thickness rotator cuff tears. My methods will probably change over the next 1600 repairs of full-thickness tears. We are constantly presented with new materials, fixation devices, sutures, and tools that have the potential to allow us to produce better repairs with less trauma to the patient. More important, newer concepts of rotator cuff pathophysiology and fixation evolve from our present level of knowledge. The technique I will describe below is used for the vast majority of the full-thickness rotator cuff tears that I encounter but cannot be performed in all patients for all lesions. Some tears are irreparable; tendon substance loss or retraction requires a medial repair in others; and a few patients need tendon-to-tendon repair without any suture anchors. However, most of my patients have, at operation, a repairable full-thickness tear of the supraspinatus that I repair as described below.

9.1. Indications and Contraindications

The indication for an arthroscopic rotator cuff repair is a patient who has continued symptoms after an attempt at more conservative options. There is often a feeling that the arthroscope is less invasive and therefore can be applicable to borderline patient situations. A surgical repair is a major investment from a patient's perspective, whether it is preformed via an arthroscope or through an incision. Through a series of skin punctures, the deltoid maintains its attachments to the acromion as the rotator cuff is reattached. Patients need to be able to tolerate surgery and perform the postoperative rehabilitation and restrictions.[3] Poor tendon quality, musculo-tendinous retraction, and muscular atrophy are not improved with arthroscopic fluid or magnification. Only if the patient has symptoms consistent with acromioclavicular joint arthritis on preoperative history and examination do I perform an acromioclavicular joint resection.

9.2. Preoperative Planning

The three central issues are passive range of motion, tendon retraction, and muscle viability. It is rare for the patient to have a profound loss of motion, such as seen in adhesive capsulitis, and most minor losses of motion are corrected with a gentle manipulation under anesthesia prior to making the skin incision. The amount of tendon retraction is best estimated with magnetic resonance imaging (MRI) or diagnostic ultrasound. Muscle quality is determined on physical examination by estimating the amount of infraspinatus and supraspinatus atrophy on ultrasound and by the size and appearance of the muscles on MRI.

9.3. Operative Technique

9.3.1. Anesthesia

Patients are operated with interscalene blocks combined with general anesthesia. Regional anesthesia reduces the amount of medication for analgesia during the surgery and initial post operative period. General anesthesia maintains desirable blood pressure and prevents patient movements during the procedure.[3]

9.3.2. Positioning

I prefer the sitting position as the orientation of the shoulder is similar to that seen during open procedures and easy access is afforded to the anterior, lateral, and posterior aspects of the shoulder.

9.3.3. Portals

Three portals are used. The posterior portal is 1.5cm medial and 1.5cm inferior to the posterolateral acromial border. The lateral portal is made 1cm posterior to the anterior acromial border and approximately 2 to 4 centimeters lateral to the acromion; the anterior portal is made 2cm anterior to the anterolateral acromion. The posterior portal is made superior to the traditional point of entry in the "soft spot" so that the arthroscope enters the subacromial space parallel to and just underneath the acromial undersurface. This maximizes the distance between the arthroscope and the rotator cuff tear and improves the surgeon's ability to determine tendon tear size and geometry. The lateral portal should allow the cannula (8mm) to enter midway between the humeral head and the acromion. This location facilitates acromioplasty and also enables the surgeon to tilt the cannula inferiorly towards the humeral head so that the surgeon may easily place suture anchors in the greater tuberosity for rotator cuff repair.

9.3.4. Glenohumeral Joint

I first determine the range of motion and stability of the shoulder with an examination under anesthesia and then perform an arthroscopic glenohumeral joint inspection to determine if there are any intra-articular abnormalities that could alter the diagnosis, treatment, or prognosis. I correct these as needed.[4]

9.3.5. Subacromial Space

The cannula and trocar are then redirected through the same posterior skin incision into the subacromial space. I palpate the acromial undersurface with the cannula and sweep the cannula medially and laterally to make certain that no portion of the rotator cuff is adherent to the acromion. The camera is oriented so that the acromion appears horizontal and parallel to the floor; I try to maintain this orientation throughout the procedure. The lateral portal is located with a spinal needle. I insert the needle percutaneously and direct it so that it is 1 cm posterior to the anterior acromial border and positioned midway between the acromion and the greater tuberosity. A cannula is then inserted. Once the bursa is removed, the acromion and coracoacromial ligament are examined for signs of impingement, such as erythema, fraying, and fibrillation.

9.3.6. Tear Classification

It is critical to appreciate tear geometry in order to properly repair the cuff. Small and medium tears are most commonly crescent shaped and may have variable amounts of medial retraction. I use a tissue grasper to pull on the tear edge, attempting to determine the repair site location. Varying both the direction of pull and the arm positions of elevation, abduction, and rotation is often required. Typically, the arm is positioned in 20° of elevation, 15° of abduction, and 10° of internal rotation.

9.3.7. Acromioplasty

My experience is that acromioplasty does not appear to alter patient outcome. Therefore, I do not routinely perform an acromioplasty during repair of a full-thickness rotator cuff tear. I perform an acromioplasty if the subacromial space is small and I cannot see the tear or maneuver the instruments.[5]

9.3.8. Cuff Mobilization

Optimizing cuff edge mobility is important to allow for a low tension repair. This may include release of adhesions to the acromion and deltoid, as well as anterior and posterior releases. The anterior release from the corocoid and coracohumeral ligament is best performed with electrocautery.[6] Posterior adhesions can be achieved with blunt manipulation of the lateral cannula with a sweeping motion clearing the bursae in a posterior direction. After proper releases, tears that may have initially appeared as irrepairable, can be restored.[3]

9.3.9. Repair Site Preparation

A 4-mm round bur is used to prepare a cancellous bed for the tendon. From 1 to 2mm of cortical bone is removed until the cancellous bone is visible. The tendon tear length determines the length of the bone preparation site in its anterior-to-posterior dimension. The width is the distance from the articular cartilage of the humeral head to the medial margin of the greater tuberosity. If anatomical repair is not possible without excessive tendon tension, then I move the repair site. I prefer to repair the tendon up to 10mm medially without tension rather than anatomically under excessive tension.

9.3.10. Anchor Selection

The ideal suture anchor should have the following characteristics:

1. It should allow firm fixation in the greater tuberosity.
2. The surgeon should be able to select which suture type is loaded on the anchor.
3. The anchor should be inserted manually without the need for predrilling or power instruments.
4. The suture should slide through the anchor.
5. The anchor should be removable from the bone in case of suboptimal placement or suture breakage.
6. The anchor must be attached securely to the inserting device so that it does not become dislodged during placement within the tight confines of the subacromial space.
7. The anchor must be able to penetrate the bone at an acute angle.
8. It should be biodegradable without any adverse effects.

No currently available suture anchor meets all these criteria. Each available anchor offers relative advantages and disadvantages when compared to the others, and the surgeon should select the anchor based on personal preference. Presently, I use 5-mm metal anchors (Smith & Nephew Endoscopy, Andover, MA) for rotator cuff repair. These anchors have excellent pullout strength. The handle design and shaft length of the inserter are appropriate. The anchors are attached to the inserter shaft sufficiently so that they do not dislodge as the surgeon manipulates the anchors within the subacromial space. The anchors have a trocar tip so that predrilling is not necessary. I do not like to predrill during rotator cuff repair because the area lateral to the tuberosity is covered with soft tissue, making it difficult to find the screw hole.

The Smith & Nephew anchor has two preloaded #2 sutures. One suture is green and the other white. The anchor eyelet is large enough to allow the sutures to slide freely during knot tying.

9.3.11. Suture Selection

As the management and identification of sutures within the subacromial space can be difficult, it is advantageous to use different colored sutures. This allows the surgeon to more easily identify which suture corresponds to each suture anchor. I prefer braided, nonabsorbable #2 Ethibond (Ethicon, Johnson & Johnson, New Brunswick, NJ).

9.3.12. Anchor Placement

The number of anchors is dependent upon the length and geometry of the rotator cuff tear. For all but the smallest tears, I place two anchors. I place the anchors lateral to the greater tuberosity for the following reasons:

1. The anchor is placed in bone with an intact cortical surface as compared to the prepared cancellous bed of the repair site.
2. Bone density is greater in this distal location than in the more proximal bone.
3. The angle of anchor insertion between the anchor and the bone is minimized allowing a "straight in" anchor insertion.
4. The anchor can be inserted through the cannula without the need for a percutaneous insertion.
5. Lateral anchor position places the vector of tendon pull approximately 90° to the longitudinal axis of the anchor, minimizing anchor pullout.
6. The tendon can be repaired anatomically.

I position the anchor trocar tip against the humeral cortex approximately 5 mm distal to the greater tuberosity. After I insert each anchor, I pull on the suture strands to test anchor fixation. After the anchors are inserted, I then pass the anchor sutures through the tendon. Passing the sutures independently of the anchor insertion allows me to more easily determine the precise location of suture penetration through the tendon.

9.3.13. Suture Placement

Following the placement of suture anchors, the braided sutures are placed from anterior to posterior approximately five to eight millimeters proximal to the tendon edge. A soft tissue grasper is passed through the lateral canulla to estimate the proper placement of the sutures to create an ideal repair.[3]

9.3.14. Suture Passing

I insert a crochet hook through the lateral cannula and withdraw the green suture from the anterior anchor and load it into the jaws of the Elite suture punch (Smith & Nephew Endoscopy, Andover, MA). I then insert the Elite through the lateral cannula and grasp the tendon at the point that I believe should be translated to the anterior anchor. I then pull the tendon towards the anterior anchor and determine if this is indeed an anatomical repair. Once I have assured myself that I have identified the appropriate site for the first suture, I deploy the needle and pass the suture through the tendon. An assistant then reaches in through the anterior cannula and grasps the suture with a grasping forceps and pulls it out the anterior cannula. These steps are repeated as necessary until all the sutures have been passed and are exiting from the anterior cannula.

9.3.15. Knot Tying

Knot tying generally begins posteriorly and proceeds anteriorly, though the surgeon may modify this as determined by tear geometry. Using a crochet hook, each pair of posterior anchor sutures is transferred from the anterior cannula to the lateral cannula and tied individually. The anterior sutures are retrieved from the anterior cannula, brought out the lateral cannula, and tied in similar fashion. I have tried various suture techniques (mattress, modified Mason–Allen), but find them cumbersome and time consuming. I prefer to use simple (rather than mattress) sutures to repair all sizes of rotator cuff tears and have not experienced problems with suture pullout. Simple sutures pass over the tendon edge and hold it firmly against the bone.

After the repair is completed, I remove the arm from the arm holder and move it through a range of motion. This allows me to document repair security and examine the amount of clearance between the rotator cuff and the acromion. Each incision is closed with a single, subcutaneous, inverted 3-0 monocryl suture and steri-strips. An absorbent sterile dressing is placed over the shoulder.

9.4. Postoperative Management

The postoperative management is identical to that of an open repair. I remove the dressing the morning after the operation and allow showering without any protection for the surgical wounds. The patient is placed in a sling except for those periods when the continuous passive motion machine moves the arm in elevation and then into external rotation. The safe limits of movement are determined at the time of surgery and documented. I have the patient use the continuous passive motion chair for 2 weeks. I evaluate the patient in the clinic after 2 weeks and obtain an anterior–posterior radiograph to evaluate anchor position. I discontinue the continuous passive motion chair and have a physical therapist instruct the patient in a home program of passive range of motion exercises for elevation and external rotation with a dowel or pulley. The patient continues to wear the sling and is cautioned to avoid active range of motion with the operated shoulder. I next see the patient at 6 weeks after surgery. Passive range of motion continues, but active elevation and external rotation are allowed. Strengthening is instituted after 3 months, and the rehabilitation continues for 12 months.

9.5. Results and Complications

Our experience is that the results are equal to those of open repairs or mini-open repairs. I found that the average postoperative University of California at Los Angeles (UCLA) score was 31 out of 35 and that 84% of patients were rated as good to excellent. Moreover, the UCLA, American Shoulder and Elbow Surgeons, and Constant rating systems all demonstrated an improvement in shoulder function. When the results were analyzed in terms of patient self-reporting, we found improvement in all the parameters of the SF-36.[7]

The most common complications following arthroscopic rotator cuff repair are stiffness and re-tear or failure of the repair to heal. The treatment of these complications is no different than if they occur after open rotator cuff repair. If stiffness persists 6 months after operation, then I perform an arthroscopic contracture release. If the patient has persistent pain and weakness, then I obtain an MRI with gadolinium. Unfortunately, this often results in a false-positive study due to artifacts from the prior surgery. Diagnostic ultrasound appears to be more reliable. Nonetheless, persistent pain and weakness 6 months after surgery is a relative indication for revision operation. If a tear is identified at re-operation, then it is repaired again. Occasionally, adhesions in the subacromial space produce a tethering effect and are responsible for the pain. The adhesions are usually easily removed. Most patients will elect a second surgery but some, who are improved but have moderate pain and good function, will accept their condition and decline further surgery.[8]

9.6. Conclusions

I have been pleased with the results of my technique but realize it differs very little from the methods of others. Lateral fixation is a small technical variation that I use for the following reasons:

1. The anchor is placed in bone with an intact cortical surface as compared to the prepared cancellous bed of the repair site.
2. Bone density is usually greater in this distal location rather than in the more proximal bone.
3. The angle of anchor insertion between the anchor and the bone is minimized allowing a "straight in" anchor insertion.
4. The anchor can be inserted through the cannula without the need for a percutaneous insertion.
5. Lateral anchor position places the vector of tendon pull approximately 90° to the longitudinal axis of the anchor, minimizing anchor pullout.
6. The tendon can be repaired anatomically.

References

1. Gartsman, GM. Shoulder arthroscopy. Philadelphia: Harcourt Brace; 2003: 197–229.
2. Gartsman GM, Khan M, Hammerman SM. Arthroscopic repair of full-thickness rotator cuff tears. J Bone Joint Surg Am 1998;80:832–840.
3. Gartsman GM. Arthroscopic rotator cuff repair. Clin Orthop 2001;390: 95–106.
4. Gartsman GM, Taverna E. The incidence of glenohumeral joint abnormalities in patients with full-thickness, reparable rotator cuff tears. Arthroscopy 1997; 13:450–455.
5. Gartsman GM, O'Connor D. Arthroscopic rotator cuff repair with and without arthroscopic subacromial decompression: a prospective, randomized study of one-year outcomes. J Shoulder Elbow Surg 2004;13:424–426.
6. Gartsman GM. Arthroscopic assessment of rotator cuff tear reparability. Arthroscopy 1996;12:546–549.
7. Gartsman GM, Brinker MR, Khan M. Early effectiveness of arthroscopic repair for patients with full-thickness tears of the rotator cuff. J Bone Joint Surg Am 1998;80:3340.
8. Gartsman GM, Hasan SM. Pearls and how to avoid pitfalls of arthroscopic rotator cuff repair. Operative Techn Orthop 2002;12:176–185.

10
Tendon-to-Tuberosity Repair: Double Row Fixation

James C. Esch and Sarah S. Banerjee

The technique of double row fixation for rotator cuff tears involves two rows of suture anchors. A medial row of anchors is placed close to the articular surface, and a second, lateral row is placed at the lateral aspect of the rotator cuff "footprint" or the greater tuberosity. Different variations on the technique have been described in the recent literature, with Burkhart describing his method in detail in 2003.[1] Typically, one to two suture anchors are used in the medial row and two to three suture anchors in the lateral row. The medial row fixation sutures are mattress sutures, and the lateral row may be simple, mattress, or T-type sutures. Double row fixation has evolved as an arthroscopic technique based on two principles: increased coverage of the footprint should lead to better healing, and healed rotator cuffs have superior clinical results.

The insertion of the rotator cuff tendons, called the *footprint*, has been examined in several anatomical studies.[2–4] Curtis and other authors have defined the size of the rotator cuff footprint and outlined the footprints specific to the supraspinatus, infraspinatus, and subscapularis.[5] In a study of 48 cadavers, Nottage and colleagues found the average antero-posterior dimension of the supraspinatus insertion to be 25 mm and the distance from the articular cartilage margin to the tendon insertion to be a mean of 1.7 mm.[4] Traditionally, the landmark used for placing suture anchors in most arthroscopic repairs has been the articular margin. With the additional lateral row of anchors in a double row repair, more of the footprint is covered by tendon, creating a larger surface area for healing.

In 2002, Apeleva, Warner, and other authors used three-dimensional reconstruction in a cadaver study to look at restoration of the footprint with different techniques of rotator cuff repair.[2] No technique adequately restored the entire footprint. The more medially based single row repair restored only 67% of the supraspinatus footprint; transosseous simple suture repair restored 85%. The authors proposed that restoration of the original insertion of the rotator cuff provides a larger tendon-to-bone contact area, allowing more fibers to "participate in the healing process

(p. 525)." They also felt that it could improve mechanical strength and function of the repair.

Several other studies have also looked at the footprint in double row repairs. Meier and colleagues, in a cadaver model, observed that the double row repair reproduced 100% of the original footprint.[6] This was in contrast to the single row repair that reproduced 46% of the original footprint and the transosseous suture repair that restored 71% of the original footprint. They, too, felt that recreating the original footprint should enhance the tendon–bone interface and accelerate healing.

Costic and colleagues looked at both footprint coverage and initial bio-mechanical properties after double row repair.[7] Using a cadaver model, they created a 3-cm supraspinatus tear, which they cyclically loaded to produce a typical crescent tear. They performed single and double row repairs with four anchors placed in each row. The medial row was placed inside the footprint and fixed with mattress sutures, and the lateral row was placed just proximal to the footprint. After the repairs, a digitization system was used to measure the area of the new footprint. They found that the single row repairs restored only 40% of the footprint versus 90% in the double row repairs. It remains to be proven that increased coverage of the footprint actually leads to better healing, but most authors believe this will be borne out in future studies.

In addition to better healing, the double row repair should provide stronger fixation by means of improved load distribution over a greater number of anchors. A greater number of anchors generally leads to a stronger repair. This is, of course, limited by the area of the humeral head available for suture anchors and the surface area of available cuff tissue for suture. Burkhart, in 1997 and in several later studies, used the cross-sectional area of the supraspinatus muscle and its force capacity to estimate its pulling force to be 180 N. Using this number, a perfectly balanced three anchor, double row repair with six sutures should be expected to reduce the stress to 30 N per suture, from 45 N per suture with a two anchor, single row repair.[8] Using a double row repair technique should therefore reduce the incidence of suture breakage and failure. The double row illustrates the principle of "spot welding," where a greater number of fixation points leads to greater fixation strength of the repair overall. When introducing his method in 2003, Burkhart suggested that using double row repair might result in greater strength in healing of the rotator cuff. Many recent studies have attempted to evaluate this scientifically.

Kim and coworkers presented a biomechanical analysis of single versus double row repairs at Orthopaedic Research Society (ORS) 2005 showing a 48% increase in ultimate load to failure and a 46% increase in stiffness with the double row repair.[9] They showed that the gap formation at the repair site was significantly smaller with cyclic loading of the double row repair. Perhaps their most significant finding was that the strain over the footprint area in the double row repair measured one third the strain in the single row repair.

In another study, also at ORS 2005, Ma and coworkers reported higher ultimate tensile load with the double row compared to three varieties of single row fixation.[10] They also found decreased motion at the repair site with the double row. Their "massive cuff stitch," a stitch combining a horizontal and a vertical loop that they had presented in their previous studies, was shown to have cyclic load and load-to-failure properties similar to the double row.

Not all studies, however, have shown the double row repair to offer biomechanical advantages. Millett and colleagues, in 2004, found that biomechanical testing of their double row technique showed no difference between single and double row repairs.[11] Their MDA (mattress double anchor) method is unique, however, and depends on the sliding capability of a suture linking the medial and lateral anchors. Thus, their results may not be representative of more traditional double row repairs.

In a study published in the *American Journal of Sports Medicine* in 2005, Mazzocca and Millett found no differences in load to failure, gap formation, and displacement with cyclic loading when testing single row versus double row repairs.[12] They evaluated three types of double row repairs: diamond, their MDA, and a modified MDA. They did find that a greater supraspinatus footprint was recreated with the double row repair.

Costic and colleagues presented at Arthroscopy Association of North America (AANA) 2005 a biomechanical load-to-failure analysis, in addition to their investigation of the footprint.[7] Their data showed that the double row and single row had similar ultimate loads and stiffness. They concluded that the double row repair did not improve the initial structural properties of the single row rotator cuff repair but felt that this might be due to their placing the lateral row outside of the footprint. The main mode of failure in their study was suture cutting through the tendon, indicating too much tension within the repair. Still, they suggested that healing might be improved with the double row repair.

Pedowtiz, Tamberlane, and Esch, in 2005, compared a single row repair with two types of double row repair in bovine shoulder specimens.[13] The single row repair consisted of two lateral, double-loaded anchors. Both of the double row repairs groups had two double-loaded anchors medially, but one group had two double-loaded anchors laterally while the third group had single-loaded anchors laterally. Cyclic loading and load-to-failure testing were carried out, which showed no difference between single row and double row repairs for peak-to-peak elongation or load to failure. The conclusions were that double row repairs have better tendon contact, that the strength of the repair may or may not be better, but that the disadvantages are the cost, complexity, and time involved. In addition, they felt that an advantage with the double row might exist in repairs of degenerative tissue that was not seen in the repairs of young, healthy bovine tissue performed in this study.

In 2005, Rodosky presented at American Orthopaedic Society for Sports Medicine (AOSM) his work that also indicated no difference in initial biomechanical properties of the double row versus the single row repair.[14] It is worth noting, however, that many of the authors who found no difference in initial strength of the repair in their cadaver studies still believe that the double row repair may lead to more successful healing over time.

The goal of better footprint coverage and a stronger cuff repair is to maximize the potential for vascularization and healing. This is particularly important because of the suboptimal setting in which healing needs to take place. The tendon–bone interface has often been thought of as the weak link in the repair situation. We know that the quality of the rotator cuff tissue decreases with age, and the majority of patients with cuff tears are middle aged or older. Kumagi, in 1994, studied 27 rotator cuff tendons from cadavers aged 30 and greater and found that all of the tendons from elderly cadavers showed changes, including microtears, calcifications, and scar formation.[15] None of these were found in the younger subjects. Clearly, one of the challenges with rotator cuff repair is one of biology: trying to aid a compromised, degenerative tissue in healing to the point where it can resist normal physiological loads. While advances have been made with the development of stronger suture material and suture anchors with greater pull-out strength, the problem of attaining actual tissue healing at the bone–tendon interface still remains. In the future, it is likely that products will be engineered and used to alter the environment at the tendon–bone junction for more successful healing.

Healing is even more of a challenge in the case of delayed repairs, in which muscle atrophy and decreased bone density become problematic. Meyer and Gerber showed in 2004 that bone density in the humeral head decreased by 50% in patients with full-thickness rotator cuff tears.[16] In another recent study of tendon repairs done in rats, an acute repair group was compared to a group that underwent repair 3 weeks after creation of a tear.[17] The animals in the delayed repair group had developed both markedly decreased bone density and stiffening of the tendon over 3 weeks. Both of these properties have negative implications for achieving tendon healing, making the challenge even greater.

Even if the double row repair is shown over time to lead to better healing, this is only significant if healed cuffs yield superior clinical results. It is well proven that the incidence of nonhealing rotator cuffs after repair is high, and increases with the age of the patient population. Re-tear rates in the literature have ranged from 16% to 68%. A recent study by Galatz in patients with an average age of 61 years showed 17 out of 18 cuff repairs failed, with re-tears identified by ultrasound at minimum follow-up of 1 year.[18] Although only 72% of patients had ASES scores of ≥90, all patients were satisfied with their surgery. This reflects the trend in the literature, that despite the high incidence of repair failures, most patients are satisfied with the result of their surgery.

Flatow and Bishop in 2004 reviewed 32 open repairs with postoperative magnetic resonance imaging (MRI) at a minimum of 1 year and measured

Constant scores and American Shoulder and Elbow Surgeons (ASES) scores in the healed versus nonhealed groups.[19] They did not find postoperative cuff integrity to have a significant effect on outcomes and reported that "those with a re-tear still had a significant improvement in all clinical areas assessed, including strength (p. 1721)."

However, other recent studies with longer follow-up have provided evidence that patients with healed rotator cuff tears do indeed function better. In 2002, DeBeer examined the incidence of nonhealing after arthroscopic cuff repair and its significance at an average of 15 months.[20] He noted a definite correlation between integrity of the rotator cuff on ultrasound at an average of 15 months, and clinical results assessed by Constant scores. All patients with good to excellent results (Constant scores ≥60) had intact rotator cuffs on ultrasound. He noted that the patients with re-tears identified on ultrasound had been documented intraoperatively as having markedly poor tissue quality.

In 2005, Boileau reported a 70% healing rate in his study of 65 patients with follow-up arthrograms and MRI after arthroscopic rotator cuff repair.[21] Follow-up in his study measured 2 to 4 years. Both groups of patients, with healed and nonhealed cuffs, had a 95% satisfaction rate. However, the patients with healed rotator cuffs had 7.1 kg strength of elevation, versus 4.7 kg in the nonhealed group.

Even in Galatz' study, with 95% patient satisfaction in both groups,[18] the authors made note that with longer follow-up they noticed a concerning trend toward decline in function in their patients. Thus, when results are examined more critically in longer term studies, we may find more consistently a difference in healed versus nonhealed repairs.

10.1. Indications and Contraindications

The double row repair can be performed for tears of any size that are able to be mobilized to the footprint without undue tension. This includes small and medium tears and even some larger, more chronic tears. Burkhart reported that less than 10% of tears were massive, chronic, and retracted to the point of not being amenable to double row repair.[1] This percentage is likely related to the surgeon's ability to mobilize a chronic tear, which is key to the success of this technique. A particularly good case for a double row repair is a large, acute tear where the supraspinatus and infraspinatus tendons are pulled off of the tuberosity but can be reduced anatomically. We expect that as further evidence proves better healing rates with this type of repair, more surgeons will use this technique for tears of increasing size. However, the principle of avoiding tension must not be violated, or the vascularity of the tendon is compromised.

There are no true contraindications to the double row repair, but certainly there are some drawbacks and some limitations associated with the technique. One important limitation is the availability of space in the humeral head for all the anchors required. Cost is an issue with this technique as well. Both the number of anchors required and the time needed to place them and pass the sutures can be double that of a typical rotator cuff repair. Another consideration is the surgeon's skill level. This is a technique for the experienced arthroscopist and one that requires planning for proper placement of the suture anchors. Often, this can be done only after the tear has been visualized intra-operatively.

10.2. Preoperative Planning

We obtain plain radiographs, including a true anterior–posterior view in the plane of the scapula, an axillary lateral, and an outlet view, on all patients preoperatively. The outlet view allows the surgeon to best assess the shape and width of the acromion and the condition of the acromioclavicular joint. In addition, it is important to look for signs of rotator cuff arthropathy on the anterior–posterior view, including superior migration of the humeral head, osteophyte formation, and glenohumeral joint space narrowing.

Preoperative MRI can give the surgeon a general idea of the size of the cuff tear, the amount of retraction of the tendon, and any other pathology present in the shoulder. In particular, the sagittal views are helpful in assessing the size of the muscle bellies and any atrophy. The T2 sequences are best for illustrating the amount of fatty infiltration in long-standing tears. Severe fatty infiltration seen on preoperative MRI has been associated with failure of the cuff repair.[22] If this is found, it should be discussed with the patient that the tear may be irreparable or the repair unsuccessful over the long term.

10.3. Surgical Procedure

10.3.1. Positioning and Setup

The author employs the lateral position with 10-lb traction on the arm in all cases. It is preferred that the table be turned 180° away from the anesthesiologist to allow the surgeon full access to the shoulder. Standard draping technique is used. The anesthesiologist is asked to keep the systolic blood pressure under 100 mm Hg to help to control bleeding.

10.3.2. Instrumentation

In addition to the standard equipment for shoulder arthroscopy, the surgeon must have a variety of tools available to facilitate suture passage in the double row repair. Suture shuttles with varying degrees of curve, as well as a selection of penetrator–grabber type of instruments are essential. A direct suture passer, such as the E-Pass™ (Smith & Nephew Endoscopy, Andover, MA), is particularly useful for quickly placing the lateral row sutures.

The surgeon should check before the procedure that there are adequate numbers of the preferred type of suture anchor and cannulas at hand. We use nonabsorbable metal titanium screw-in anchors double loaded with high strength Ultrabraid® suture (Smith & Nephew Endoscopy). Clear plastic cannulas allow visualization of the suture during knot tying. Most often, two 7.5-mm clear cannulas, through which curved instruments may be passed, are used for the anterior and posterior portals, and a 5.5-mm cannula is used laterally.

10.3.3. Surgical Technique

The shoulder is entered through the standard posterior portal, and a switching stick is used to create the anterior portal in the rotator interval. After inspection of the glenohumeral joint, debridement of the undersurface of the cuff tear is carried out. It is even possible to decorticate the footprint at the greater tuberosity from inside the joint, if desired. The subacromial space is then entered and the bursa debrided thoroughly. For this part of the procedure, the shaver is used first in the lateral portal and then switched with the camera and used in the posterior portal. Acromioplasty is carried out if needed for visualization; otherwise this is done at the end of the repair, when more time can be taken to control bleeding.

The shape and extent of the tear is then assessed, and a grasper is used to determine tear mobility in both the anterior/posterior and medial/lateral directions. This is the crucial time when the surgeon must be able to form the operative plan quickly, that is, the sequence and location of the anchors to be placed. The shaver is used to mobilize the tear further if needed, via release of the rotator interval and/or an anterior release about the coracoid. Only the peripheral 1 to 2 mm of cuff must be debrided. The footprint is then abraded using rotation of the arm to bring the entire tuberosity into view. Figure 10.1 shows the anatomy of the footprint on a shoulder model, as it lies below the torn rotator cuff. The goal of this step in preparation for the repair is *decortication*, and creation of a deeper bony trough is not necessary.[16]

One to two medial anchors are then drilled and placed, according to our technique, at the articular margin (Figure 10.2). As Meyer showed, the best bone for fixation is medially, under the articular surface, or in the lateral cortex of the humerus.[16] The sutures are passed using a pierce-and-grab type of instrument, a direct suture passer, or a shuttle technique to create a double medial mattress configuration (Figures 10.3, 10.4, 10.5). Suture management requires constant attention in the double row repair. It is often helpful to use a superior portal behind the acromioclavicluar

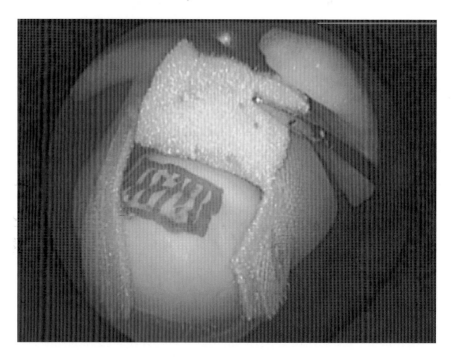

FIGURE 10.1. The rotator cuff footprint.

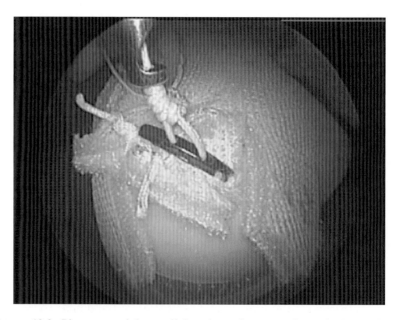

FIGURE 10.2. Placement of the medial anchor adjacent to the articular cartilage.

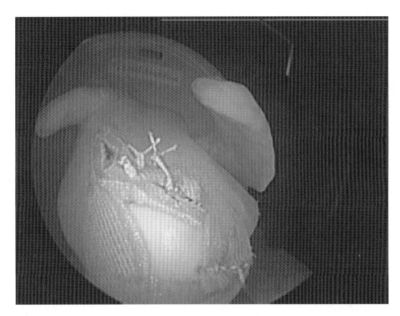

FIGURE 10.3. A pierce-and-grab instrument, such as the Arthropierce™ (Smith & Nephew Endoscopy, Andover, MA), can be used to pass the medial sutures.

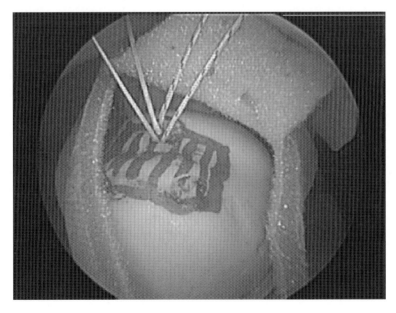

FIGURE 10.4. Alternatively, a direct suture passer may be used.

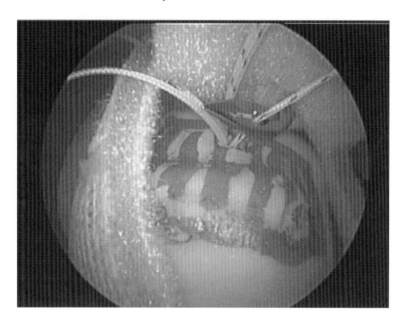

FIGURE 10.5. The mattress configuration of the medial sutures.

joint to place the medial anchors and store their sutures until they are ready to be tied. It is important that there is little or no tension at the sutures of the medial row, and that after they are placed, the lateral edge of the tendon rests at the tuberosity.

The lateral row anchors are then drilled and placed (Figure 10.6). Again, the number of anchors needed is determined by the size and configuration of the tear as it is seen at the time of surgery. Anchors should generally be placed 1 cm apart to preserve a bony bridge between them. A direct suture passer (E-Pass, Smith & Nephew Endoscopy) is often used to pass the lateral sutures as simple sutures. Alternatively, a suture shuttle or a Twinfix™ Quick T device (Smith & Nephew Endoscopy) can be used to pass the sutures in a simple fashion and complete the repair (Figures 10.7–10.10). This T–bar type of anchor system is especially helpful in flattening a broad area of cuff that rides high after the medial row has been secured. In order to obtain the best visualization for each step of the repair, it should be noted that we switch the location of the camera frequently.

There continues to be controversy about the best location for placement of the anchors in rotator cuff repair, even in the double row repair. The traditional location has been at the articular margin, as suggested by Snyder. This is where we place our medial row. Our lateral row of suture anchors is placed at the proximal, lateral aspect of the footprint. The proximal aspect of the tuberosity has been shown to have the highest bone

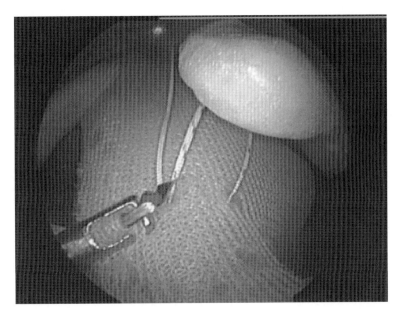

FIGURE 10.6. Placement of a lateral anchor at the lateral aspect of the footprint.

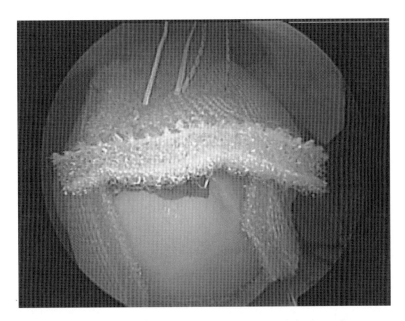

FIGURE 10.7. A suture shuttle is used to pass one of the lateral sutures.

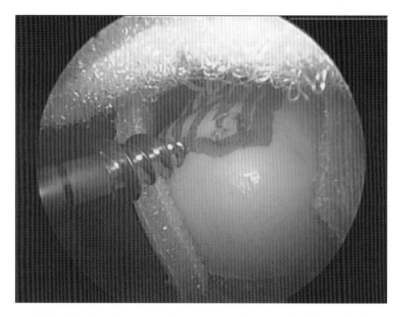

FIGURE 10.8. The lateral sutures from one anchor are tied in a simple suture configuration.

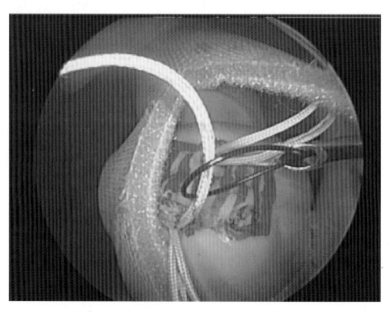

FIGURE 10.9. A Quick-T™ (Smith & Nephew Arthroscopy, Andover, MA) bar anchor is used for lateral fixation.

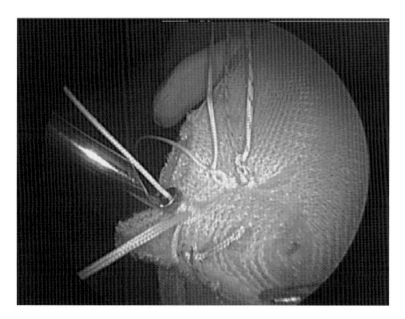

FIGURE 10.10. The final, double row repair of the rotator cuff.

density, yielding the greatest pull-out strength for suture anchors placed within the area of the tuberosity.[23]

Boileau and others recommend placing the anchors even more laterally, in a tension band type of single row repair.[21] He advocates his technique for repair based on studies like Rossouw's in 1997, which showed the dense bone of the lateral cortex to provide the biomechanically strongest repair.[24] In Rossouw's study, the lateral cortex–based repair measured 363 N (±120) versus 147 N (±74). Boileau asserted at the 2005 San Diego Shoulder meeting that the lateral insertion allows a large area of supraspinatus contact, compressing the tendon against the footprint and restoring the normal smoothness of the upper surface of the cuff. He and others have felt that the double row repair involves "double cost and double trouble."

Alternately, Millett and colleagues advocate their MDA or mattress double anchor technique, a unique type of double row repair mentioned earlier in this chapter. In 2004, they presented their technique, which is designed to simulate a traditional transosseus technique with linking of the medial and lateral anchors for load sharing. A preloaded suture loop is placed through the lateral anchor eyelet, and one of the medial anchor sutures is threaded through this loop. This technique requires anchors with anchor eyelets that allow suture passage in situ and allow sutures to slide well. It is therefore somewhat more technically demanding.

DeBeer's method of double row repair involves interlocking the medial row mattress sutures with simple sutures from the lateral row.[20] He believes that this allows for better load distribution and prevents a "quadregia phe-nomenon" from occurring with the more tensioned suture. He places his medial and lateral anchors in a location similar to ours and contends that his method achieves a good reconstruction of the footprint.

10.4. Postoperative Management

Immoblization of the shoulder is paramount in achieving successful healing of the repaired tendon. This is accomplished by having the patient wear an abduction sling, with no active therapy for 6 weeks. Patients are allowed to do pendulums in the sling, and passive range of motion exercises limited to 90° of forward flexion, 10° of external rotation. This protocol is supported both by the high incidence of nonhealed rotator cuffs and also by mechanical studies such as those done by Thomopoulos.[25] He showed in a study of rat shoulders that the repairs in animals immobilized after surgery demonstrated superior collagen structural properties and visco-elastic properties to those that were exercised. This was contrary to his expectations.

Rossouw's biomechanical evaluation of suture anchor repairs in the rotator cuff also supports our belief in delayed mobilization. In his study, the repairs were loaded cyclically and failed at low loads by cutting into bone and tendon. His findings caused him to question the benefits of early mobilization after surgery. Especially in the case of massive rotator cuff repairs, we find that the evidence supports immobilization rather than early motion, for a better chance of healing at the repair site. In addition, we avoid the use of nonsteriodal anti-inflammatory drugs (NSAIDs) in the postoperative period. Both traditional NSAIDs and cyclooxygenase-2 (COX-2) inhibitors decreased rotator cuff healing in one recent study in rats.[26] The treatment group had inferior results based on gross inspection of the repair, load-to-failure testing, and analysis of collagen organization and composition.

10.5. Results and Complications

The results of the double row repair are still in the early stages of collec-tion. However, thus far, they appear equal to or better than the results of arthroscopic repair in the literature.

DeBeer has provided perhaps the best analysis of results after double row repair.[20] He began using a double row repair in 1998 and has performed approximately 260 arthroscopic repairs with his technique. In 2002, his report on 58 patients with an average follow up of 15 months showed 90% good to excellent results. As discussed earlier in this chapter, the 8% inci-dence of nonhealing cuffs he found on ultrasound correlated with the 10%

patients in his study who had moderate to poor results. Still, a 90% rate of healing, if sustained over time, represents a significant increase when compared to healing rates in previous studies, such as those of Galatz.[18]

Lo and Burkhart acknowledged the high rate of healing DeBeer appeared to achieve with his technique in the 2003 description of their own double row repair.[1] They reported that, although they had not been gathering postoperative imaging data on their patients, their clinical impression of their results was similar.

In summary, the double-row repair does an excellent job of restoring the rotator cuff footprint and affording a biological environment for tendon-to-bone healing. The stronger fixation with this repair should reduce the chance of early failure of the anchor, suture, bone, and tendon reconstruction during the time of healing. Ongoing study of these repairs is needed to demonstrate that a higher rate of healing is achieved and maintained with the double row repair. Studies in the literature with longer follow-up demonstrate a significant difference in the strength of healed versus non-healed rotator cuffs. In addition, the future will likely involve some type of biological enhancement of tendon-to-bone healing, which remains the primary challenge in rotator cuff repair.

References

1. Burkhart SS, Lo IKY. Double-row arthroscopic rotator cuff repair: re-establishing the footprint of the rotator cuff. Arthroscopy 2003;19:1035–1042.
2. Apreleva M, Ozbaydar M, Fitzgibbons PG, et al. Rotator cuff tears: the effect of the reconstruction method on three-dimensional repair site area. Arthroscopy 2002;18:519–526.
3. Dugas JR, Campbell DA, Warren RF, et al. Anatomy and dimensions of rotator cuff insertions. J Shoulder Elbow Surg 2002;11:498–503.
4. Ruotolo C, Fow JE, Nottage WM. The supraspinatus footprint: an anatomic study of the supraspinatus insertion. Arthroscopy 2004;20:246–249.
5. Curtis AS, Burbank KM, Tierney JJ, Scheller AD, Curran AR. The insertional footprint of the rotator cuff: an anatomic study. Arthroscopy 2006; 22:609.e1.
6. Meier SW, Manigrasso MB. Rotator cuff repair: the effect of double-row fixation on initial repair strength. Paper presented at: ORS Annual Meeting, Washington, DC, 2005.
7. Costic RS, et al. Biomechanical properties of arthroscopic rotator cuff repair: single and double row of suture anchors. Paper presented at: AANA Annual Meeting, Vancover, BC, 2005.
8. Burkhart SS, Diaz-Pagan JL, Wirth MA, et al. Cyclic loading of anchor-based rotator cuff repairs: confirmation of the tension overload phenomenon and comparison of suture anchor fixation with transosseous fixation. Arthroscopy 1997;13:720–724.
9. Kim DH, et al. A biomechanical analysis of an arthroscopic footprint rotator cuff repair technique. Paper presented at: ORS Annual Meeting, Washington, DC, 2005.

10. Ma CB, et al. Biomechanical analysis of arthroscopic rotator cuff repairs — double row vs. single row. Paper presented at: ORS Annual Meeting, Washington, DC, 2005.
11. Millett PJ, Mazzocca AD, Guanche CA. Mattress double anchor footprint repair: a novel, arthroscopic rotator cuff repair technique. Arthroscopy 2004; 20:875–879.
12. Mazzocca AD, Millett PJ, Guanche CA, et al. Arthroscopic single-row versus double-row suture anchor rotator cuff repair. Am J Sports Med 2005;33: 1861–1868.
13. Pedowitz RA, Tamborlane J, Esch JC. Strength of double row arthroscopic rotator cuff repair in bovine cadaveric humerus model. In press.
14. Rodosky M. Does increasing the attachment footprint of the repaired rotator cuff improve the initial biomechanical properties? Paper presented at: AOSSM Annual Meeting, Keystone, CO, 2005.
15. Kumagai J, Sarkar K, Uhthoff HK. The collagen types in the attachment zone of rotator cuff tendons in the elderly: an immunohistochemical study. J Rheumatol 1994;21:2096–2100.
16. Meyer DC, Fucentese SF, Koller B, et al. Association of osteopenia of the humeral head with full-thickness rotator cuff tears. J Shoulder Elbow Surg. 2004;13:333–337.
17. Galatz LM, Rothermich XY, Zaegel M, et al. Delayed repair of tendon to bone injuries leads to decreased biomechanical properties and bone loss. J Orthop Res 2005;23:1441–1447.
18. Galatz LM, Ball CM, Teefey SA, et al. The outcome and repair integrity of completely arthroscopically repaired large and massive rotator cuff tears. J Bone Joint Surg Am 2004;86:219–224.
19. Klepps S, Bishop J, Lin J, et al. Prospective evaluation of the effect of rotator cuff integrity on the outcome of open rotator cuff repairs. Am J Sports Med 2004;32:1716–1722.
20. DeBeer J, Berghs B, Van Rooyen K. Arthroscopic rotator cuff repair by footprint reconstruction. 19th Annual San Diego Shoulder meeting syllabus. 2002:425–431.
21. Boileau P. Arthroscopic cuff repairs: How well do they heal? 22nd Annual San Diego Shoulder meeting syllabus. 2005:494–502.
22. Goutallier D, Postel JM, Bernageau J, et al. Fatty infiltration of disrupted rotator cuff muscles. Rev Rhum Engl Ed 1995;62:415–422.
23. Tingart MJ, Apreleva M, Zurakowski D, et al. Pullout strength of suture anchors used in rotator cuff repair. J Bone Joint Surg Am 2003;85: 2190–2198.
24. Rossouw DJ, McElroy BJ, Amis AA, et al. A biomechanical evaluation of suture anchors in repair of the rotator cuff. J Bone Joint Surg Br 1997;79: 458–461.
25. Thomopoulos S, Williams GR, Soslowsky LJ. Tendon to bone healing: differences in biomechanical, structural, and compositional properties due to a range of activity levels. J Biomech Eng 2003;125:106–113.
26. Cohen DB, Kawamura S, Ehteshami J, et al. Indomethacin and celecoxib impair rotator cuff tendon-to-bone healing. Am J Sports Med 2006;34: 362–369.

11
Partial Articular-Sided Tendon Avulsion Transtendon Rotator Cuff Repair

Jeffrey S. Abrams

Articular tears of the rotator cuff are common and may be problematic. Histological studies have shown anatomical differences that make the articular portion of cuff tendons more vulnerable to tension. Codman used the term *rim rents* in his original thesis on why rotator cuff tears begin on the articular side of the tendon. The partial articular-sided tendon avulsion (PASTA) repair is an arthroscopic technique used to repair the articular-sided tear without disrupting the intact bursal tendon fibers.

The PASTA lesion is a term created by Snyder to represent *partial articular-sided tendon avulsion.*[1] Before the arthroscopic PASTA technique was available, surgeons had the choice of debridement or completing the tear and creating a full-thickness tendon repair. Open surgical techniques included subacromial decompression, palpating thin tendons and excising damaged tendons, followed by reattachment to the greater tuberosity. The arthroscope allows the surgeon to identify and quantify the problem while visualizing the pathology from an articular view.

The natural history of articular-sided tears was studied via arthrograms. When patients had a follow-up study 1 year later, approximately half of the patients had larger defects, and one quarter went on to full-thickness tears.[2] The current belief is that an active patient with a painful articular-side partial tear is at risk for tear extension, possibly a full-thickness tear. Many patients have minimally symptomatic partial tears. Patients who have a painful tear extension include delaminations and tears that extend along the greater tuberosity. Articular avulsions expose medial portions of the greater tuberosity. This "footprint" has been quantitated by measuring the amount of tendon detachment, which reflects the size of tear.[3-5] Dr. Ellman and others have recommended surgical repair of tears approaching 50% of the thickness of the tendon or approximately 6mm of footprint.

The etiology of PASTA lesions can be multifactorial. A tear can result from a single traumatic event as in a dislocation, or from multiple subluxations. Internal impingement results from excessive compression of the articular-side of the tendon against the glenoid and labrum. Degenerative tears are common and may be caused by the relatively poor blood supply within the crescent of the supraspinatus.

Patients can develop associated lesions that may require treatment. Labral pathology may occur as a result of internal impingement or instability. Shoulders can be stiff, and adhesive capsulitis can be a painful coexistent condition. Patients can become concerned that assisted stretching to reverse stiffness may possibly cause tear extension.

There exists some controversy on the role of impingement in producing shoulder pain. Most would agree that bursal-sided partial tears may result from abrasion of the exterior of the cuff on the subacromial arch. Articular-sided tears may have normal bursae on arthroscopic evaluation. It is possible that impingement is secondary to a poorly functional cuff, not creating adequate shoulder depression during arm elevation. This may be why partial pain relief occurs from a cortisone injection within the subacromial space.

11.1. Treatment Classification

Patient selection is based on patient lifestyle and demands, the location and dimensions of the tear, and the response to conservative treatment. Most patients should attempt a course of nonoperative treatment that includes flexibility and strengthening exercises. Those patients that fail to improve are candidates for surgical treatment.

Lifestyle needs may be a significant motivation for patients seeking medical advice. Heavy-demand patients, including worker's compensation cases, may be at greater risk for failure. When a time-dependent recovery is important, surgical repair of the PASTA lesion is easier to explain to patients than telling them to "wait and see."

The anatomical considerations of the tear are important. The most common tendon involved is the supraspinatus. The anterior third of the tendon is commonly involved in instability and trauma, and the posterior third is associated with internal impingement. Patients can tolerate greater sized tears in the posterior third, adjacent to the junction of the infraspinatus. These tears include the tuberosity attachment and extend medially into the crescent of the tendon. The depth of the tear can be measured by measuring exposure of the footprint and using arthroscopic instruments of a known size adjacent to or into the tear.

Tear patterns include degenerative tears, longitudinal split tears, T-shaped tears extending through the thickened cable, and cuff avulsions (partial and near complete; Figure 11.1). The degenerative tears with tissue loss can be debrided. If the tissue is thin following debridement, a side-to-side closure can be performed. Tendon splits and delamination may be repaired with side-to-side full-thickness closure. Tears with footprint exposure require a suture anchor repair to restore the tendon attachment to the greater tuberosity. As tears approach full thickness, it may be more practical to divide the remaining thin bursal tissue and create a full-thickness repair.[6]

11.2. Patient Evaluation

A history and physical examination is important to appreciate the level of dysfunction an individual is experiencing. Reproduction of pain, range of motion, strength deficits, and loss of function are important. It is not unusual to find mild degrees of atrophy along the posterior scapula. An understanding of the mechanism of injury, activity demands, and response to treatment should be ascertained. A history of an event that has resulted in instability is important to appreciate because corrective approaches may include stabilization.

Imaging of the shoulder includes plain radiographs, possibly an arthrogram or magnetic resonance imaging (MRI) study. Articular dye may be helpful in viewing defects and delaminations. Unfortunately, many tears can be missed for a variety of reasons. The arthroscopic evaluation is the most efficient way to visualize the articular-side tear. Debridement of devitalized tissue, followed by quantitating depth and dimensions of the tear, are important steps in deciding on how to proceed.

11.3. Surgical Repair

11.3.1. Percutaneous Side-to-Side Repair

The indications for this repair include tears or delaminations that overlie the articular surface with minor detachment from the tuberosity. The scope is in the posterior viewing portal; an anterior portal has a cannula placed; and a shaver is introduced to debride the tear. A needle is placed in the tear for later identification on the bursal side. The scope is removed and reintroduced through the posterior portal into the bursae. A lateral portal is created to create a bursectomy and to palpate adjacent to the needle to estimate the significance of the tear. An acromioplasty is performed in patients with bursal findings that are consistent with impingement.

The arthroscope is placed back within the glenohumeral joint. A spinal needle is percutaneously placed anterior to the tear, and a shuttle is placed through the needle. The free end is retrieved out the anterior

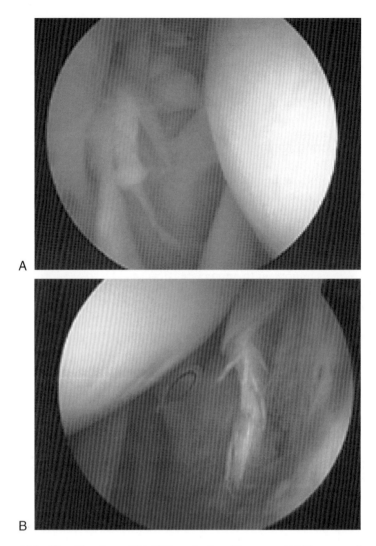

FIGURE 11.1. Classification of PASTA articular-side tears. (A) Degenerative tear: diffuse loss of tissue within the crescent. (B) Supraspinatus split tear: linear tear over the articular surface. (C) T-crescent tear: combined avulsion and linear split. (D) Articular avulsion: crescent tendon detachment from tuberosity.

portal, and a braided #2 suture is retrieved. A second pass with the spinal needle posterior to the tear, advance a shuttle, and retrieve out the anterior cannula to retrieve the prior suture. This creates a mattress suture on the articular side. The process is repeated until the tear is reduced. The arthroscope is placed in the bursae, and the sutures are tied (Figure 11.2).

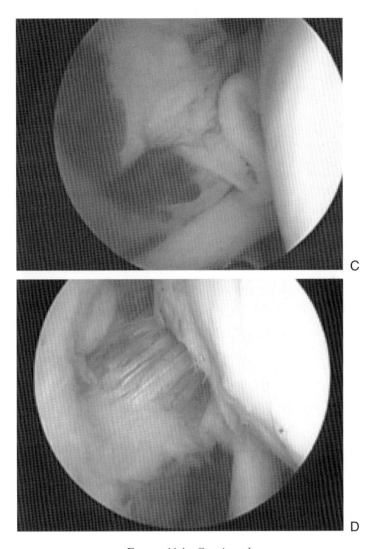

FIGURE 11.1. *Continued*

11.3.2. PASTA Suture Anchor Repair

After debridement of the articular tear, the scope is placed in the bursa. Bursae debridement and decompression are carried out, if indicated. The arthroscope is placed in the glenohumeral joint through the posterior portal. A spinal needle is placed adjacent to the lateral acromion through the defect into the medial margin of the footprint. Arm abduction may need to be adjusted to create a favorable angle of entry. A small stab wound

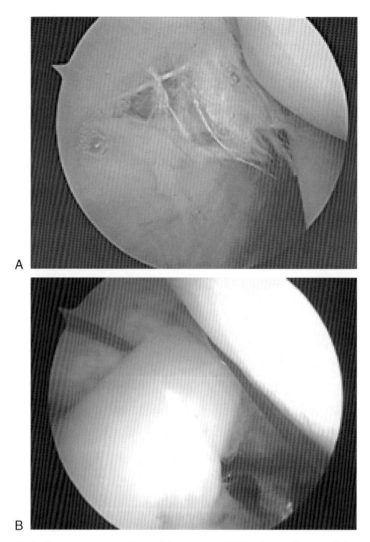

FIGURE 11.2. Percutaneous side-to-side repair. (A) Tendon split tear. (B) Percutaneous needle placement to introduce shuttle. (C) Side-to-side sutures transversing the tear. (D) Knots tied in the subacromial bursa.

will allow a suture anchor to be placed without using a cannula. After the anchor is placed, arm abduction can be increased to open the tear. The anchor eyelet should allow mattress suture placement.

A spinal needle is then placed 1 cm anteriorly to the anchor and passed through the intact tissue anterior to the tear. The anterior cannula allows

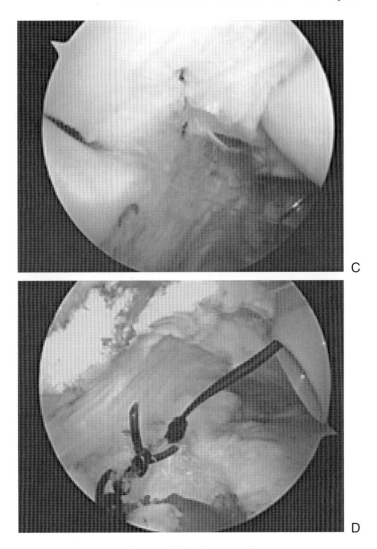

C

D

FIGURE 11.2. *Continued*

for retrieval of the suture shuttle (Linvatec, Largo, FL). A suture from the anchor is also retrieved out the anterior cannula. A knot-tier can be used to assist suture management, allowing for easy retrieval. The spinal needle is replaced 1 cm posterior to the tear, and the shuttle is reintroduced (Figure 11.3). Again, the shuttle is retrieved out the anterior cannula, along with

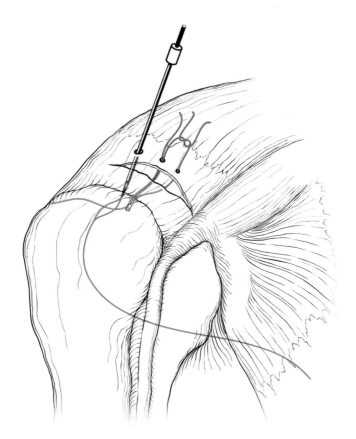

FIGURE 11.3. A spinal needle can percutaneously pass the shuttle and retrieve the braided sutures to create a series of mattress sutures.

the second colored stitch. After securing the stitch within the shuttle, the shuttle is drawn up into the bursae (Figure 11.4).

The arthroscope is placed within the bursae, and the sutures are tied securely. Arm abduction of 30° or less is ideal for tying these knots. Place the scope within the joint to confirm the repair side of the PASTA anchor repair.

11.3.3. Conversion to Full Tear

Following tear debridement, a needle is placed through the tear. The scope is reintroduced into the bursa through the posterior portal. A lateral portal is developed 3 cm lateral to the lateral margin of the acromion. After bursectomy, a probe can be used to palpate tissue superficial to the articular tear. In patients with near full-thickness articular-sided tears (75% thickness defect or greater), surgeons may consider converting to a full-thickness defect, prior to repair.

Subacromial decompression is completed in patients with appropriate preoperative symptoms and confirmative arthroscopic findings. A beaver blade is placed through the lateral portal, and the bursal tissue is divided perpendicular to the tuberosity insertion. A shaver blade can further debride the tissue, creating a V-shaped defect. A Caspari punch (Concept division, ConMed Linvatec, Largo, FL) is used to place a monofilament suture through the edge of the supraspinatus. The tear can be repaired arthroscopically with double-row or offset anchor technique, or a mini-arthrotomy can be performed.

The arthrotomy can be created by extending the skin incision anteriorly and posteriorly approximately 4 cm. After undermining a flap superiorly, a deltoid split without detachment is created to the lateral margin of the acromion. Full-thickness retracting sutures are placed along the deltoid incision. The free suture in the cuff tear is mobilized, and a reinforced braided #2 suture is woven through the free edge in a Mason–Allen technique.

A bidirectional repair combines suture anchor(s) medially with tuberosity sutures laterally.[7] A suture anchor (or two) is placed medially along the articular margin of the greater tuberosity. The sutures are passed through the cuff in a mattress fashion. The free suture in the tendon edge is placed through drill holes in the greater tuberosity, repairing the lateral margin of the tear. The advantages of double-row fixation are combined with increased greater tuberosity surface area coverage, and reparative vectors angled 90° apart (Figure 11.5). In the past 12 years, this technique was among the earliest reports of a double-row repair.

11.4. Postoperative Management

Patients are protected in a sling for 4 to 5 weeks. On the first postoperative day, passive external rotation is started. Pendulum exercises can be started early as well. Supine forward flexion begins after 4 weeks. Internal rotation is delayed 6 to 8 weeks. Strengthening exercises are started after 10 weeks. This would include external rotation strength and scapular stabilizing exercises. Return to activity may be seen 3 to 6 months after surgery, depending on the required activities.

11.5. Results

A series of 56 patients underwent PASTA repairs between 1998 and 2005. These patients were unique due to their activity demands. Sixteen patients were worker's compensation cases (29%), eight played sports on a competitive level, five patients were revision surgeries of failed open and arthroscopic procedures, and four were elderly (over 60 years). All patients presented with pain and loss of function. Five patients had moderate

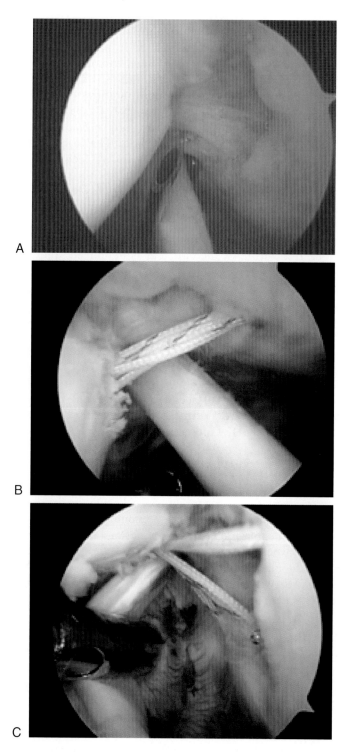

FIGURE 11.4. PASTA suture anchor repair. (A) Supraspinatus articular avulsion. (B) Percutaneous anchor placed adjacent to articular surface. (C) Sutures retrieved with shuttle anterior and posterior along supportive cuff cable.

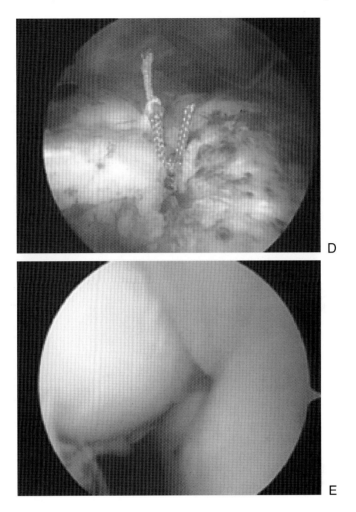

FIGURE 11.4. *Continued* (D) Knots tied in subacromial space. (E) Articular view
of repair.

restricted passive motion at the time of surgery and were released at the
time of surgery.

Relief of pain was good or excellent in 50 patients (89%). Three patients
admitted to significant relief but continued with limitations preventing a
return to the same level of work. Three patients continued to experience
loss of sleep but returned to an active or athletic lifestyle. One patient had
continued arm symptoms from a ruptured biceps tendon 2 years after
rotator cuff repair.

Return to sports and work was accomplished in 94%. Activity returns began after 12 weeks, but in some overhead sports took as long
as 10 months. Three patients had follow-up arthrographic MRIs due
to delay in return to work, and one tennis player 6 months after

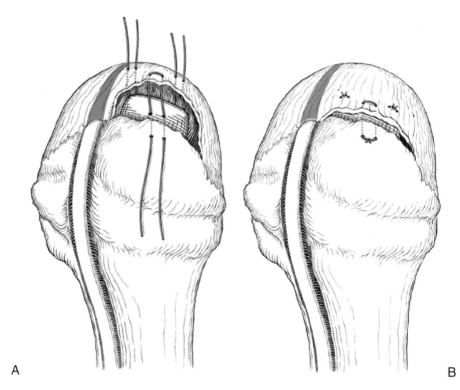

A

B

FIGURE 11.5. Bidirectional double-row repair. (A) Suture anchors medially, tuberosity fixation laterally. (B) Final repair.

surgery. All MRI studies demonstrated a satisfactory restoration of the footprint.

Strength deficits were uncommon. Many patients with preoperative weakness or atrophy had improvement after repair. Most weakness was felt to be related to discomfort and avoidance of activity. As pain relief was achieved, most patients had symmetrical strength. Patients subjectively felt their strength return occurred approximately 6 months following surgery. The average University of California at Los Angeles (UCLA) score improved from 9 preoperatively to 32 following repair.

11.6. Conclusions

The arthroscope provides an excellent technique to visualize and treat partial-thickness articular rotator cuff tears. Partial articular-sided tear avulsion lesions are common, and traditional open techniques most likely underestimated their occurrences. Imaging studies may be helpful in detection and have shown tear extension in many active patients.

Partial articular-sided tendon avulsion lesions can become painful due to tear extension and loss of rotator cuff function. Tear patterns include degenerative tears with tissue loss, T-shaped tears that extend through the crescent, and cuff avulsions of varying thickness. Tear pattern visualization includes the footprint along the greater tuberosity and the medial components of the tear overlying the humeral head articular surface. Anatomical repairs include suture anchor repairs of the tendon avulsion or split, and side-to-side repairs of the medial tear extension and delaminations.

Activity demands are important criteria for patient selection for surgical repair of a PASTA lesion. Many patients may do well with debridement of small lesions and possibly decompression in cases where impingement findings are present. A select group of patients with increased activity demands should be considered for PASTA repair, if patients fail to respond to a conservative program. Additional pathology, including stiffness, and biceps pathology may need treatment. Currently, the preoperative decision of impingement findings and confirmative arthroscopic bursal pathology may indicate a subacromial decompression to be performed in addition to treatment of the tear. Failure of rotator cuff depression of the humeral head during arm elevation may lead to subacromial impingement. Many of these patients are middle aged, athletic, or worker's compensation cases, and correction of pain generators may be the difference between success and failure. I have chosen the decompression approach over the risk of need for further surgery.

The PASTA repair maintains the collagen scaffold of the lateral rotator cuff attachment. This maintains the anatomical length of the supraspinatus. The repairs emphasize the medial attachment to the greater tuberosity of the footprint. Suture anchors are placed with mattress sutures to reapproximate tendon to tuberosity direct repair (Figure 11.6). Tears that extend further medially into the crescent or crossing the cable should be repaired with side-to-side techniques. These tears should not be advanced to the tuberosity to avoid over tensioning of the repair. Restoring normal flexibility is often coexistent with patients' pain relief.

The indication to complete the tear prior to repair is when patients' tear depth is near full thickness. A double row allows for medial and lateral fixation. This can be achieved arthroscopically with offset suture anchor fixation (Figure 11.7) or open with a bidirectional repair through lateral tuberosity bone tunnels.

The surgical results have been extremely promising and have been a better option in active and high-demand individuals. The rules of half-thickness tears may not apply to all patients. A tear that extends into the tendon (25% or greater) may create a delamination and should be considered for surgical repair in a high-demand patient. Shoulders are at risk for tear extension, and symptomatic patients unresponsive to conservative

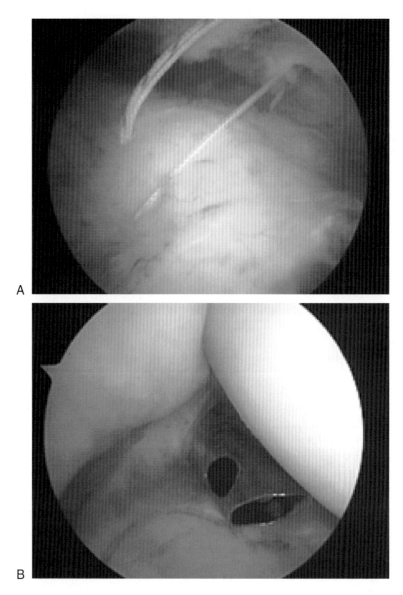

FIGURE 11.6. Mattress sutures along the medial aspect of greater tuberosity. (A) Sutures passed 1 cm medial to edge of tendon in a mattress fashion. (B) Articular view of repair.

treatment may benefit from arthroscopic repair. Restoring tendon thickness followed by specific rehabilitation may correct functional stabilization of the humeral head during arm elevation. Satisfactory pain relief, return of function, and limiting progression of the tear can be achieved in a high percentage of patients.

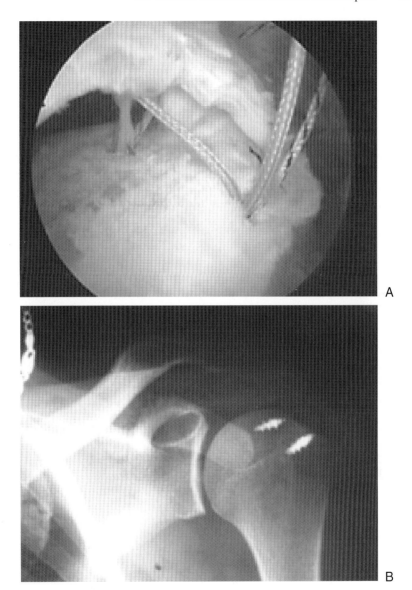

A

B

FIGURE 11.7. Offset suture anchor fixation. (A) Lateral anchors placed obliquely to medial anchor to create triangular repair. (B) Radiograph of double-row anchors medial and lateral.

References

1. Dunteman RC, Fukuda H, Snyder SJ. Surgical treatment of partial-thickness tears. In: Norris TR, editor. Orthopaedic knowledge update, shoulder and elbow, 2nd ed. American Academy of Orthopaedic Surgeons; Rosemont, IL: 2002:163–170.

2. Yamanaka K, Matsumoto T. The joint-side tear of the rotator cuff. Clin Orthop 1994;304:68–73.
3. Ellman H. Diagnosis and treatment of incomplete rotator cuff tears. Clin Orthop 1990;254:64–74.
4. Ruotolo C, Fow JE, Nottage WM. The supraspinatus footprint: an anatomic study of the supraspinatus insertion. Arthroscopy 2004;20:246–249.
5. Tierney JJ, Curtis AS, Kowalk DL, Scheller AD. The footprint of the rotator cuff. Arthroscopy 1999;15:556–557.
6. Weber SC. Arthroscopic debridement and acromioplasty versus mini-open repair in the treatment of significant partial-thickness rotator cuff tears. Arthroscopy 1999;15:126–131.
7. Abrams JS. Arthroscopic assisted mini-open rotator cuff repair: revo anchors and tuberosity tunnels. In: Gazielly DF, Gleyze P, Thomas T, eds. The cuff. Paris: Elsevier; 1997:289–291.

12
Suture Anchor Repair of Small and Medium Supraspinatus Tears

Robert H. Bell

Arthroscopic rotator cuff repair, once the domain of a select group of surgeons, is quickly becoming the standard of care employed by more and more orthopedists. This transformation is due in great part to the advent of improved anchors, stronger suture material, and enhanced suture passing devices, resulting in enhanced success rates.[1-4] However, the most significant advances have come about due to constant improvement in our teaching of new techniques. What was once an operation done by few is now one that even the general orthopedist might well consider for his or her occasional rotator cuff repair. This chapter is directed to those individuals far enough along on the learning curve to be comfortable with an all-arthroscopic repair and ready to tackle some of the small and medium tears they may encounter during routine decompressions. Other chapters will deal with more advanced techniques such as mobilization and interval releases; this chapter describes my technique for the simple, mobile, small and medium tears from room setup to suture passing, knot tying to rehabilitation. After all, these are not only the lesions best suited for a surgeon's first all-arthroscopic repairs but also are the most common tears the average orthopedist will encounter.

12.1. Indications and Contraindications

The principal indication for rotator cuff surgery is pain. Lack of mobility and diminished strength, while often of concern to the patient, are secondary to that of pain relief. Patients should understand that the intent of the surgery is to remove the offending acromial prominence and repair the damaged tendons. It is important that they realize the results of such surgery depend upon many factors, including tear size, retraction, tissue quality, preoperative mobility, and their overall health. Furthermore, they should understand their role in the postoperative rehabilitation and the length of time required for recovery.

Relative and absolute contraindications to this surgery are rare but should include active infection or a recent history of such, significant medical problems, advanced degenerative joint disease requiring arthroplasty, and advanced cuff arthropathy. Those patients with fixed superior migration of the humeral head on anterior–posterior films, an absent acromiohumeral interval, fatty infiltrates, or atrophy and marked retraction of tendon edges on magnetic resonance imaging (MRI) are not candidates for an arthroscopic rotator cuff repair, much less an open one, and should be recognized preoperatively.

12.2. Surgical Procedure

12.2.1. Operating Room Setup

For a case to go well it must start well, beginning with room setup. I do all rotator cuff surgery with the patient in the lateral decubitus position. This allows ready access to posterior, anterior, and superior aspects of the shoulder while holding the arm in an appropriate position of slight abduction, and facilitates approximation of the tendon edge to the region of the greater tuberosity.

Cannulas are used in nearly every case to provide optimal suture management and to simplify knot tying without the risk of capturing soft tissue in a knot. Cannulas facilitate fluid management, ensuring less extravasation and edema and better hemostasis. Prior to cannula placement, determine the size needed and the location for insertion with "outside-in" needle localization.

As with many orthopedic procedures, arthroscopic rotator cuff repair is an instrument-dependent procedure, and its success is often determined by the availability and appropriate use of special devices. I use a basic set of instruments that are necessary for every case. They include: a simple knot pusher, a ring grabber or crab claw device for retrieving individual sutures, a set of Spectrum pig tail suture passers (Linvatec, Key Largo, FL), and a Liberator knife (Linvatec, Key Largo, FL) for mobilization. An ExpresSew suture passer (Depuy Mitek Inc., Norwood, MA) and Innovasive suture snare are available but not appropriate for every case. Other instruments are available to facilitate suture passing; the surgeon needs to investigate and test each of these as they become available. It is important that she has an armamentarium of tools that are comfortable and facile. The operating room is not the place to first try a new instrument; that should be done in the laboratory or on a model.

12.2.2. Portals

All arthroscopic repairs require three principal portals and, occasionally, an additional anterior ancillary portal. The viewing portal is located 1 cm

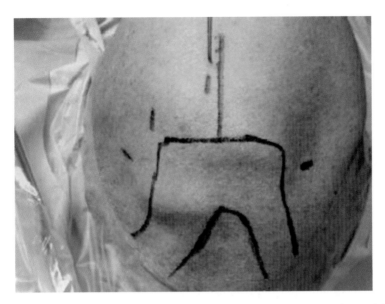

FIGURE 12.1. Standard portals for repairs: viewing portal 1 cm medial and 2 cm inferior to the posterior corner of the acromion, working portal for acromioplasty and suture passing 2 cm lateral and 2 cm posterior to anterior corner acromion, and anchor portal, just off the anterior corner acromion.

medial and 2 cm inferior to the posterolateral corner of the acromion (Figure 12.1). The working portal is located immediately anterior to the "finish line," a line drawn perpendicular to the lateral margin of the acromion beginning at the posterior extent of the acromioclavicular joint (Figure 12.1). The working portal is just anterior to this line, 2 to 3 cm inferior to the lateral margin of the acromion. The anchor portal is determined using needle localization technique in the subacromial space. This portal is typically positioned at the anterolateral corner of the acromion (Figure 12.1). An additional fourth portal, called the *waiting room*, may be made anterior to the acromion. I utilize this in large tears in which three or more anchors and six or more sutures are used. This portal allows me to store sutures after passing them, thereby freeing the remaining subacromial space, improving visualization and facilitating knot tying. As each knot is tied, the next suture limbs are grasped from the waiting room portal and brought into either the anchor or working portal for subsequent tying. This aids greatly in suture management.

12.2.3. Glenohumeral Inspection

All rotator cuff repairs begin with a thorough inspection of the glenohumeral joint to identify and treat other associated pathology, such as labral lesions, capsulolabral disruptions, biceps tears, and loose bodies. Additionally, partial-thickness tears of the rotator cuff can be assessed, localization sutures placed, and repair performed.

12.2.4. Acromioplasty

All chronic full-thickness rotator cuff tears and the majority of acute full-thickness rotator cuff tears undergo a concomitant arthroscopic subacromial decompression utilizing standard technique. The decompression provides additional clearance for the repair, prevents further impingement, and improves the area of the subacromial space for viewing and instrumentation. I will avoid a decompression in younger patients in whom there are no apparent changes consistent with prior impingement.

12.2.5. Mobilization

As in open repairs, mobilization of the rotator cuff tendons may be necessary to facilitate a tension-free repair; this is accomplished by a technique similar to that used during open procedures. Traction sutures, if needed, are applied to the tendon edges, a shaver or Liberator knife (Linvatec, Key Largo, FL) is employed, and subacromial adhesions are gently released. Intra-articular adhesions are released by applying traction to the tendon edge while releasing the capsulolabral junction. Care should be taken to preserve the biceps insertion and to avoid medial excursion in the region of the suprascapular nerve posteriorly.

12.2.6. Anchor Placement

With the acromioplasty complete, the tendon edges mobilized, and the repair planned, anchors should be placed in a position that affords minimal tension on the tendon margin at the time of repair. In the majority of cases, anchors are placed immediately medial to the greater tuberosity, in the sulcus between it and the articular surface. In small and medium tears, requiring no more than three anchors, all anchors can be placed before suture passing. Anchor choice and orientation is dependent upon the surgeon's preferences; however, most are double loaded with variations of the most current, enhanced strength suture material. My preference in anchors has been double-loaded metallic devices for a number of reasons: ease of insertion without need to predrill or tap, postoperative X-ray confirmation of location, optimal pullout strength, and limited risk of inflammatory reaction.

Before the first anchor is placed, the anchor portal is established. Viewing from the posterior portal, looking up at the anterolateral corner of the acromion, a spinal needle is introduced percutaneously, making certain to clear the edge of the acromion and ensure the appropriate angle for anchor

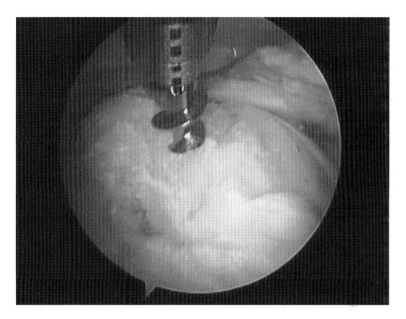

FIGURE 12.2. Viewing from the posterior portal, the anchor is introduced from the anterior portal, beginning at the posterior extent of the tear.

insertion. A 6.5-mm cannula is placed. I place the first anchor at the posterior extent of the tear and then pull all four strands of this anchor out the lateral working portal to clear the anchor portal for the second anchor (Figure 12.2). The second anchor is inserted in similar fashion. The next step is dictated by the anticipated technique for suture passing. If I plan to use a snare device, I will move all the sutures to the anterior portal, freeing the lateral portal for the arthroscope. If, however, I plan to use a suture passing device such as the ExpresSew (Depuy Mitek Inc., Norwood, MA), I will move sutures to the anterior portal and bring them one by one to the lateral portal, load them into the passer, pass them, and move them back to the anterior portal. This process is repeated for each suture on each anchor.

12.2.7. Suture Passing

12.2.7.1. Snare Retrieval Technique (Depuy Mitek Inc., Norwood, MA)

Having placed all the anchors, I move the arthroscope from the posterior to the lateral working portal. This position gives me the optimal view of the tear and a perspective for suture passing. The suture snare is introduced from either the posterior or, if needed, an additional anterior medial portal near the acromioclaviclar (A-C) joint. Under direct visualization, the snare penetrates the tendon 1 to 2 cm medial to its margin

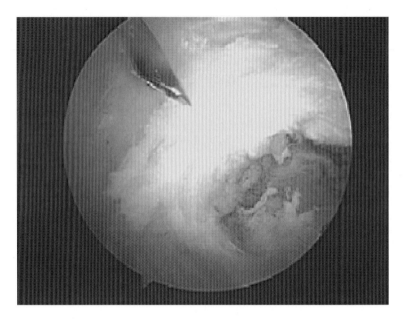

FIGURE 12.3. The snare is introduced from the posterior portal, penetrates the tendon 1 to 2 cm from its edge, and is directed towards the anchor sutures.

(Figure 12.3). Once through the tendon, the snare is opened and a suture limb is isolated and captured. The snare is closed only enough to contain the suture but not so as to impede its motion through the snare eyelet (Figure 12.4). The retriever is backed out, bringing the suture limb along and creating a simple stitch ready for tying. This process is then repeated for each subsequent double-loaded anchor.

12.2.7.2. ExpresSew Suture Passer (Depuy Mitek Inc., Norwood, MA)

Several devices allow direct passing of the anchor suture through the free tendon edge from articular to bursal side. One such device is the ExpresSew suture passer. After the anchors have been placed, the lateral working portal is cleared. The arthroscope is maintained in the posterior viewing portal, and one limb of the suture is retrieved from the anchor portal and brought out the lateral portal to be coupled to the device. The ExpresSew has a flexible tine with an eyelet at its tip, into which the suture is loaded. The jaws are closed, the passer introduced into the subacromial space, jaws opened, and the tendon edge is engaged and closed, holding the tendon to allow suture passage (Figure 12.5) As the device is fired, the tine, with coupled suture, is driven from the articular to bursal side of the tendon edge and then retracted, leaving the free suture to be retrieved

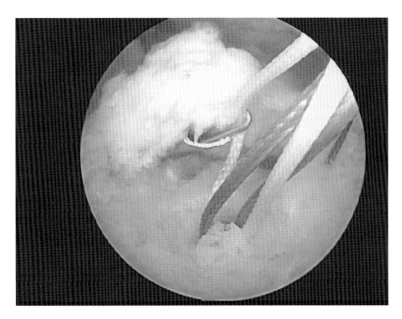

FIGURE 12.4. With the eyelet open, one limb of the anchor suture is isolated, captured, and drawn retrograde back through the tendon.

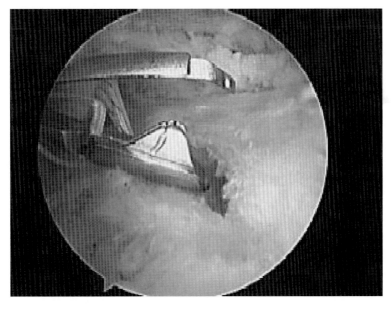

FIGURE 12.5. The ExpresSew (Depuy Mitek Inc., Norwood, MA) passer is introduced into the subacromial space, the jaws are opened, and the tendon edge is engaged to allow suture passage.

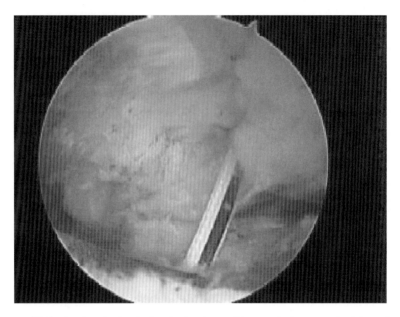

FIGURE 12.6. As the device is fired, the tine, with coupled suture, is driven from the articular to the bursal side of the tendon edge and then retracted, leaving the free suture to be retrieved.

(Figure 12.6). This process is repeated for each subsequent anchor suture.

12.2.7.3. Pulling Stitches

The pulling suture is a monofilament O-PDS, which is passed using a Spectrum pigtail Conmed (Linvatec, Key Largo, FL). The pigtail device has the advantage of various degrees of offset (45° and 90° both right and left), which allows optimal placement of the suture. Before being inserted in the shoulder, the device is loaded with a strand of the monofilament suture. Using a twisting motion, the suture passer penetrates the articular side of the tear [Figure 12.7(A)] and passes through the tendon, exiting the bursal side, where the suture is deployed [Figure 12.7(B)]. The suture is retrieved along with one limb of the anchor suture [Figure 12.7(C)] tied with a half hitch to the anchor suture and pulled back through the tendon, creating a simple stitch ready for tying [Figure 12.7(D)]. This process is repeated for each subsequent anchor suture.

12.2.7.4. Opus Auto Cuff (Opus Medical, San Juan Capistrano, CA)

The Opus system employs an automated suture passer, the Smartstitch (Opus Medical, San Juan Capistrano, CA), which facilitates the passage of an inclined horizontal mattress suture [Figure 12.8(A–C)]. The suture is then coupled to the Magnum anchor [Figure 12.8(D)], a cinching mechanism draws the tendon edge into the anchor site, and an internal locking mechanism secures the suture to the anchor, maintaining loop tension without the need for knot tying [Figure 12.8(E)]. This system is ideal for the surgeon just beginning to incorporate an all-arthroscopic approach to repairs, for whom knot tying is still somewhat challenging.

12.2.8. Procedure Completion

Once the repair is complete, stability is assessed with rotation and gentle flexion. If the patient has had a long-acting intrascalene block, all portals are closed and a light compressive dressing is applied. If no block has been used, a pain catheter is inserted in the subacromial space under direct visualization. This catheter will deliver 2 mL of long-acting anesthetic per hour with the capability to self-bolus another 2 mL/h. The patient will remove the catheter on the second postoperative day and begin a gentle passive range of motion program that allows external rotation to 30° with the elbow at the side.

12.3. Postoperative Management

12.3.1. Week 1

For the first 24 h following surgery, I ask the patient to perform gentle active assisted range of motion exercises elbow and wrist to decrease the risk of venous stasis and deep vein thrombosis (DVT). If a subacromial pain catheter has been used, it is removed by the patient after 2 days. The remainder of the week the patient is encouraged to perform gentle pendulum exercises that had been taught preoperatively and to continue the exercises for the elbow and wrist. The patient is further instructed to wear the immobilizer at all times while out in public and in bed.

12.3.2. Weeks 2 to 4

This constitutes phase I of the exercise program and is passive in nature. I teach a passive range of motion (ROM) program for forward elevation and external rotation to be performed in a supine position. If there is any question about a patient's ability to participate in this program, formal supervised therapy is employed. During the first month, the patient must avoid extension and internal rotation. No resistive exercises are performed at this time; however, I do add scapular rotation exercises.

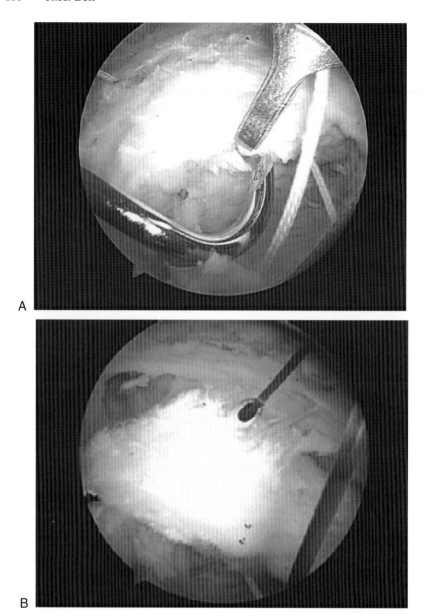

FIGURE 12.7. (A–D) Viewing from the lateral portal, the passer is introduced from the posterior portal; it penetrates the articular side of the tear, and the suture is deployed. A ring grasper retrieves the pulling suture along with one limb of the anchor suture; they are tied together and pulled back through the tendon, creating a simple stitch ready for tying.

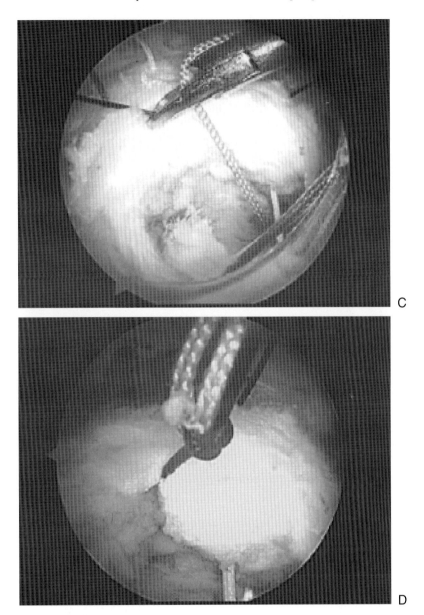

FIGURE 12.7. *Continued*

12.3.3. Weeks 5 to 10

Phase II consists of active and active assisted ROM. These are begun in a supine position, progressing to a seated or standing position. Patients are asked to use their normal limb or a cane to assist with the early active motion program. All planes of motion are incorporated, including forward elevation, abduction, external rotation, as well as gentle internal rotation.

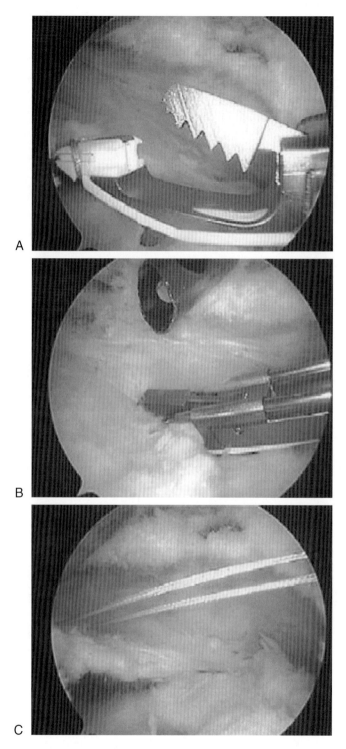

A

B

C

FIGURE 12.8. (A–E) The Opus Medical device is introduced from the lateral portal; it grasps the tendon edge and passes an inclined mattress stitch. The suture is coupled to the Magnum anchor, the anchor is inserted into a predrilled hole and deployed; a cinching mechanism draws the tendon edge into the anchor site, and an internal locking mechanism secures the suture to the anchor.

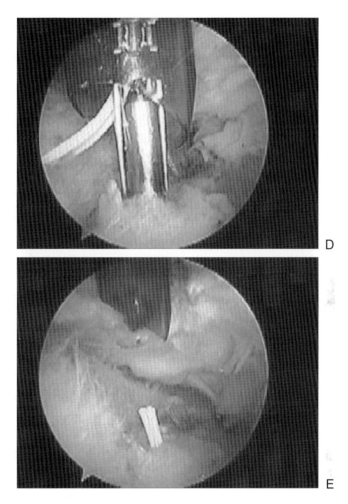

FIGURE 12.8. *Continued*

12.3.4. Week 10

There is some controversy as to when resistive exercises may be safely added to a rehabilitation program. Clearly, size of the tear, quality of repair, and patient's compliance will factor into the decision. However, for most small- and medium-sized tears can be started at the 10- to 12-week mark postoperatively when a comfortable range of active motion has been achieved.

The time for a return to athletic endeavors and/or manual labor will differ from patient to patient, depending upon the size of the tear as well as rehabilitation potential and individual motivation. Most patients are told that discharge should be anticipated at the 4- to 6-week mark, but that ultimate return to athletic endeavors and/or heavy manual work may take 6 to 9 months. Furthermore, they are instructed that full maturation of their repair and ultimate return of strength can take greater than 12 months and that they should not be frustrated by some residual discrepancy in strength relative to their normal contralateral shoulder.

12.4. Complications

12.4.1. Pain

The etiology of residual or persistent pain following an arthroscopic rotator cuff repair is no different from that seen after an open repair and may be due to any one of a number of sources.[5] An inadequate decompression must be considered in those patients in whom motion and strength seem to be improved from the preoperative status, yet pain relief has been only partial.

Occasionally, the A-C joint may be painful following a repair. Clearly, careful preoperative planning and treatment of symptomatic A-C problems during the initial surgery should avoid later trouble. For postoperative pain, selective injections may provide adequate relief, if not, an arthroscopic resection maybe needed.

A painful biceps tendon is not uncommon following both open and arthroscopic rotator cuff repairs. This is seen during the early phase of strengthening exercises and will usually pass. However, additional modalities, such as phonophoresis and/or injections, may be helpful. Once again, preoperative recognition of a painful biceps may warrant it being addressed at the time of the initial procedure with either a tenodesis or tenotomy.[6]

12.4.2. Re-Tear

Re-tear following an arthroscopic repair of a small- or medium-sized tear is uncommon but may be seen more commonly in the larger tears and those with poor quality tissue and/or significant retraction.[7] Often patients with suspected re-tears will note an improvement in their postoperative pain to the point where nothing further is needed. In those individuals with confirmed re-tears and ongoing symptoms, repair is warranted if the tissue quality at the time of the initial repair was adequate.

12.4.3. Stiffness

Each and every patient undergoing rotator cuff surgery will note a different rate of recovery both in terms of pain relief as well as return of motion.

Occasionally, patients may develop postoperative adhesive capsulitus. More often than not I see this in those patients with preoperative stiffness and patients with acute tears repaired in the first few weeks following their injury. As in anterior cruciate surgery, there seems to be a greater likelihood of arthrofibrosis if surgery is performed during the initial postinjury inflammatory phase. Therefore, I have begun to delay the repair in those patients for 3 weeks, to regain motion and allow the postinjury inflammatory component to resolve. This delay has not been a problem in terms of reparability of even large tears and their postoperative stiffness has been less. If motion remains limited after 4 to 5 months, a gentle manipulation with concomitant arthroscopic release is performed.

References

1. Murray TF Jr, Lajtai G, Mileski RM, Snyder SJ. Arthroscopic repair of medium to large full-thickness rotator cuff tears: outcome at 2- to 6-year follow-up. J Shoulder Elbow Surg 2002;11:19–24.
2. Wilson F, Hinov V, Adams G. Arthroscopic repair of full-thickness tears of the rotator cuff: 2- to 14-year follow-up. Arthroscopy 2002;18:136–144.
3. Gartsman GM. Arthroscopic rotator cuff repair [review]. Clin Orthop 2001; 390:95–106.
4. Wolf EM, Pennington WT, Agrawal V. Arthroscopic rotator cuff repair: 4- to 10-year results. Arthroscopy 2004;20:5–12.
5. Weber SC, Abrams JS, Nottage WM. Complications associated with arthroscopic shoulder surgery. Arthroscopy 2002;18(suppl 1):88–95.
6. Walch G, Edwards TB, Boulahia A, et al. Arthroscopic tenotomy of the long head of the biceps in the treatment of rotator cuff tears: clinical and radiographic results of 307 cases. J Shoulder Elbow Surg 2005;14:238–246.
7. Galatz LM, Ball CM, Teefey SA, Middleton WD, Yamaguchi K. The outcome and repair integrity of completely arthroscopically repaired large and massive rotator cuff tears. J Bone Joint Surg Am 2004;86:219–224.

13
Arthroscopic Repair of Subscapularis Tears

Laurent Lafosse and Reuben Gobezie

Rupture of the subscapularis tendon, especially from isolated tears, is a rare finding that was first described by Hauser in 1954.[1] This special pathology, its epidemiology, and the clinical and radiological findings were evaluated by Gerber and Krushell in 1991.[2] As with many pathologies, it appears to be more and more common as soon as it becomes well known. Lift off and belly press tests should now be part of all physical exams of the shoulder as soon as a rotator cuff tear is suspected. Subscapularis tear may be isolated or associated with posterior superior cuff tear, but symptoms, clinical signs, and natural history are very different. The treatment of subscapularis lesions has been neglected despite studies with satisfying results with open subscapularis repair.[3–5]

Arthroscopic treatment of rotator cuff lesions has developed during the last two decades and has become a successful approach even for large tears. But despite rapid progress of arthroscopic rotator cuff repair techniques, the subscapularis tendon seemed inaccessible until recently. In 2002, Burkhart and Tehrany[6] reported encouraging preliminary results in 25 cases with arthroscopic repair of subscapularis tears. The proposed technique demonstrated the feasibility of arthroscopic subscapularis repair, but the short follow-up of the patients and the heterogeneity of the series did not permit valid conclusions about the success of arthroscopic subscapularis repair. The only other author who reported on isolated arthroscopic subscapularis repair is Bennet; his series included eight cases, including two partial tears but no extended tear, and he proposed a new classification.[7]

We started all-arthroscopic repairs of subscapularis tears in 1995, but our series starts in 2000. We present the surgical technique and review of clinical results.

13.1. Anatomy and Endoscopy

The subscapularis is a large muscle that contributes 50% of the strength of the rotator cuff and is attached to the surface of the scapula medially. Its humeral attachment at the lesser tuberosity is made up of two parts

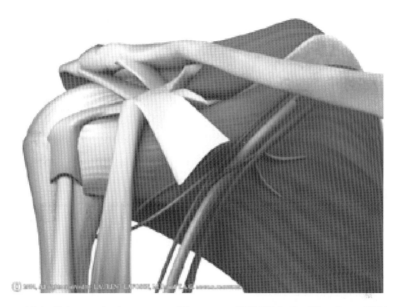

Figure 13.1. Subscapularis anatomy. (Courtesy of TAG Medical Products, Kibbutz Gaaton, Israel.)

(Figure 13.1): the superior two third is a big, strong tendon and the inferior third is a weak, direct attachment of the muscle. The surface of insertion of the lesser tuberosity has a large foot print (3 × 2 cm). Its anterior limit is the bicipital grove, and the subscapularis superficial fibers are connected to the facia of the sulcus grove as the end of the superior glenohumeral (SGHL) and coracohumeral (CHL) ligaments. This fibrous area is considered as the anterior restraint of the long head of the biceps (LHB) at its entrance in the groove, thereby preventing subluxation of the LHB, especially during external rotation.[8]

The arthroscope allows one to visualize the intra-articular side, which is the superior third only, as the remaining two thirds is covered by the capsule. The upper part of the LHB pulley is formed by the conjoint attachment of the SGHL and CHL back to the subscapularis tendon attachment. Stability of the biceps is assessed by external rotation of the humeral head. The intra-articular subscapularis tendon has a long sliding distance (3 cm) and passes in the concave part of the glenoid rim when the humeral head is internally rotated. The rotator interval goes from the superior part of the subscapularis tendon to the CHL. These weak aponeurotic fibers are used for easy access of instruments to the joint for Bankart repair and for the intra-articular part of the subscapularis tendon repair. A probe passed through this portal can go under the tendon and shows the deep fibers, while some internal rotation and flexion of the humerus decreases the tension of the muscle in order to have good visualization.

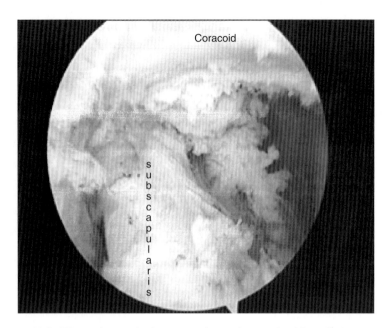

FIGURE 13.2. The subscapularis runs along the underside of the coracoid process.

As the inferior two thirds are covered by the capsule, there is no intra-articular access and the endoscopic visualization must be done from the subacromial area. All of the extra-articular side of the subscapular lateral part can be assessed: the superior third by sliding under the coracoid; the inferior two thirds are crossed medially to the coracoid by the plexus, the most medial element of which is the musculocutaneus nerve going to the conjoint tendon, and the artery (Figures 13.2 and 13.3). The inferior part and border of the muscle is crossed by the axillary nerve, which goes under the glenohumeral capsule to the posterior deltoid (Figure 13.4).

The enervation of the muscle comes from two main roots. Both are direct branches of the plexus: one goes to the superior third just medial to the coracoid; the other goes to the inferior two thirds much more medially. Other accessory branches go directly into the muscle. This point is crucial and explains why the subscapularis muscle is never involved when the suprascapular nerve is damaged at the suprascapular notch. As the plexus is very close to the muscle and the enervating branches are very short, it is easy to understand that when the muscle is retracted due to a large tear, reduction becomes dangerous and difficult in chronic cases when the plexus is stuck to the muscle. Release must be done carefully, especially at the superior level of the muscle, in order to avoid destruction of this essential enervation. When the release is not done during the repair, it may cause

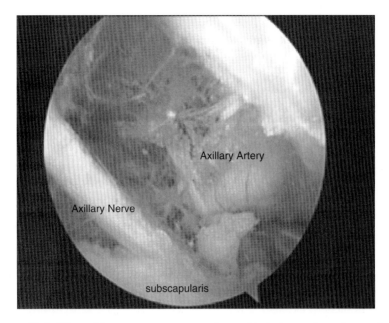

FIGURE 13.3. The axillary artery runs anterior and inferior to the subscapularis.

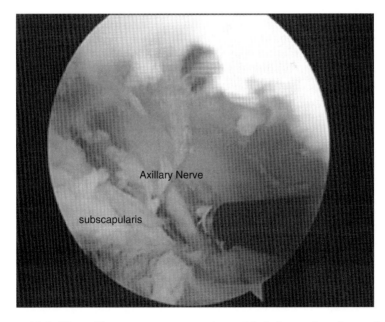

FIGURE 13.4. The axillary nerve runs anterior and inferior to the subscapularis.

pain after surgery going to the forearm and the hand with a feeling of weakness and heavy arm. The ability to release the suprascapular nerve may be one of the most interesting advantages of arthroscopic release compared to open surgery.

The subscapularis tendon is an essential part of the anterior wall of the shoulder and keeps the head and the lesser tuberosity behind the coracoid during internal rotation.

13.2. Causes of Subscapularis Tendon Tear

Subscapularis tendon tears generally occur on degenerative tendons, but they quite often result from traumatic injury by a muscular contraction of the subscapularis to resist an overrotation while the arm is in abduction external rotation. Partial tears are generally purely degenerative, and massive tears are mainly traumatic.

The tear starts in the superior third and may be partial or retracted. When the tear extends to the inferior two thirds, the superior third is always detached. Detachment may be in the deep layer only, and when the superficial layer is still attached it is not possible to diagnose this form by open surgery unless the bicipital groove is opened to expose the border of the subscapularis attachment.[8] Usually, the mechanism of detachment goes vertically from superior to inferior and horizontally from the articular to the superficial layer.

When the superior third of the tendon is detached, often the anterior sling of the biceps is stretched or torn and the LHB may be subluxated or dislocated.[8] When the biceps is intact and reattachment of the subscapularis tendon is performed, it is not uncommon that it shrinks the entrance of the groove and squeezes the biceps. This concept of proximity of the biceps and the subscapularis attachment is essential to avoid LHB problems after subscapularis repair, whether arthroscopic or open. As the supraspinatus is inserted on the greater tuberosity, its superficial fibers are linked with the distal part of the CHL, SGHL, and the upper part of the subscapularis tendon. Often, the complete complex is detached from the bone and is retracted medially. This creates an appearance of a "comma," as described by Burkhart,[9] and the reattachment often needs a medial release of the superior structures to reconstruct the anatomical insertion.

When the entire tendon is torn, there is no more active anterior wall. There is a marked increase in external rotation and the humeral head has no resistance to superior and anterior subluxation while the deltoid is pulling superiorly and anteriorly, mainly during maximum internal rotation. The head is translated and the elbow is fixed when the hand is placed against the belly. As the humeral head and the lesser tuberosity go forward, it creates a coracoid impingement that is initially dynamic but becomes permanent in chronic tears.

When the tear becomes chronic, the muscle atrophies and undergoes fatty infiltration, according to the Goutallier classification[10] initially described for computerized tomography (CT) scanning, and then for magnetic resonance imaging (MRI).[11] The atrophy may be reversible but not the fatty degeneration that can occur after a very variable delay. Stage III on the four-stage classification means that at least 50% of the muscle is fat and functional outcome is poor.[12]

13.3. Diagnosis and Evaluation

Subscapularis tear should be suspected when a shoulder is painful and/or weak, with or without associated supraspinatus or infraspinatus tear. It may even be suspected in traumatic injury that results in an acute, very painful and weak shoulder or at least in the case of a spontaneous LHB tear. Physical examination should focus on external hyperrotation and should include the lift off and belly press tests. The bear hug test recently described by de Beer and Burkhart[6] is done in the same position as the Yocum test, but the test is performed by pulling on the hand applied on the opposite shoulder. This creates pain the strength of which can be measured. When only the belly press test is positive, it is usually because the inferior part of the tendon is intact. Use the standard anterior–posterior view and profile outlet view to look for a lesser tuberosity fracture.

Diagnosis is accomplished by arthro-CT scan as resolution is better, the number of slices per centimeter is much higher, and the injection of contrast gives a perfect view of the tendon attachment at the anterior part of the LHB groove than in MRI. The size of the tear and the level of retraction are evaluated, as is the fatty degeneration. Furthermore, it is important to document the position of the humeral head, noting the presence of anterior subluxation and the distance between the coracoid and the lesser tuberosity. Anterior subluxation, coracoid impingement, and fatty degeneration make a successful repair less likely.

13.4. Surgical Procedure

13.4.1. Positioning, Portals, and Visualization

The beach chair position with 3-kg traction gives a shoulder positioning of the arm with slight flexion and internal rotation that allows more room for the subscapularis arthroscopic surgery.

Arthroscopy starts with the classic intra-articular posterior portal, and the following portals will be effective, depending on the lesion. As no cannula is used, portals are created from outside to inside, and a needle is used to visualize the portal and the access that the instrument can get. At

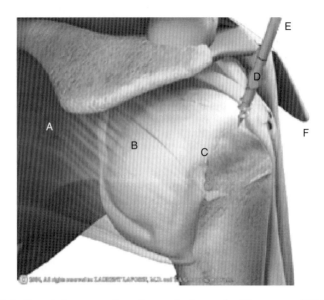

FIGURE 13.5. Portal placement for subscapularis repair. (Courtesy of TAG Medical Products, Kibbutz Gaaton, Israel.)

least three portals are used, depending on the size of the lesion (Figure 13.5). A 30° arthroscope is introduced into the glenohumeral joint through the posterior "soft-spot" portal (portal A, Figure 13.5). Using this posterior portal, adequate visualization of tears involving the superior two thirds of the subscapularis tendon without retraction can be achieved. The stability at the entrance of the groove and the shape of the LHB are evaluated while rotating the humeral head. By opening the rotator interval, it is possible to have good access to the superior tendon under the coracoid process and to see the extra-articular part of the superior third, especially when a 70° scope is used. If the LHB is torn or if biceps tenodesis or tenotomy is needed, access to the subscapularis becomes easier. The deep layer of the tendon can be visualized by pulling the superficial part with a probe introduced by the anterior portal.

When the tear extends inferiorly and is retracted, extra-articular visualization is needed. In such cases, a lateral (portal C, Figure 13.5) or anterolateral portal (portal D, Figure 13.5) may be used. Both of these portals allow an enhanced view of the anterior aspect of the shoulder, including the coracoid, subscapularis muscle, subscapularis nerves, plexus, axillary artery, and axillary nerve. This visualization is necessary to perform the release before the repair. After visualization of the coracoid and conjoint tendon, the other anterior portals are established before release of the plexus and artery. The scope is swished from portal C to portal D, according to the lesion and the working portals. Two anterior working portals (portals D and E, Figure 13.5) are used to perform the debridement, place the anchors, and pass the sutures through the torn tendon. The anterosuperior portal lateral to the coracoid (portal E, Figure 13.5) is used to pass the sutures through the torn tendon edge, and an anterolateral (portal D, Figure 13.5) portal in the rotator interval is used to release the subscapularis, debride the subcoracoid space and lessen the tuberosity, and to place the suture anchors. In larger and retracted tears, an anteroinferior portal (portal F, Figure 13.5) is used to perform the subscapularis release circumferentially. This portal gives a good access for inferior anchor placement and suture management through the inferior subscapularis tendon.

13.4.2. Classification

In general, ruptures of the subscapularis are readily identified once a careful diagnostic arthroscopy is performed. We use a new classification scheme in order to further characterize the subscapularis tears arthroscopically and to guide our operative approach to repair these lesions. Because most prior studies and techniques for evaluating subscapularis tears were based on principles correlating to open tendon reconstruction, we believe the incidence of partial tears to the subscapularis tendon is underreported. In addition, the current classification schemes do not differentiate between complete retracted tears of the subscapularis tendon that result in an eccentrically positioned humeral head and those with a completely congruent glenohumeral joint. In our experience, this distinction is important because the outcomes of the patient populations differ markedly. According to our classification, subscapularis tears may be divided into five types (Table 13.1).

- Type 1 tears are localized to the superior third of the subscapularis tendon and are partial tears of the deep fibers at the insertion onto the lesser tuberosity. These tears never display tendon retraction as a feature of their presentation because the superficial fibers of the subscapularis remain intact.
- Type II tears are complete ruptures limited to the superior third of the tendon affecting both the superficial and deep fibers [Figure 13.6(A)].
- Type III tears are complete tears of the superior two thirds of the subscapularis tendon. The intact inferior third of the subscapularis tendon

TABLE 13.1. Subscapularis Tear Classification.

Type	Lesion	Cases
I	Partial lesion of superior third	2
II	Complete lesion of superior third	5
III	Lesion of superior two thirds	6
IV	Complete lesion of the tendon, but head centered and fatty degeneration < type III	4
V	Complete lesion of tendon but excentric head with coracoid impingement and fatty degeneration > type III	0

Source: Reproduced with permission from Lafosse et al., Structural integrity and clinical outcomes after arthroscopic subscapularis repair. J Bone Joint Surg Am. 2007, in press.

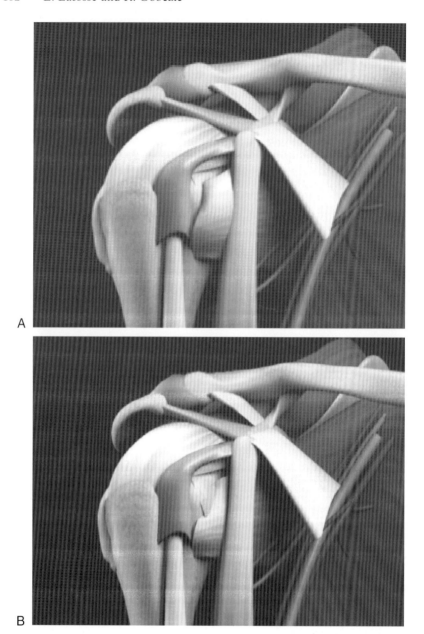

FIGURE 13.6. (A) Type II, subscapularis tendon avulsion (superior third). (B) Type III, subscapularis tendon avulsion (two thirds). (Courtesy of TAG Medical Products, Kibbutz Gaaton, Israel.)

insertion limits the degree of retraction that may occur with these lesions [Figure 13.6(B)].

- Type IV tears are complete tears of the entire subscapularis tendon from its insertion and are combined with retraction of the tendon edge to the level of the glenoid rim without anterior eccentricity of the humeral head on the glenoid [Figure 13.7(A)].
- Type V tears are complete tears of the subscapularis with retraction and an eccentric humeral head that is displaced anteriorly on the glenoid due to a disruption of the force-couple of the rotator cuff. These tears often result in coracoid impingement and in a fatty degeneration grade IV [Figure 13.7(B)].

Tears of the superior third of the subscapularis are often covered by a synovial membrane or, less often, by an intact anterior pulley and can be clearly identified after debridement and positioning of the arm in flexion and internal rotation. More extended ruptures with a retracted tendon are frequently combined with a detachment of the superior glenohumeral and coracohumeral ligaments from their insertion on the humerus. These ligaments are usually still attached to the superolateral border of the subscapularis tendon, creating the comma described by Burkhart and Tehrany.[6] Although this structure can aid in localizing the superior border of the torn subscapularis tendon, none of the patients in this study had supraspinatus tears so that debridement of the lesser tuberosity from the subacromial view is often required to correctly identify the tendon edge.

13.4.3. Surgical Technique

The release is performed as soon as the subscapularis becomes retracted, initially superiorly and intra-articularly. The upper part of the tendon is released from the glenoid and coracoid by shaving the soft tissues and adhesions between the superficial surface of the tendon and the deep surface of the coracoid. The intra-articular release of the subscapularis requires debridement of the middle glenohumeral ligament from the posterior subscapularis. Superiorly and anteriorly, the subdeltoid and sub-coracoid adhesions are released. To improve visualization and assist in mobilizing the tendon, we also routinely release the origin of the coraco-humeral ligament from the coracoid process. A traction suture is placed through the anterolateral portal to facilitate the release of the subscapularis tendon. The anatomical structure limiting the release of the subscapularis tendon in type III tears is the axillary nerve. However, in order to mobilize some type III and IV subscapularis tears, adhesions between the brachial plexus and the retracted tendon are released and careful dissection is performed in order to avoid damage to the two branches of the subscapular nerve on the anterior surface of the muscle belly.

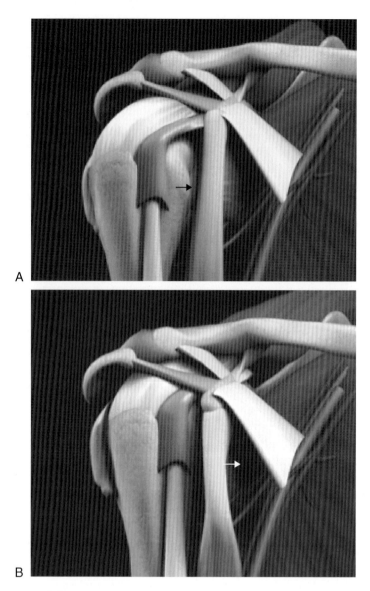

FIGURE 13.7. (A) Type IV, complete avulsion with retraction to the conjoined tendon. The arrow points to the lateral edge of the subscapularis. (B) Type V, complete avulsion with retraction medial to the conjoined tendon. The arrow points to the lateral edge of the retracted subscapularis. (Courtesy of TAG Medical Products, Kibbutz Gaaton, Israel.)

Release should be managed from a superior to inferior direction, and the shaver should not be used other than at the medial part of the coracoid and conjoint tendon. A smooth arthroscopic trochar is usually used gently to recreate an anatomical sliding space between the plexus and the subscapularis muscle. When the inferior part of the muscle is retracted, the axillary nerve is released following its pathway from the superior direction in order to be sure not to injure it.

13.4.3.1. Reduction

Reduction is managed with a grasper and/or a suture passed through an anterolateral portal that allows one to check the reduction and to move the tensioning of the tendon during the reattachment. The key is to perform a release sufficient to allow an easy reduction without excessive tensioning in a neutral position. Once the tendon edge is released, a burr or shaver is used to decorticate the lesser tuberosity in preparation for anchor placement and to optimize the environment for tendon healing.

13.4.3.2. Coracoplasty

Coracoplasty is performed when the humeral head is dynamically eccentrically positioned and associated with retracted subscapularis tears, mainly in type IV, when posterior relocation is possible by restoring the subscapularis muscle sling.

13.4.3.3. Fixation

Portals for fixation are variable and adapted to the tear but always lateral to the coracoid and the conjoint tendon. They may be very inferior when the tear is extended. Fixation always starts with the most inferior and medial anchor. Reconstruction of the footprint always proceeds from the most inferior aspect of the torn tendon working proximally. Anchors are always placed along the anterior border of the bicipital groove in order to achieve an anatomical footprint repair. In type III and IV tears, a mattress suture is used inferiorly and medially and a more lateral simple suture laterally over the footprint to perform a double row suture anchor repair. We believe that this repair technique maximizes the contact area for tendon healing and results in a more stable reconstruction.

We use metallic Fastin (Smith & Nephew Endoscopy, Andover, MA) and, more recently, Spiralok (Smith & Nephew Endoscopy, Andover, MA) absorbable anchors because we have been convinced that they are reliable. We use the Twinfix (Smith & Nephew Endoscopy, Andover, MA) metallic anchors. What appears to be important is the quality of the suture; we always use two strong Orthocord™ (Depuy Mitek, Westwood, MA) sutures per anchor in order to decrease the risk of failure by damaging the sutures during knot tying. We try to avoid sliding knots and perform a simple nonsliding knot as in open surgery.

For a superior lesion of types I and II (Figure 13.8), the anchor is placed through the anterosuperior portal just under the superior tendon insertion on the lesser tuberosity. The sutures are retrieved through the lateral portal and positioned under the subscapularis tendon in order to let a retriever penetrating grasper (Clever hook, Mitek Depuy) pass through the

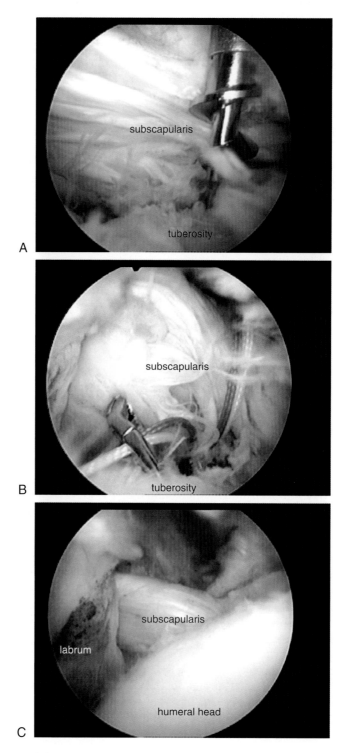

FIGURE 13.8. (A). Suture anchor placement in superior lesser tuberosity. (B) The suture grasper retrieves braided sutures through subscapularis tendon. (C) The subscapularis is firmly attached to the lesser tuberosity.

anterosuperior portal and the upper part of the tendon. The four ends of sutures are passed, two in one shot and the two others in two alternative tendon penetrations in order to create a mattress for both sutures. Knots are tied by grasping the two ends of the same suture in one shot through the portal in order to avoid a soft tissue interposition as no canula is used.

For more extended lesions, as in types III and IV, the D portal is used for visualization, and two E and F anterior portals are used for instrumentation (Figure 13.9). After placement of the most inferior anchor though the most medial and inferior F portal, the suture is retrieved through E, the more anterolateral one, in order to give room in F for the penetrating grasper to be in the best position, as perpendicular as possible, to go through the tendon and to catch the suture previously positioned behind the articular surface of it.

When the extension of the tear goes inferiorly, reattachment starts with a very inferior anchor and the footprint is re-created using a W (Cassiopeia) technique of re-insertion.

13.4.3.4. Associated Lesions

Before and after repair, as it may reduce an anterior subluxation, it is very important to check that there is no impingement between the lesser tuberosity and the coracoid process by subacromial visualization of the tendon during internal rotation. If needed, coracoplasty may be indicated to avoid the impingement.

When the supraspinatus and infraspinatus are torn, subscapularis repair should be performed first as the tear of the superior cuff allows good access for subscapularis release and reattachment. In a few cases when supraspinatus and subscapularis are both detached from the bone but still attached together, the more inferior subscapularis is reattached first, then fixation of both subscapularis and supraspinatus is managed on the same superior anchor. When the biceps is involved, we perform a tenodesis with a specific technique of reattachment on an anchor.

13.4.4. Postoperative Management

Postoperatively, patients are immobilized in a sling for isolated subscapularis repair, or with a small resting pillow with around 30° abduction and flexion for a supraspinatus repair, for 6 weeks. During this period, only passive motion is allowed with internal rotation to the belly but not behind the back, external rotation to 0°, nonrestricted forward flexion in internal rotation. After 6 weeks, nonrestricted active-assisted forward flexion and rotation is allowed. Muscle reinforcement starts after 3 months.

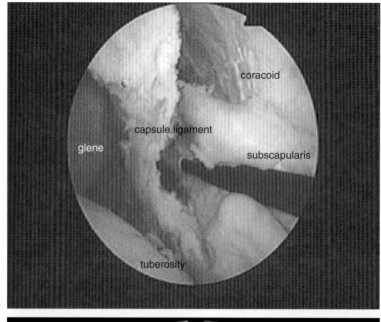

A

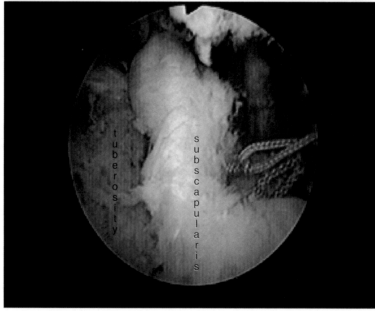

B

FIGURE 13.9. (A) Subscapularis retracted tear Type III. (B) Anterior view of repaired subscapularis tendon.

13.4.5. Results

In order to assess specifically the subscapularis arthroscopic repair, we studied a series of patients who had isolated subscapularis tears repaired arthroscopically.

13.4.6. Patient Selection

Between May 2000 and July 2002, 17 patients underwent arthroscopic repair of isolated, full-thickness subscapularis tears.[14] The 13 men and 4 women had an average age of 47 years (range, 29–59 years) at the time of surgery. The dominant side was involved in 94% (16 of the 17 patients). The mean duration of symptoms until surgery was 24 months (range, 3–44 months).

Thirteen patients had a traumatic tear, caused by combined forced abduction and external rotation in six cases, by direct heavy trauma or blow to the shoulder in four cases, by heavy lifting in two cases, and by severe traction on the arm in one case. Six of these traumas were work injuries. In the remaining four cases, symptoms developed progressively over a mean of 15 months without any traumatic shoulder event in the history.

13.5. Preoperative and Postoperative Clinical and Radiological Assessment

Pre- and postoperatively, all were clinically assessed with the Constant score and the University of California at Los Angeles (UCLA) score. Postoperatively, all were reviewed by an examiner independent from the operating surgeon. Preoperatively, the specific diagnosis of a subscapularis tear was made clinically with the lift off test. Pain was evaluated by Constant score from 0 to 15 and strength from 0 to 5 according to the international strength evaluation in neurological classification. A subscapularis tear was clinically diagnosed with the help of the lift off and the belly press tests in 94% (16 of 17) of the patients. Additionally, four patients had positive tests for the long head of the biceps tendon. In two patients, the long head of the biceps tendon was ruptured at the time of diagnosis with the typical clinical appearance of a distalized bulky muscle belly.

Radiographically, all 17 patients had pre- and postoperative standard radiographs (true antero-posterior and axillary lateral) and arthro-CT scan. On radiographs and CT scan, pre- and postoperative centralization of the humeral head in antero-posterior and supero-inferior direction was assessed.

13.6. Classification

On preoperative arthro-CT scan, the subscapularis tear was confirmed and the size of the rupture classified in the different types: two type I, five type II, six type III, and four type IV.

Pre- and postoperative fatty infiltration of the subscapularis, supraspinatus, and infraspinatus muscles was assessed according the classification of Goutallier.[10] All cases still had centered head, and no coracoid impingement was noticed. None had fatty infiltration greater than II. There were no type V lesions.

There was no additional full-thickness tear of the other rotator cuff tendons, but four patients had an additional articular partial tear of the supraspinatus tendon that was confirmed under arthroscopy. Because the partial tear involved less than one third of the tendon thickness and did not need treatment, the four patients were included in this series.

The 17 patients were reviewed after an average follow-up of 29 months (range, 24–34 months).

13.7. Clinical Results

- Subjectively, at final follow-up, 12 patients were very satisfied with their results, 4 were satisfied, and 1 was not satisfied.
- At follow-up, the relative Constant score averaged 96% (range, 68%–106%) and improvement compared to before surgery was statistically significantly ($p<0.001$; relative Constant 58%; range, 19%–80%). All patients had improved compared to their preoperative condition (Table 13.2).
- The mean pain was at 5.9 points before and at 13.5 points after the operation. Only one single patient continued to suffer from a painful shoulder after a long term. The median active forward flexion increased

TABLE 13.2. Average Result According to Constant and UCLA Score.

	Preoperative	Revision	Statistical significance
Pain (15 points)	5.9	13.5	$p < 0.001$
Active anterior elevation	145.6°	174.7°	$p = 0.005$
Active external rotation	50°	60.3°	$p = 0.03$
Internal rotation (10 points)	4	7.6	$p < 0.001$
Strength (25 points)	7.4	15.6	$p < 0.001$
Constant score (100 points)	52	84.9	$p < 0.001$
Constant score relative	58%	96.4%	$p < 0.001$
UCLA (35 points)	16.2	32.1	$p < 0.001$

Source: Data from Lafosse et al., Structural integrity and clinical outcomes after arthroscopic subscapularis repair. J Bone Joint Surg Am. 2007, in press.

TABLE 13.3. Change in Pain and Strength for Lift Off Test before Surgery and at Revision.

Lift off	Preoperative	Revision	Statistical significance
Pain (15 points)	3.3	12.6	$p < 0.001$
Strength (5 points)	2.3	4.1	$p < 0.001$

from 145.6° (70°–95°) to 174.7° (150°–180°) and the active external rotation in adduction from 50° (10°–80°) to 61° (10°–80°).

- Preoperatively, eight patients had an increased passive external rotation, in connection with an extended subscapularis rupture. Postoperatively, this was only found in one patient. Preoperative active internal rotation was median to the level of the sacrum (4 points); postoperatively, the patients reached the level of L12 (7.6 points).
- Strength was at median 7.4 points (0–12 points) before and 15.6 points (6–24 points) after the refixation. The UCLA score increased to 32.1 points postoperatively. The clinical results were excellent in 10 patients, good in 5, medium in 1, and poor in 1 patient.
- In order to assess specifically the subscapularis clinically, we compared the strength and the pain during the modified lift off and the belly press test before surgery and at revision (Tables 13.3 and 13.4). The mean gain of the force in belly press and lift off test was 2 points. In total, the clinical evaluation reflects the quality of our repair. Before the repair, five patients were not able to perform the lift off test for pain and restricted internal rotation. At follow up, all patients could perform this test, and we observed a significant improvement in pain and force (Table 13.3). Eight patients regained the same force as on the contralateral shoulder. Four patients stayed on force level ≤3; one of them had a subluxated LHB, another a rerupture of the upper two thirds of the tendon. In two patients, the control arthro-CT scan did not reveal any anomaly to explain the loss of force.
- The belly press test could be performed by all patients pre- and postoperatively. At the time of follow up, we noticed a significant improvement in pain and force in this test (Table 13.4). Ten patients had force comparable to the contralateral shoulder. Two patients reached ≤3 points,

TABLE 13.4. Change in Pain and Strength for Belly Press Test before Surgery and at Revision.

Belly press	Preoperative	Revision	Statistical significance
Pain (15 points)	5.6	14.1	$p < 0.001$
Strength (5 points)	2.5	4.4	$P < 0.001$

one of them had a subluxation of the LHB, the other rerruptured the upper two thirds of the tendon.

- We did not find a correlation between the results and age at the time of the operation, period between start of complaints and date of operation, follow-up period, and Constant Morley Score (CMS) values. The factors work injury, kind of injury, preoperative status of the LHB, and size of the rupture had no influence on the outcome. The influence of a persistent fatty degeneration ≥ degree 2 or a rerupture of the subscapularis tendon could not be statistically evaluated because of limited patient numbers.

13.8. Radiological Results

Standard X rays showed that all inserted anchors were in place. The radiographic arthro-CT scan before surgery was ≤ grade I in 15 shoulders and grade 2 in 2 cases. The control revealed no progression of fatty degeneration. Fifteen patients (88.3%) in the series were watertight after injection, which meant no recurrent tear and was good evidence of perfect healing.

13.9. Complications

There was no infection. A rerupture of the repaired subscapularis tendon was observed in two patients. Despite the structural failure, one had a good clinical result. One patient had postoperatively on the arthro-CT scan an anterior subluxation of the long head of the biceps tendon, but with an intact subscapularis repair. The clinical result at follow-up was unsatisfactory with pain but the patients refused further treatment.

13.10. Comparison of Results with the Literature

It looks as though our series has had good results comparable to the arthroscopic repair of Burkhart and better results than open surgery as arthroscopy avoids stiffness and lack of external rotation. It is difficult to compare our results with those in the literature (Table 13.5), because method, number of patients, follow-up period, size of rupture, and degree of tendon retraction vary a lot. In our study, 94% of the arthroscopically treated shoulders are not painful at the first follow-up after 6 weeks, compared to 63% of open treated patients for the series by Gerber[4] and 71% for Deutsch.[3] The median postoperative CMS increased in our series up to 94%.

All our patients had an arthro-CT scan control after long term, which in 11.7% of them revealed a leaking repair. Other studies judged only the

TABLE 13.5. Comparison between Results in Literature and Our Series.

Study	Follow-up (months)	Technique	No pain	Constant relative	UCLA	Stiffness	Leakage Postoperatively
Gerber[2] (16 cases)	43	Open	63%	82%	—	18.7%	—
Deutsch[3] (14 cases)	24	Open	71%	—	—	35.7%	—
SOFCOT (43 cases)	38	Open	—	76%	—	2%	19%
Burkhart[6] (8 cases)	10.7	Arthroscopic	—	—	32.8 points	—	—
Our series (17cases)	24	Arthroscopic	94%	96.4%	32.1 points	0%	11.7%

Source: Reproduced with permission from Lafosse et al., Structural integrity and clinical outcomes after arthroscopic subscapularis repair. J Bone Joint Surg Am. 2007, in press.

repair quality clinically with the lift off and belly press test. We also used these tests and evaluated separately pain and loss of force. In the literature there is no uniformity in classifying these tests negative or positive and there is no agreement in considering pain and/or loss of force.

In spite of the obvious superiority of our results, we are convinced that the arthroscopic treatment of isolated subscapularis ruptures could bring at least the same good results as open procedures with the advantage of no postoperative stiffness. The arthroscopic treatment of isolated subscapularis ruptures is a technically demanding method, presupposing a good experience in arthroscopic shoulder surgery. In contrast to Nové-Josserand,[13] we believe that arthroscopy makes possible a better intraoperative analysis of lesions, especially the small ones. In open techniques, the lesions of the superior third often are not detected because they are covered by a fibrous fascia of the attachment of the distal part of the CHL and SGHL that is inserted on the external part of the biceps sulcus and needs to be open in order to detect the subscapularis lesion.[13] Arthroscopy also allows better evaluation of the stability of the LHB. The subacromial view allows perfect assessment of the all tendon insertions and permits repair in a way that is as reliable as open surgery.

13.11. Indications

According the classification, types I, II, III, and IV are repaired arthroscopically. Complementary treatment as coracoplasty is done according the impingement after repair, and biceps tenotomy or tenodesis should be performed every time the LHB may be involved by the pathology or the subscapularis reattachment.

Type V, in which the humeral head is in a permanent position subluxated anteriorly with an irreparable subscapularis due to the fatty degeneration of the muscle, is an indication for a tendon transfer in young people or a reverse arthroplasty for elderly patients.

13.12. Conclusions

The results of our study show for the first time that arthroscopic treatment of isolated of subscapularis lesions brings the same good results that have been obtained with open procedures but without the postoperative restriction of mobility. This series with more than 2 years' follow-up of arthroscopic repair for isolated subscapularis tears shows not only good clinical results but even establishes the excellent quality of the reattachment by arthro-CT scan, which was performed for all patients after surgery.

References

1. Hauser ED. Avulsion of the tendon of the subscapularis muscle. J Bone Joint Surg Am 1954;36:139–141.
2. Gerber C, Krushell RJ. Isolated rupture of the tendon of the subscapularis muscle. Clinical features in 16 cases. J Bone Joint Surg Br 1991;73:389–394.
3. Deutsch A, Altchek DW, Veltri DM, Potter HG, Warren RW. Traumatic tears of the subscapularis tendon. Clinical diagnosis, magnetic resonance imaging findings, and operative treatment. Am J Sports Med 1997;25:13–22.
4. Gerber C, Hersche O, Farron A. Isolated rupture of the subscapularis tendon. J Bone Joint Surg Am 1996;78:1015–1023.
5. Gerber C, Schneeberger AG, Perren SM, Nyffeler RW. Experimental rotator cuff repair. A preliminary study. J Bone Joint Surg Am 1999;81:1281–1290.
6. Burkhart SS, Tehrany AM. Arthroscopic subscapularis tendon repair: technique and preliminary results. Arthroscopy 2002;18:454–463.
7. Bennett WF. Arthroscopic repair of massive rotator cuff tears: a prospective cohort with 2- to 4-year follow-up. Arthroscopy 2003;19:380–390.
8. Walch G, Nove-Josserand L, Boileau P, Levigne C. Subluxations and dislocations of the tendon of the long head of the biceps. J Shoulder Elbow Surg 1998;7:100–108.
9. Burkhart SS. Shoulder arthroscopy. New concepts. Clin Sports Med 1996;15:635–653.
10. Goutallier D, Postel JM, Bernageau J, Lavau L, Voisin MC. Fatty muscle degeneration in cuff ruptures. Pre- and postoperative evaluation by CT scan. Clin Orthop 1994;304:78–83.
11. Ticker JB, Warner JJ. Single-tendon tears of the rotator cuff. Evaluation and treatment of subscapularis tears and principles of treatment for supraspinatus tears. Orthop Clin North Am 1997;28:99–116.
12. Goutallier D, Postel JM, Gleyze P, Leguilloux P, Van Driessche S. Influence of cuff muscle fatty degeneration on anatomic and functional outcomes after simple suture of full-thickness tears. J Shoulder Elbow Surg 2003;12:550–554.
13. Nove-Josserand L, et al., [Isolated lesions of the subscapularis muscle. Apropos of 21 cases]. Rev Chir Orthop Reparatrice Appar Mot 1994;80:595–601.
14. Lafosse L et al. Structural integrity and clinical outcomes after arthroscopic subscapularis repair. J Bone Joint Surg Am. 2007, in press.

14
Tendon Mobilization in Large Rotator Cuff Tears

Felix H. Savoie III and Larry D. Field

Rotator cuff tears are one of the more common injuries.[1,2] Most managing physicians agree that symptomatic tears require repair.[3,4] Although traditionally repairs have been performed by open techniques, the advent of arthroscopic technique has increased our understanding of tear patterns and the need for anatomical restoration of the insertional footprint of the rotator cuff.[5]

Many factors influence the success or failure of a rotator cuff repair.[6–13] Factors inherent to the patient include size of the tear, the presence of atrophy of the muscle tendon unit, intraoperative adhesions or contractures, healing potential, and compliance with postoperative rehabilitation. Factors inherent to the surgeon include adequate preoperative assessment of the patient factors, evaluation of the tear patterns during preoperative imaging with reassessment during diagnostic arthroscopy, adequate releases to allow a tension-free repair of the tendon without undue pressure on the supplying neurovascular structures, elimination of tear-instigating factors (spurs, labral/biceps tears, etc.) while preserving the blood supply to the damaged cuff tissue, stable repair of the tendon with restoration of the normal footprint anatomy, and adequate postoperative immobilization and rehabilitation specific to both the tear and the patient.

In this chapter, we will detail the specific techniques of releases to allow a tension-free repair. Most of the techniques have been adapted from the open measures previously described by masterful surgeons and educators, including Codman, Neer, Rockwood, Fukada, Resch, and many others. The arthroscopic techniques were pioneered by Elman and Caspari, then modified and modernized by Esch, Snyder, Warren/Dines, Gartsman, Burkhart, and many others.[14]

14.1. Indications and Contraindications

The indications for releases around the rotator cuff vary by patient and surgeon. One of the key components of a successful repair is the ability to restore the footprint without tension on the repaired tissues.[15–17]

This usually necessitates the need to release the nonessential attachments of the muscle tendon units of the rotator cuff. As a minimum, the coracohumeral ligament almost always requires release, while the rest of the techniques described in this chapter may be applied on an individual basis.

Contraindications to release primarily relate to technical considerations. The lack of appropriate equipment or technical skills to release the tissue without damaging the muscle, tendon, or neurovascular structures is a contraindication not only to releases but to the repair itself.

14.2. Preoperative Planning

14.2.1. Anatomy

The structures that may produce tension on the rotator cuff repair include the capsule, the coracohumeral ligament, the subacromial and subdeltoid bursa, the venous plexus beneath the acromioclaviclar (A-C) joint, the suprascapular nerve and artery, and the anterior and posterior rotator interval tissue. The tissue released is dependent on the specific tear patterns and may be different in each case.

As a general guide, in small tears the coracohumeral ligament may be released from the base of the coracoid on the bursal side of the cuff. In medium tears without cleavage planes, the subdeltoid and subacromial bursa should also be released, in addition to the coracohumeral ligament. In medium-sized tears of the supraspinatus and infraspinatus tendons with cleavage planes, release of the capsular tissue beneath the undersurface component is required in addition to the previously detailed releases of the coracohumeral ligament, subdeltoid, and subacromial bursa.

Large (2+ tendon) tears without superior migration of the humeral head on the glenoid require release of the entire subtendon capsule, that is, the capsule beneath the supraspinatus, infraspinatus, and teres minor tendons, the coracohumeral ligament, the subdeltoid and subacromial bursa, as well as the plexus of veins and bursa beneath the A-C joint. For both the large tear with superior migration of the humeral head on the glenoid and the massive tear, we recommend a 360° capsular release just outside the labrum to improve mobilization of the subscapularis, supraspinatus, infraspinatus, and teres minor and to allow the humeral head to descend on the glenoid. The coracohumeral ligament should be released both within the joint and in the subacromial bursa, along with the subdeltoid/subacromial bursa, the sub–A-C joint venous plexus and bursa, the bursa from the entire undersurface of the acromion anterior to the spine, as well as on the spine and just posterior to the spine. In addition, in the massive tear selective release of the suprascapular nerve from the suprascapular notch may be indicated. In specific cases, the anterior or posterior rotator interval may be further released using the techniques described by Tauro and Burkhart, respectively.[18–20]

14.3. Surgical Procedure

14.3.1. Positioning and Setup

The patient may be placed in either the lateral decubitus or beach chair position. In the lateral decubitus position, the trunk should be rolled posteriorly 30° to allow access to the anterior aspect of the shoulder. A sterile arm suspension unit should be utilized so that the arm may be removed and replaced in traction as necessary. In the beach chair position, an arm-holding device is most useful in positioning the arm for repair.

The authors prefer the lateral decubitus position because it allows easier and safer access to the inferior capsule during release techniques.

14.3.2. Instrumentation

A standard 5-mm arthroscope and shaver with resector and abrader blades is required. It is advantageous to have one with an interchangeable cannula se, which allows the arthroscope and shaver to be switched back and forth without removing and re-establishing the portals. A series of duck bill punches or a needle tip cautery are useful in the capsular release part. The needle tip cautery may also be used if bleeding occurs. A suture-passing instrument may also be used to place a traction suture into the rotator cuff tendon during the releases to determine if adequate mobilization has been performed.

14.3.3. Surgical Technique

Specific techniques for releases about the shoulder and rotator cuff tears are based on tear patterns and on the anatomy of the patient. On the initial intra-articular diagnostic arthroscopy, the capsule should be assessed for tightness. If the capsule seems to be contracted, it should be released using a punch, knife, or cautery [Figure 14.1(A)]. Adequate release of the anterior capsule should allow the coracoid to be visualized from the posterior portal in the depth of the release [Figure 14.1(B)]. If the entire capsule is contracted, the release should continue until the entire inferior capsule has been released. This release then continues up the posterior capsule between the labrum and the infraspinatus tendon, releasing the entire capsular attachment of the infraspinatus (Figure 14.2). Once adequate intra-articular release has been accomplished, attention may then be directed toward the bursal tissues.

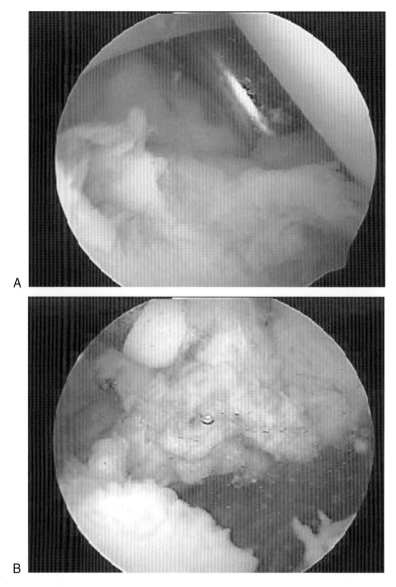

FIGURE 14.1. (A) Arthroscopic view of the anterior capsule. (B) Arthroscopic view of the coracoid as seen from the posterior portal in the depth of the release.

The scope is removed from the glenohumeral joint and placed into the subacromial bursa by removing it from the posterior portal, pulling the skin over the posterior deltoid superiorly and laterally, and placing the canula directly beneath the acromion. A lateral instrument portal is

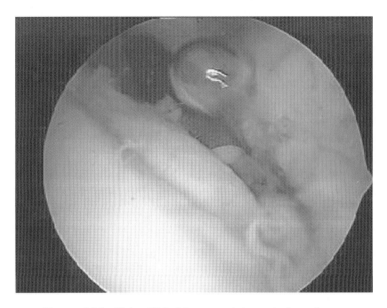

FIGURE 14.2. This will finish a complete posterior release.

established approximately 3 cm distal to the anterolateral corner of the acromion. The shaver is introduced initially into the subacromial area and then placed into the subdeltoid bursa on the lateral humerus. The deep layer of the subdeltoid bursa is then resected off the humerus, preserving the layer covering the inferior deltoid. This subdeltoid bursal release functionally elevates the deltoid away from the rotator cuff as well as the humerus. This is continued anteriorly and posteriorly around the humerus until the entire subdeltoid bursal release has been accomplished (Figure 14.3). The improved visualization provided by the elevation of the deltoid allows the shaver to be shifted anteriorly toward the coracohumeral ligament. The coracoacromial ligament is used as a guide, leading the surgeon down to the base of the coracoid [Figure 14.4(A)]. Once the coracoid has been visualized, the shaver is placed posterior to the coracoid process and tracked medially into the coracohumeral ligament [Figure 14.4(B)]. The coracohumeral ligament is resected off the coracoid, allowing increased mobilization of the supraspinatus tendon. The medial aspect of the coracoacromial ligament is then followed superiorly until the A-C joint is encountered. Following the ligament superiorly allows one to place a shaver directly beneath the A-C joint, releasing the venous plexus and subacromial bursa down toward the rotator cuff and away from the overlying bone of the acromion and distal clavicle (Figure 14.5). This release is then continued beneath the acromion, allowing the subacromial bursa to be released from the overlying acromion and scapular spine and drop

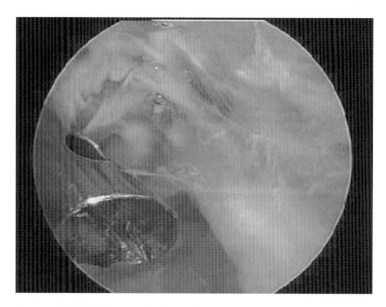

FIGURE 14.3. Arthroscopic view of the subdeltoid bursa contractures.

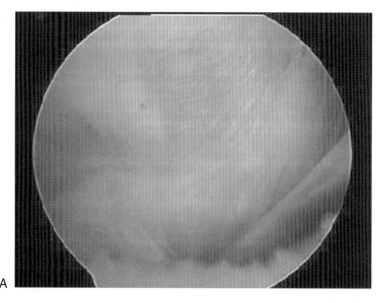

A

FIGURE 14.4. (A) The coracacromial ligament is used as a guide leading down to the base of the coracoid. (B) The shaver is then placed posterior to the coracoid process and tracked medially into the coracohumeral ligament.

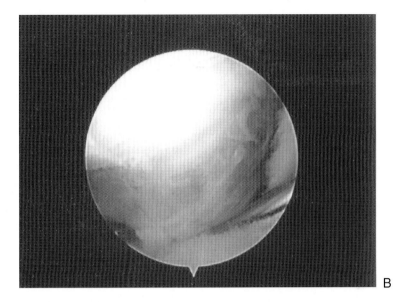

B

FIGURE 14.4. *Continued*

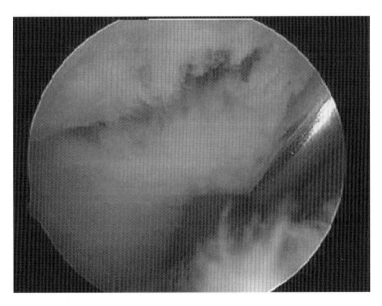

FIGURE 14.5. Here, the release of the venous plexus and subacromial bursa down toward the rotator cuff is accomplished.

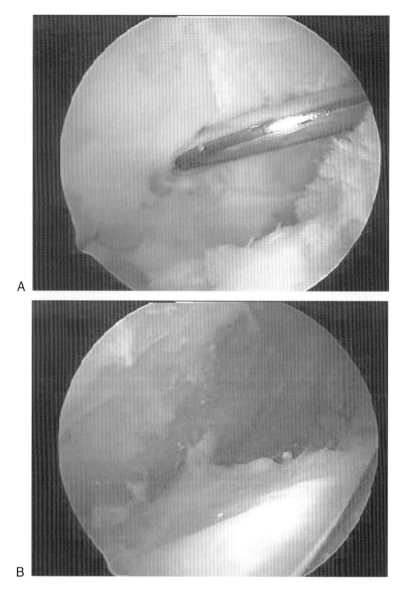

A

B

FIGURE 14.6. (A) The release is continued beneath the acromion, allowing the subacromial bursa to be released. (B) Arthroscopic view of the underside of the acromion post–bursa release.

down onto the rotator cuff. This is done in soft tissue by utilizing a back-and-forth as well as an in-and-out motion of the shaver [Figure 14.6(A,B)]. Once the scapular spine is encountered, the soft tissue should be released anteriorly, laterally, and posteriorly off the scapular spine to prevent contractures of the normal posterior rotator interval to the scapula spine [Figure 14.7(A,B)]. The scope is then directed more inferiorly and the shaver is swept around the posterior aspect of the remaining rotator cuff, staying just beneath the deltoid and completing the subdeltoid bursa release from the underlying rotator cuff tissues.

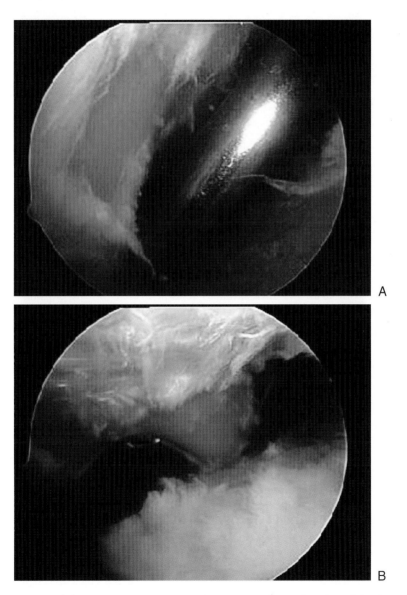

A

B

FIGURE 14.7. (A) View of the scapular spine from the posterior view. (B) View of the scapular spine from the lateral view.

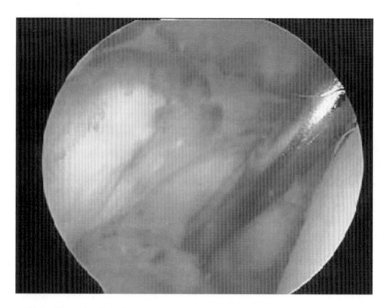

FIGURE 14.8. Bursal view in the posterior portal showing the shaver under the rotator cuff but above the labrum.

The basic release technique is completed by placing the shaver beneath the supraspinatus and infraspinatus tendons, releasing the capsule from these tendons and completing the capsular release initially performed from within the joint (Figure 14.8).

14.3.4. Special Release Techniques

There may be situations where further release techniques are necessary. In certain cases the entire anterior rotator interval, including the coracohumeral ligament, may be released by using scissors and by taking this down just anteriorly to the supraspinatus tendon, as described by Tauro.[19] In certain specific tear patterns in which the tear is directly displaced medially, the posterior rotator interval may be adherent to the scapular spine. Though in most cases an adequate inferior and superior release of the cuff allows mobilization of this interval, occasionally one may have to actually incise the normal confluence between the supraspinatus and infraspinatus tendons to adequately relieve pressure in this area, as described by Burkhart.[20]

In certain retracted subscapularis tears, the capsule may need to be released off the anterior and posterior aspects of the subscapularis. This is in addition to the release of the capsule off the anterior labrum, which is required in many large rotator cuff tears. This specific release of the capsule anteriorly and posteriorly allows mobilization of this tendon and placement back into its insertional footprint (Figure 14.9).[21]

Another technique that may be used is release of the suprascapular nerve (Lafosse L, personal communication, 2005, and Ref. 22). When there is significant medial displacement of the supraspinatus tendon or preoperative electromyographic (EMG) analysis of contracture, the arthroscope may be tracked from the lateral portal over the labrum anterior to the supraspinatus and the suprascapular artery. Once the artery is encountered, the suprascapular notch, suprascapular nerve, and overlying ligament can be well visualized. Utilizing a Neviaser portal and a blunt switching stick, careful retraction and analysis of these structures can be completed. Then using a punch or knife to protect the nerve and artery, the ligament itself may be incised and the suprascapular notch deepened or the nerve mobilized out of the notch.

Completion of all these release techniques may allow a large or massive rotator cuff repair to be easily repaired while centering the humeral head on the glenoid and minimizing any tension of the repair (Figure 14.10).

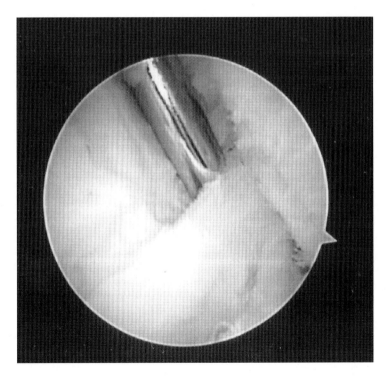

FIGURE 14.9. Special technique, release of capsule off subscapular.

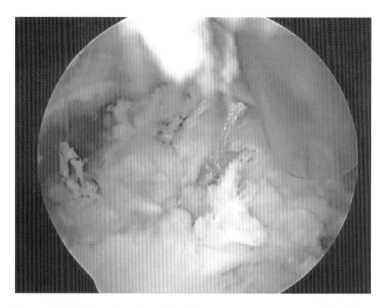

FIGURE 14.10. Completed repair with convergence sutures and anchors.

14.4. Conclusions

Arthroscopic rotator cuff repair has become the gold standard in the management of all types of rotator cuff tears. As with all surgeries, the techniques are constantly being advanced and modified. Adequate release of the tendon tissue with preservation of the neurovascular supply through meticulous dissection allows tension-free repair of all sizes of rotator cuff tears. This tension-free repair is one important factor in providing a successful result after rotator cuff repair surgery.

References

1. Bokor DJ, Hawkins RJ, Huckell GH, et al. Results of nonoperative management of full thickness tears of the rotator cuff. Clin Orthop 1993;294: 103–110.
2. Itoi E, Tabata S. Conservative treatment of rotator cuff tears. Clin Orthop 1992;275:165–173.
3. Ellman H, Hanker G, Bayer M. Repair of the rotator cuff. J Bone Joint Surg Am 1986;68:1136–1144.
4. Ellman H, Kay SP, Wirth M. Arthroscopic treatment of full thickness rotator cuff tears: 2 to 7 year follow-up study. Arthroscopy 1993;9:195–200.
5. Tauro JC. Arthroscopic rotator cuff repair: analysis of technique and results of 2 and 3 year follow-up. Arthroscopy 1998;14:45–51.
6. Bigliani LU, Cordasco, FA, McIlveen SJ, et al. Operative repair of massive rotator cuff tears: long term results. J Shoulder Elbow Surg 1994;1:120–130.

 7. Ha'eri GB, Wiley AM. Advancement of the supraspinatus in the repair of the rotator cuff. J Bone Joint Surg Am 1981;63:232–238.
 8. Millstein ES, Snyder SJ. Arthroscopic evaluation and management of rotator cuff tears. Orthop Clin North Am 2003;34:507–520.
 9. Gerber C, Meyer DC, Schneeberger AG, et al. Effect of tendon release and delayed repair on the structure of the muscles of the rotator cuff: an experimental study in sheep. J Bone Joint Surg Am 2004;86:1972–1982.
10. Codd TP, Flatow EL. Anterior acromioplasty, tendon mobilization, and direct repair of massive rotator cuff tears. In: Burkhead WZ Jr, ed. Rotator cuff disorders. Baltimore: Williams and Wilkins; 1996:323–334.
11. Gerber C. Massive rotator cuff tears. In: Ianotti JP, Williams GR, eds. Disorders of the shoulder: diagnosis and management. Phildelphia: Lippincott, Williams & Wilkins; 1999;62–63.
12. Goutallier D, Postel JM, Bernageau J, et al. Fatty infiltration of disrupted rotator cuff muscles. Rev Rhum Engl Ed 1995;62:415–422.
13. Jones CK, Savoie FH. Arthroscopic repair of large and massive rotator cuff tears. Arthroscopy 2003;19:564–571.
14. McGinty JB. Operative arthroscopy. Philadelphia: Lippincott, Williams & Wilkins; 2003.
15. Burkhart SS, Danaceau SM, Pearce CE. Arthroscopic rotator cuff repair: analysis of results by tear size and by repair technique. Margin convergence versus direct tendon to bone repair. Arthroscopy 2001;17:905–912.
16. Gartsman GH, Khan M, Hammerman SM. Arthroscopic repair of full-thickness tears of the rotator cuff. J Bone Joint Surg Am 1998;80:832–840.
17. Cordasco FA, Bigliani FA. Large and massive tears: technique of open repair. Orthop Clin North Am 1997;28:179–193.
18. Tauro JC. Arthroscopic repair of large rotator cuff tears using the interval slide technique. Arthroscopy 2004;20:13–21.
19. Tauro JC. Arthroscopic "interval slide" in the repair of large roator cuff tears. Arthroscopy 1999;15:527–530.
20. Brady PC, Burkhart SS. Mobilization and repair techniques for the massive contracted rotator cuff tear: technique and preliminary results. Techniques Shoulder Elbow Surg 2005;6:14–25.
21. Worland RL, Arredondo J, Angeles F, et al. Repair of massive rotator cuff tears in patients older than 70 years. J Shoulder Elbow Surg 1999;8:21–36.
22. Greiner A, Golser K, Wambacher M, et al. The course of the suprascapular nerve in the supraspinatus fossa and its vulnerability in muscle advancement. J Shoulder Elbow Surg 2003;12:256–259.

15
Arthroscopic Rotator Cuff Repair with Interval Release for Contracted Rotator Cuff Tears

Joseph C. Tauro

As experience has been gained in the arthroscopic repair of small and moderate rotator cuff tears, there has been a natural progression toward the repair of larger tears.[1-3] There is now considerable experience in the arthroscopic repair of these larger tears. The most significant advantage of an all-arthroscopic approach in the repair of large and massive rotator cuff tears is the elimination of deltoid morbidity that often occurs after open surgery.[4-6] Many patients will not recover full function of the cuff despite attempts at repair, and so loss of deltoid function is an even more significant complication in this group. The larger the cuff tear (and the more extensile the surgical exposure), the greater the potential benefit of an arthroscopic repair.

Some large rotator cuff tears may be quite mobile and therefore do not require soft tissue release. Other tears are contracted and cannot be repaired without mobilizing the tendon from contracted capsule or, in the case of revision repairs, scar tissue.[2,7-9] In this chapter, we will discuss the indications and the techniques for soft tissue release for contracted cuff tears and revision repairs.

15.1. Surgical Procedure

Arthroscopic repair of large rotator cuff tears is technically challenging but possible using a systematic and stepwise approach. Experience in repairing smaller tears is mandatory before taking on this greater challenge. Loss of rotational stability (not only superior, but anterior and posterior as well) is one of the major causes of pain and loss of function in these patients. The repair is performed to correct this problem by closing as much of the cuff as possible. However, it is much better to perform a partial repair of the cuff that will function well than to perform a high-tension repair of the cuff that will fail postoperatively. All of the concepts of arthroscopic cuff repair discussed in prior chapters need to be followed. Especially critical to success is complete exposure of the tear and the identification of its configuration.

Smaller tears of the supraspinatus are usually contained within the bursa so that exposure is not difficult. Large tears will usually extend more posteriorly and, therefore, outside the bursa. This necessitates a more difficult extrabursal debridement but one that must be performed in order to fully expose the tear. An electrosurgical ablative device is used primarily in this exposure as the extrabursal tissue is quite vascular and will bleed if debrided initially with a rotary shaver alone.

Pattern configurations of large tears are the same as those described for smaller tears, namely, crescent and longitudinal. Many tears that appear to be very large are still quite mobile. In these cases, crescent-shaped tears can be repaired directly to bone and longitudinal tears can be repaired with a combination of side-to-side repair (margin convergence) and then end-to-bone repair if necessary. Some retracted tears, however, have poor mobility. Inability to close the cuff tear due to intrinsic muscle atrophy and fibrosis is not correctable with primary repair. Poor cuff mobility secondary to attachment to contracted capsular tissue or scar tissue from prior repair attempts (open or arthroscopic) is correctable with arthroscopic releases.

In large tears, we subdivide the crescent and longitudinal patterns into nonretracted and retracted categories. Note how in Figures 15.1(A) and 15.2(A) the supraspinatus tendon is tethered by the contracted coracohumeral ligament and the attached rotator interval capsule. Retracted tears must be released from these tissues to achieve the maximum closure possible. Other special considerations need to be made when repairing large cuff tears arthroscopically, which will be outlined below.

15.1.1. Positioning and Setup

All arthroscopic cuff repairs are performed as outpatient surgeries, usually under general anesthesia. Scalene block anesthesia is used if there is a patient preference or a medical contraindication to general anesthesia. We perform the procedure with the patient in the lateral decubitus position with the arm placed in 45° of abduction and 15° of forward flexion and with 10 pounds of traction. The beach chair position is preferred by some surgeons and is certainly acceptable. Excessive abduction should be avoided because it will block access to the greater tuberosity.

15.1.2. Surgical Technique

Routine diagnostic arthroscopy is performed first in the glenohumeral joint to assess the size and shape of the tear. In revision cases, the cuff tendon may be scarred to the acromial roof and can be difficult to identify. Careful dissection of cuff tissue off the acromion, starting from more posterior where more normal cuff tissue can be identified, is necessary in these cases before proceeding with any further work. This is best accomplished

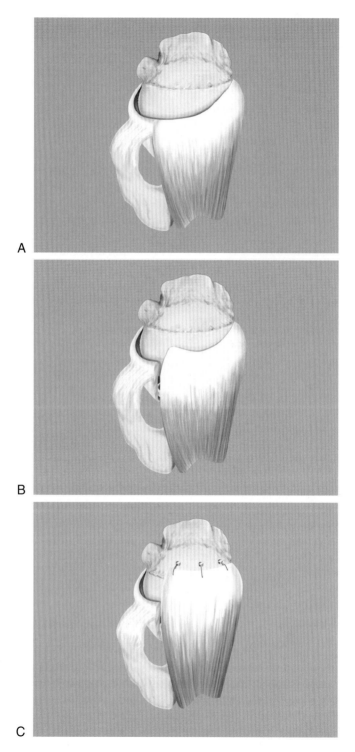

FIGURE 15.1. (A) Retracted crescent-shaped tear. (B) Completed interval slide release, crescent-shaped tear. (C) End-to-bone repair after interval slide of a crescent-shaped tear.

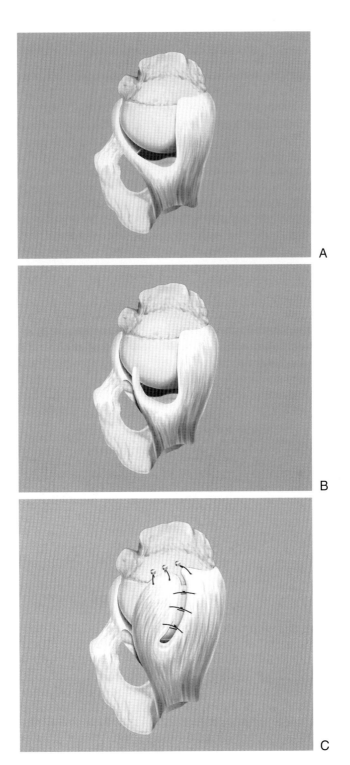

FIGURE 15.2. (A) Retracted longitudinal tear. (B) Completed interval slide release, longitudinal tear. (C) Completed repair of an oval-shaped tear. Some of the anterior–superior humeral head that may still be exposed after tendon rotation in very large tears.

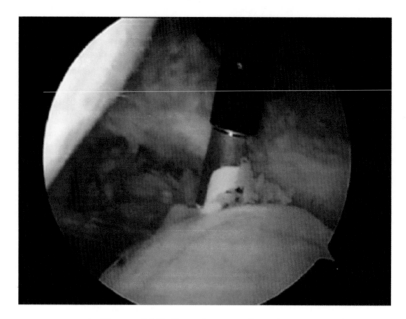

FIGURE 15.3. Superior capsular release.

with an electrosurgical (RF) cutting device inserted through the lateral subacromial portal. We have found RF devices to be much better at controlling bleeding than sharp arthroscopic elevators that have been used previously. An atraumatic grasper is then inserted through the lateral subacromial portal, and cuff mobility is assessed from the articular side. If supraspinatus tendon mobility is poor, a superior capsular release should be performed at this time. The release is carried out by cutting through the capsule with the RF probe between the cuff tendon and the glenoid rim from the biceps anteriorly to the most posterior and inferior margin of the tear (Figure 15.3). Now, manually try to close the tear again with the tissue tensioner. At this point, if a crescent-shaped tear will not reduce to bone or a longitudinal tear will not close from side to side, then an arthroscopic "interval slide" should be performed. This soft tissue release is simply an arthroscopic adaptation of the open interval slide.

The release can be performed while viewing from either the articular or bursal side. I prefer to perform the release while viewing from the posterior intra-articular portal because the interval between the cuff and the capsule is easier to identify (Figure 15.4). This interval between the anterior border of the supraspinatus and the superior capsule (rotator interval) is divided from lateral to medial. This will also release the tendon from the contracted coracohumeral ligament on the bursal side. With the biceps intact, the release is made just caudad to the tendon. If the biceps is not intact, the release is started approximately at the anterior–superior pole of the glenoid but can be judged also by the character of the tissue being cut. It is helpful in most cases to establish a small percutaneous portal, just anterior to the lateral subacromial portal, for the RF probe. Lateral traction is gradually applied to the cuff tendon with a tissue tensioner inserted through the lateral subacromial portal so that the entire interval capsule, from lateral to medial, is exposed and cut away from the supraspinatus tendon (Figure 15.5). Once the release is completed past the medial border of the capsule, mobility is generally greatly improved.

Recently, Burkhart has described an interval release "in continuity" to be used when the subscapularis is also torn.[10] This leaves a bridge of interval tissue between the supraspinatus and subscapularis to make repair of both tendons easier. This release can also be performed from the articular or bursal side. In this case, a "window" is made in the interval, releasing the capsule and the coracohumeral ligament from both tendons.

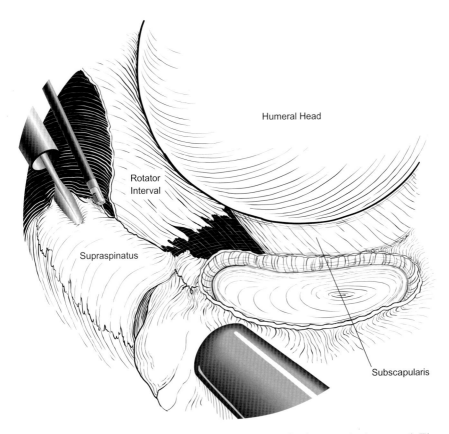

FIGURE 15.4. Interval slide as viewed from the posterior intra-articular portal. The basket punch is inserted through the tear to begin the release (biceps is absent in this case).

The arthroscope is now moved into the bursa. Acromioplasty is done routinely in these cases based on the preoperative assessment of acromial morphology determined from the magnetic resonance imaging (MRI) studies. The handling of the coraco-acromial ligament is very important. It should never be excised because it is an important restraint against superior migration of the humeral head if the tear cannot be repaired completely or if the cuff repair fails. The ligament should be elevated as an L-shaped sleeve from the anterior and lateral acromial edge. It will then heal back to the new acromial edge after acromioplasty. Complete hemostasis is mandatory before proceeding to cuff repair.

After acromioplasty, the bursa must be debrided until the entire extent of the cuff tear can be visualized. This requires viewing the cuff and bursa from the posterior, lateral, and sometimes anterior portals while performing the debridement. Any additional bursal adhesions are excised at this time. A bursal side assessment of the cuff tear is now made, once again viewing from multiple portals. The interval slide is checked to make sure the release is complete; if necessary, the release can be completed from the bursal side. If tendon mobility is still not sufficient, a release of the supraspinatus and infraspinatus off the scapular spine (described by Burkhart as the "double" interval slide) can be performed.[11] This can often result in a very small piece of supraspinatus tendon to repair, so I prefer to perform this release rarely and keep the two tendons in continuity (Figure 15.6). This is a challenging release requiring visualization of the lateral scapular spine, located directly posterior to the acromioclavicular

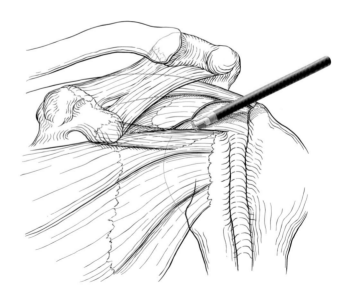

FIGURE 15.5. Basket punch inserted through the lateral subacromial portal to begin the interval release.

FIGURE 15.6. Repaired rotator cuff after the double interval slide in continuity.

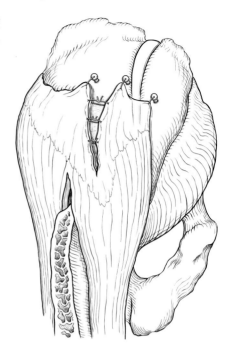

joint. Dissection must be done carefully because the suprascapular nerve is directly under the tendons in this area.

15.1.3. Special Repair Considerations

There is a large "safe zone" for portal placement in the subacromial space. Any position around the acromion from lateral to the coracoid to the posterior portal is safe as long as it is within 4 cm of the acromial margin. Needle localization for portals is very helpful. Exact portal positioning depends on the particular repair technique used and the configuration of the tear.

For the actual tendon reattachment to bone, I use an "anchor-first" technique. Screw-in anchors can be inserted percutaneously through small stab incisions. This is an advantage when repairing a broad cuff tear from anterior to posterior, because multiple large portals are not necessary. The pre-attached suture must then be pulled back through the cuff tendon using a retrograde device. The exact device used depends on the position of the tendon being repaired in relation to the desired anchoring point. For the larger grasping devices [such as a Viper punch (Arthrex, Naples, FL) or Expresso (Depuy/Mitek Providence, RI)], I use the lateral subacromial portal that was utilized during the acromioplasty. For smaller retrograde needle punches [such as a Penetrator (Arthrex, Naples, FL)], a small stab incision is all that is normally needed. Knot delivery, however, must always be done after transferring suture limbs to a cannula to avoid soft tissue entanglement.

Tears of the infraspinatus must be repaired first. This tendon is usually mobile and can be reduced fairly easily to the posterior–superior corner of the greater tuberosity. Repair of the tendon is generally performed while viewing from the lateral or posterior–lateral portal with instruments inserted through posterior accessory portals as needed.

Once released, retracted supraspinatus tears that were initially crescent-shaped tears can be pulled down to the tuberosity and repaired directly to bone, without a side-to-side repair [Figure 15.1(A,B,C)]. Tears that were longitudinal are repaired as follows: Lateral traction is applied to the released supraspinatus tendon's lateral edge with an atraumatic grasper. The posterior edge of the muscle/tendon unit is then rotated adjacent to the anterior edge of the infraspinatus. The tendon is then anchored to bone, followed by a side-to-side repair to the infraspinatus. The specific techniques of end-to-bone and side-to-side repair are the same as those discussed earlier in this and previous chapters. In very large tears, this may leave an exposed area on the anterior–superior humeral head [Figure 15.2(A,B,C)]. This conforms to our principle outlined initially, that a partial low-tension repair is better than a complete high-tension repair that will fail. In these cases, it is very important that the coraco-acromial ligament be left intact, that the interval release is from the supraspinatus and not from the humeral head (as is done in releases for frozen shoulder), and that the subscapularis be intact or repaired. Otherwise, anterior–superior instability of the humeral head can occur.

15.2. Postoperative Management

If general anesthesia was employed, 0.5% bipivicaine is injected into each of the portals and the subacromial space at the conclusion of the procedure. Patients are placed in a shoulder immobilizer and a continuous cold therapy cuff is applied over the shoulder. Hydrocodone with acetaminophen is prescribed for pain control for the first postoperative week or two, as needed.

Patients are instructed to remove the immobilizer starting the first post-operative day when in a safe environment. They may then move the hand, wrist, and elbow, but not the shoulder. Formal physical therapy begins on the third postoperative day and consists of pain and edema modalities, passive range of motion (ROM) of the shoulder to full and a para-scapular mobilization and strengthening program. Depending on the size and security of the repair, progression to active ROM of the shoulder takes place at 6 weeks postoperatively. Light resistive exercises can be added at 10 weeks with a very gradual increase in intensity until maximum improvement is achieved, usually by 6 months.

References

1. Tauro JC. Arthroscopic rotator cuff repair: analysis of technique and results of 2 and 3 year follow-up. Arthroscopy 1998;14:45–51.
2. Tauro JC. Arthroscopic repair of large rotator cuff tears using the interval slide technique. Arthroscopy 2004;20:13–21.
3. Gartsman GM, Khan M, Hammerman SM. Arthroscopic repair of full-thickness tears of the rotator cuff. J Bone Joint Surg 1998;80:832–840.
4. Bigliani LU, Cordasco FA, McIlveen SJ, et al. Operative repair of massive rotator cuff tears: long term results. J Shoulder Elbow Surg 1994;1:120–130.
5. Cordasco FA, Bigliani FA. Large and massive tears: technique of open repair. Orthop Clin North Am 1997;28:179–193.
6. Rokito AS, Cuomo F, Gallagher MA, Zuckerman JD. Long term functional out come of repair of large and massive chronic tears of the rotator cuff. J Bone Joint Surg Am 1999;81:991–997.
7. Debeyre J, Patte D, Elmelik E. Repair of the rotator cuff of the shoulder: with a note on advancement of the supraspinatus muscle. J Bone Joint Surg Br 1965;47:36–42.
8. McLaughlin HL. Lesions of the musculocutaneous cuff of the shoulder. The exposure and treatment of tears with retraction. J Bone Joint Surg Am 1944; 26:31–51.
9. Ha'eri GB, Wiley AM. Advancement of the supraspinatus in the repair of the rotator cuff. J Bone Joint Surg Am 1981;63:232–238.
10. Lo IK, Burkhart SS. The interval slide in continuity: a method of mobilizing the anterosuperior rotator cuff without disrupting the tear margins. Arthroscopy 2004;20:435–441.
11. Lo IK, Burkhart SS. Arthroscopic repair of massive, contracted, immobile rotator cuff tears using single and double interval slides: technique and preliminary results. Arthroscopy 2004;20:22–33.

16
When and How to Do Margin Convergence Repair Versus Interval Slides

Stephen S. Burkhart and David P. Huberty

Arthroscopic techniques have revolutionized the treatment of large and massive rotator cuff tears. The arthroscopic approach has not only dramatically reduced the rate of major complications from rotator cuff surgery (infection, deltoid detachment, postoperative stiffness), it has also facilitated precise anatomical repair of complex cuff tear patterns.[1,2] Restoration of the anatomy is critically important, but the surgeon must first recognize the tear pattern in order to properly repair a given tear.[3,4] Tear pattern recognition is the essential first step that leads to anatomically accurate rotator cuff repair.

16.1. Tear Pattern Recognition

Rotator cuff tears must be repaired in the direction of greatest mobility. This allows the repair to heal in a position of minimal strain.[5] Strain reduction is a major goal of rotator cuff repair.[6]

A cuff tear can be classified into one of the following categories based on the amount of mobility and the direction of greatest mobility: (1) crescent-shaped tear; (2) L-shaped (or reverse-L) tear; (3) U-shaped tear; and (4) massive contracted immobile tear.

16.1.1. Crescent-Shaped Tears

These tears are the simplest of all tears. Crescent-shaped tears typically do not retract very far medially, even when they are massive in size from anterior to posterior. They exhibit excellent medial-to-lateral mobility, and they may be repaired directly to bone with minimal tension.

16.1.2. L-Shaped and U-Shaped Tears

L-shaped tears, reverse-L–shaped tears, and U-shaped tears [Figure 16.1(A)] are repaired by side-to-side sutures as an initial step [Figure

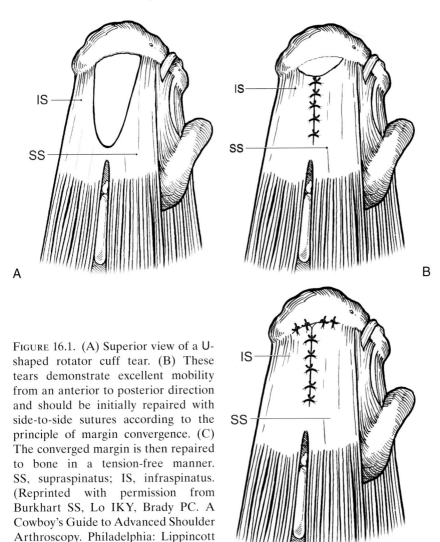

FIGURE 16.1. (A) Superior view of a U-shaped rotator cuff tear. (B) These tears demonstrate excellent mobility from an anterior to posterior direction and should be initially repaired with side-to-side sutures according to the principle of margin convergence. (C) The converged margin is then repaired to bone in a tension-free manner. SS, supraspinatus; IS, infraspinatus. (Reprinted with permission from Burkhart SS, Lo IKY, Brady PC. A Cowboy's Guide to Advanced Shoulder Arthroscopy. Philadelphia: Lippincott Williams & Wilkins; 2006.)

16.1(B)]. These sutures are sequentially tied from medial to lateral, and they progressively converge the margin of the tear laterally to the bone bed while simultaneously causing reduced strain at the new converged margin. The strain reduction feature of margin convergence is so powerful that closing 50% of a U-shaped tear side to side will reduce the strain at the converged margin by a factor of 6.[3] This greatly protects the tendon repair to bone in comparison to a U-shaped tear that is not closed by margin convergence. Once the side-to-side sutures have been tied, the converged margin is repaired to bone by means of suture anchors [Figure 16.1(C)].

16.2. Margin Convergence

The engineering definition of axial strain (ϵ) is change in length (ΔL) per initial length of a material that undergoes a uniaxial deforming force. The strain at the margin of a rotator cuff tear is related to the length of the tear and the cross-sectional area of intact tissue according to the formula:

$$\epsilon(\text{strain}) = \Delta L / L = F / AE$$

where L is the medial-to-lateral dimension of cuff tear, A is the cross-sectional area of intact cuff at level of strain measurement, F is the resultant longitudinal rotator cuff force; and E is the modulus of elasticity (Young's modulus).

As noted, side-to-side suture achieving margin convergence will dramatically decrease the strain at the converged margin of the cuff, producing a protective effect for the tendon-to-bone repair. In some cases, particularly in medium-length U-shaped tears, margin convergence to bone can be achieved by using sutures from the anchors to achieve margin convergence. When these sutures are tied, they bring the tendon tightly down to the bone bed on the greater tuberosity (Figure 16.2) for a very secure footprint reconstruction.

16.3. Massive Contracted Immobile Rotator Cuff Tears

Although most rotator cuff tears are crescent-, U-, or L-shaped, there is a category of tears that exhibits no mobility from a medial-to-lateral or from an anterior-to-posterior direction. We call these tears massive, contracted, immobile rotator cuff tears, and, in the senior author's practice, they represent 9.6% of massive tears.

We believe that massive, contracted, immobile rotator cuff tears demonstrate one of two common patterns: massive, contracted, longitudinal tears and massive, contracted, crescent tears. In general, massive, contracted, crescent tears are wider (in an anterior-to-posterior direction) than massive, contracted, longitudinal tears, and thus they are more difficult to repair. In addition, massive, contracted, longitudinal tears have a tongue of supraspinatus tendon at the anterior margin of the tear that is useful during subsequent repair of these tears.

For the massive, contracted, longitudinal tears, we perform an arthroscopic anterior interval slide similar to that initially described by Tauro.[7] This anterior interval slide improves the mobility of the supraspinatus by incising the coracohumeral ligament, which commonly becomes contracted in this tear pattern. This release generally increases the lateral excursion of the supraspinatus tendon by about 2 cm, which is usually enough to allow repair of the supraspinatus tendon to the bone bed of the greater tuberosity for this tear pattern. The posterior leaf is then advanced superolaterally, and the repair is completed by closing the residual U-shaped defect with side-to-side sutures.

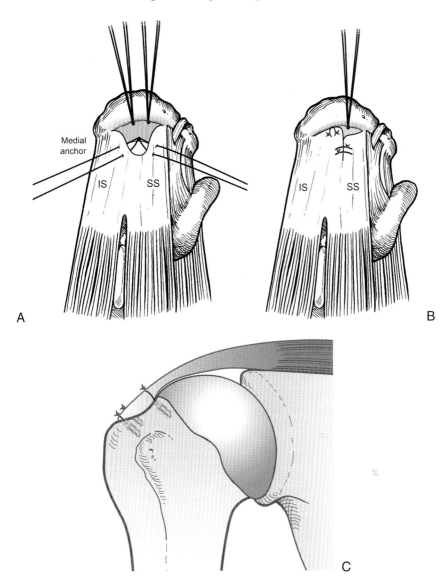

FIGURE 16.2. Margin convergence and secure footprint reconstruction can be achieved with the use of medial and lateral row anchors. (A) In this superior view of a U-shaped rotator cuff tear, sutures from medial anchor have been passed to close the longitudinal component of the rotator cuff tear (margin-convergence-to-bone technique). (B) Lateral row anchors are used to complete the repair. (C) Lateral view demonstrates the width of footprint reconstruction using margin convergence to bone. (Reprinted with permission from Place NP, © 2006.)

In the case of massive, contracted, crescent-shaped tears, insufficient mobility is obtained with a simple anterior interval slide for the rotator cuff to reach the bone bed laterally. In these cases, a double interval slide (anterior interval slide plus posterior interval slide) needs to be performed.[8] The anterior interval slide is first completed; then a posterior interval slide is performed by releasing the interval between the supraspinatus and infraspinatus tendons [Figures 16.3(A,B) and 16.4(A–D)]. The posterior slide dramatically increases the lateral excursion of both the supraspinatus and infraspinatus tendons by approximately 4 or 5 cm. Care must be taken not to injure the suprascapular nerve, which lies at the base of the scapular spine. Lateral traction on the cuff as the posterior slide is performed will help to protect the nerve. The supraspinatus is next repaired to bone, and the infraspinatus is advanced onto the bone bed as far as possible [Figures 16.3(C) and 16.4(E)]. Then side-to-side sutures are placed to close the defect between the supraspinatus and infraspinatus [Figures 16.3(D) and 16.4(F)].

16.3.1. Associated Subscapularis Tears: The Interval Slide in Continuity

Massive anterosuperior rotator cuff tears are those that involve the subscapularis in addition to supraspinatus and infraspinatus. In such cases, the subscapularis is frequently retracted. In the case of a massive retracted anterosuperior tear, the subscapularis must be mobilized and repaired prior to repairing the rest of the cuff.[9] During the course of mobilizing the subscapularis, the surgeon must release the coracohumeral ligament from the base of the coracoid by means of an arthroscopic elevator, without cutting across the free margin of the rotator cuff tear. This accomplishes an anterior interval release without disruption of the free margin of the cuff and with the coracohumeral ligament released in a different way than in a standard anterior interval slide. We call this an *interval slide in continuity*.[10] If the coracohumeral space is diminished, (to less than 6 mm as measured intraoperatively, then a coracoplasty is performed to increase the space available for subscapularis repair.[11] After doing a three-sided release of the subscapularis and an interval slide in continuity, the subscapularis tendon is repaired to the lesser tuberosity. Then the remainder of the cuff is repaired according to its tear pattern. In cases of extremely immobile, contracted tears, a posterior interval slide has to be done in addition to the interval slide in continuity to provide enough lateral excursion for a complete repair.

16.3.2. When to Release and When Not to Release

Our decision-making process on when to use margin convergence and/or releases is based on the tear pattern and mobility of the tear. We use an arthroscopic tendon grasper and test the mobility of the tear while viewing

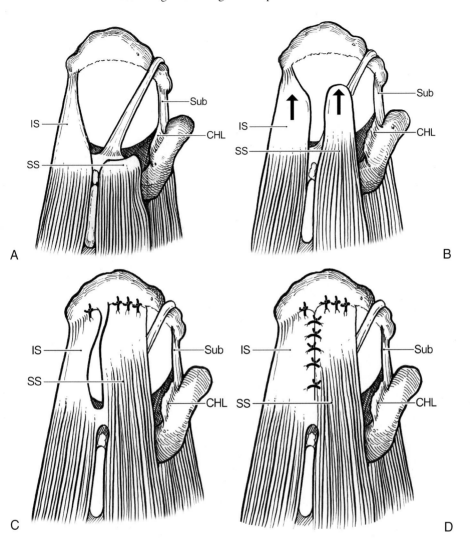

FIGURE 16.3. Repair of a massive contracted immobile rotator cuff tear. (A) A double interval slide is performed by first completing an anterior interval slide and then performing a posterior interval slide by releasing the interval between the supraspinatus and infraspinatus tendons. (B) After release, improved mobility of the supraspinatus tendon and the infraspinatus-teres minor posteriorly is seen. (C) The supraspinatus can then be repaired to a lateral bone bed in a tension-free manner, and the infraspinatus-teres minor tendons are advanced laterally and superiorly. (D) The residual defect is then closed with side-to-side sutures. SS, supraspinatus; IS, infraspinatus; Sub, subscapularis; RI, rotator interval; CHL, coracohumeral ligament; G, glenoid; H, humeral head. (Reprinted with permission from Burkhart SS, Lo IKY, Brady PC. A Cowboy's Guide to Advanced Shoulder Arthroscopy. Philadelphia: Lippincott Williams & Wilkins; 2006.)

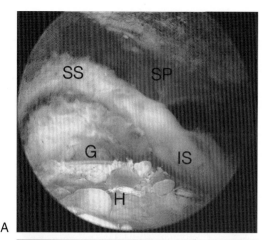

A

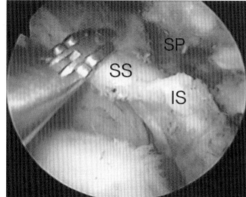

B

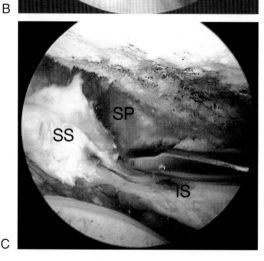

C

FIGURE 16.4. Posterior interval slide: Arthroscopic view of a left shoulder from a lateral viewing portal demonstrating a massive severely contracted rotator cuff tear. (A) This tear is not repairable with direct tendon-to-bone or margin convergence technique but instead requires an interval slide technique. (B) Traction sutures are placed in the supraspinus (SS) and the infraspinus (IS) tendons. (C) The posterior interval slide: The posterior margin of the supraspinatus tendon (SS) is released from the infraspinatus (IS) using an arthroscopic scissor.

FIGURE 16.4. *Continued* (D) Completed posterior interval slide demonstrating complete release of the infraspinatus (IS) from the supraspinatus (SS), revealing the scapular spine (SP). Tension on traction sutures elevates cuff tissue, protecting against injury to the underlying suprascapular nerve. (E) Side-to-side closure of the residual defect between the supraspinatus (SS) and in-fraspinatus (IS) tendons is performed using a hand-off technique with two Penetrator suture passers (Arthrex, Inc., Naples, FL). (F) Completed repair of the supraspinatus (SS) tendon to the infraspinatus (IS) tendon following repair of each tendon to bone. (Reprinted with permission from Burkhart SS, Lo IKY, Brady PC. A Cowboy's Guide to Advanced Shoulder Arthroscopy. Phila-delphia: Lippincott Williams & Wilkins; 2006.)

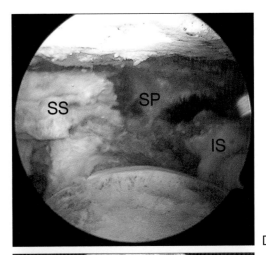

D

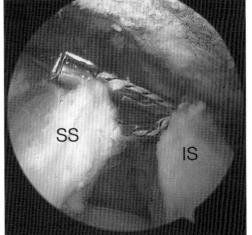

E

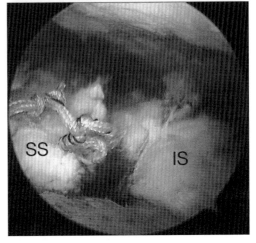

F

first through a posterior portal and then through a lateral portal in order to get a complete three-dimensional sense of the tear pattern.

If the tear is easily reducible from medial to lateral to the greater tuberosity bone bed with minimal tension, it is a crescent-shaped tear that is repaired directly to bone.

If the tear is most mobile from anterior to posterior, then side-to-side sutures are placed to achieve margin convergence and then the converged margin is repaired to bone. If side-to-side sutures do not produce tendon-to-tendon apposition of the anterior leaf to the posterior leaf in addition to lateral margin convergence, then the tear is a contracted immobile tear that is not amenable to closure by margin convergence.

If the tear is immobile in the anterior-to-posterior direction (anterior and posterior leaves cannot be brought into contact by side-to-side sutures) as well as in the medial-to-lateral direction (the cuff margin does not have enough lateral excursion to reach the bone bed of the greater tuberosity), then this is a massive, contracted immobile tear and selective releases are performed. If the subscapularis is involved, it is repaired (after mobilization, if required, by interval slide in continuity), and then the supraspinatus/infraspinatus component is repaired based on its residual tear pattern (either by direct repair, margin convergence, or posterior interval slide as dictated by tear mobility).

If the subscapularis tendon is not involved and the tear is considered to be a massive, contracted, immobile tear, then an anterior interval slide is first performed. This will typically give approximately 2 cm of additional lateral excursion of the cuff. If this is enough to accomplish repair, then the cuff is repaired with suture anchors. If additional lateral excursion of the tendon is required for repair, then a posterior interval slide is performed (completing the double interval slide). This will typically provide 4 to 5 cm of additional lateral excursion of the rotator cuff. In our experience, almost all tears will be repairable by one of the techniques described in this chapter. However, there is the occasional tear in which a double interval slide still does not provide enough lateral excursion for a complete rotator cuff repair. In such cases, a partial repair is performed.[12] The repairable portions of the tendons are repaired, the goal being to balance the force couple of the rotator cuff muscles, and a residual defect is left where the tendon does not have enough lateral excursion to reach the bone bed.

16.4. Conclusions

The logical, stepwise surgical technique described in this chapter will allow reliable recognition of tear patterns, optimized tendon excursion through selective use of margin convergence and interval releases when indicated, and precise anatomical reconstruction of the rotator cuff.

References

1. Gartsman GM, Khan M, Hammerman SM. Arthroscopic repair of full-thickness tears of the rotator cuff. J Bone Joint Surg Am 1998;80:832–840.
2. Gartsman GM. Massive, irreparable tears of the rotator cuff. Results of operative debridement and subacromial decompression. J Bone Joint Surg Am 1997;79:715–721.
3. Burkhart SS, Athanasiou KA, Wirth MA. Margin convergence: a method of reducing strain in massive rotator cuff tears. Arthroscopy 1996;12:335–338.
4. Burkhart SS, Danaceau SM, Pearce CE. Arthroscopic rotator cuff repair: analysis of results by tear size and by repair technique – margin convergence versus direct tendon-to-bone repair. Arthroscopy 2001;17:905–912.
5. Halder AM, O'Driscoll SW, Heer G, et al. Biomechanical comparison of effects of supraspinatus tendon detachments, tendon defects and muscle retractions. J Bone Joint Surg Am 2002;84:780–785.
6. Harryman DT II, Mach LA, Wang KY, et al. Repairs of the rotator cuff: correlation of functional results with integrity of the cuff. J Bone Joint Surg Am 1991;73:982–989.
7. Tauro JC. Arthroscopic "interval slide" in the repair of large rotator cuff tears. Arthroscopy 1999;15:527–530.
8. Lo IK, Burkhart SS. Arthroscopic repair of massive, contracted, immobile rotator cuff tears using single and double interval slides: technique and preliminary results. Arthroscopy 2004;20:22–23.
9. Burkhart SS, Tehrany AM. Arthroscopic subscapularis repair: technique and preliminary results. Arthroscopy 2002;18:454–463.
10. Lo IK, Burkhart SS. The interval slide in continuity: a method of mobilizing the anterosuperior rotator cuff without disrupting the tear margins. Arthroscopy 2004;20:435–441.
11. Lo IK, Burkhart SS. Arthroscopic coracoplasty through the rotator interval. Arthroscopy 2003;19:667–671.
12. Burkhart SS. Partial repair of massive rotator cuff tears: the evolution of a concept. Orthop Clin North Am 1997;28:125–132.

17
Repair of Large Anterosuperior Cuff Tears

Jeffrey S. Abrams

Anterosuperior cuff tears are less common than tears that extend posteriorly; therefore, there is less experience with their management. Rotator cuff tears begin along the anterior margin of the supraspinatus. In most instances, these tears enlarge by extending posteriorly towards the infraspinatus and anteriorly along the rotator interval. A tear can become L shaped and eventually stretch to a large U-shaped tear that may be repaired with margin convergent techniques. Cuff tears generally do not extend anteriorly due to the capsular attachments comprising the biceps pulley and the strong attachment of the subscapularis to the lesser tuberosity. Tears that extend anteriorly are most often crescent-shaped tears that include the subscapularis, rotator interval, and supraspinatus. Repairs of anterosuperior tears require direct reattachment to the lesser and greater tuberosities.

Reports in the literature of these types of tears have been few and have ranged from articular partial-thickness tears associated with biceps instability to massive tears and biceps rupture.[1,2] Anterosuperior cuff tears are often repaired with greater difficulty in visualization and access, which may have led to compromised results. Some surgeons have combined two surgical approaches to repair anterosuperior tears via the deltopectoral interval and the more common deltoid splitting approach.[1]

The long head of the biceps traverses the rotator interval and is in the middle of these tears (Figure 17.1). The rotator interval is comprised of the articular components of the superior glenohumeral capsular ligaments and the bursal component of the coracohumeral ligament. Along with the superior border of the subscapularis, the anterior margin of the supraspinatus, and the groove formed in the humerus between the tuberosities, the biceps pulley system is created. Anterosuperior tears can have a normal biceps, a subluxed biceps, or a partial or complete tear of the biceps. Surgical evaluation and treatment of the biceps needs to be considered in the treatment of this tear.

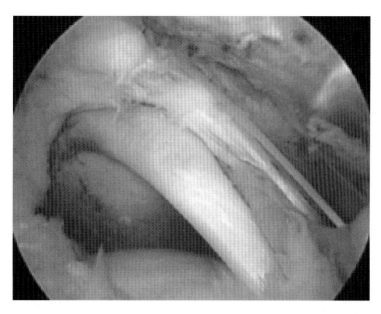

FIGURE 17.1. Rotator cuff avulsion with exposed biceps within the groove.

Several surgeons have reported on the complexity of these tears, particularly from an "open" surgical approach. Walch has popularized the term the *hidden lesion*, because the bursal view of a torn supraspinatus tendon does not always raise suspicion; therefore, surgeons should take additional time to visualize the interval, the biceps, and the superior border of the subscapularis.[3] The arthroscope provides a unique opportunity to visualize the superior subscapularis attachment to the lesser tuberosity, the articular portion of the long head of the biceps, the biceps pulley, and the articular side of the rotator cuff. Bursoscopy is used for further inspection of the cuff tendons, interval, and surrounding structural restraints to the subacromial arch.

17.1. Clinical Evaluation

Patients with anterosuperior cuff tears may have experienced a traumatic event that precipitated symptoms.[4] Tears that extend anteriorly may begin as common tendonopathy with a superimposed trauma, or from a single event, as in young athletes. The arm is often in a position of external rotation, similar to an anterior instability event. Although pain may be common following subluxation, weakness is more common when the rotator cuff is compromised. Injection tests may be useful to distinguish weakness from painful inhibition.

Clinical tests include active and passive range of motion and strength testing. Range of motion compromise may be minor or global, as found in massive tears. Careful subscapularis testing includes passive external rotation, comparison to the uninvolved side, and detection of internal rotation weakness seen in lift off tests or belly press signs. Supraspinatus and infraspinatus tears are best detected with weakness in external rotation against resistance. Abduction testing against resistance often induces a shrug to compensate for the cuff deficiency. Pseudoparalysis can be found in patients with massive tears (Figure 17.2). It is important to evaluate patients after a traumatic event to allow an early opportunity for repair. Delays in surgical treatment may allow irreversible weakness to develop that can significantly compromise postoperative strength of the shoulder.

Biceps testing should be included in the evaluation. Findings may include tenderness, biceps subluxation or "click" with rotation, radicular symptoms into the proximal muscle, or evidence of long head rupture. Preoperative discussion should include possible surgical decisions involving the biceps, that is, tenotomy, tenodesis, etc.

Imaging studies may be helpful to better identify the damaged rotator cuff (Figure 17.3). Plain radiographs include an anteroposterior view with neutral rotation, transcapular outlet view, and an axillary view. In cases of destabilization, the humeral head may be subluxed anterosuperiorly. Most patients will require additional studies, including magnetic resonance imaging (MRI) or arthrographic computerized tomography (arthro-CT) scan. The transverse cuts are best for visualizing the major portions of the subscapularis attachment to the lesser tuberosity and the biceps. The sagittal views can provide information on the rotator interval, biceps tendon, and supraspinatus. The coronal view is the most common for the supraspinatus tear but may also demonstrate rotator interval and subscapularis avulsions.

The clinical indication for surgery is pain, loss of active motion, and loss of function, particularly following a traumatic event. A short history of 3 months or less may be favorable to the outcome. Surgeries that are delayed for periods of 6 months or greater will often have permanent deficits and repairs that commonly have recurrent defects.[1] Irreparable tears are occasionally operated on to create a partial balanced repair including the subscapularis and posterior portions of the cuff crescent, as well as biceps treatment. In these cases, pain relief can be achieved, but functional gains are not predictable.

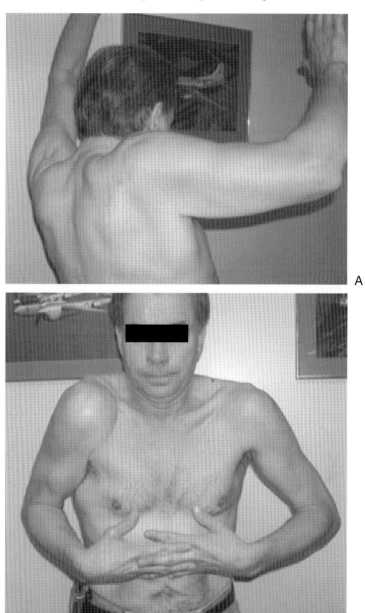

FIGURE 17.2. (A) Pseudoparalysis of the shoulder. Patient is unable to flex and externally rotate the upper extremity due to weakness. (B) Patient demonstrates weakness of internal rotation muscles due to subscapularis tear.

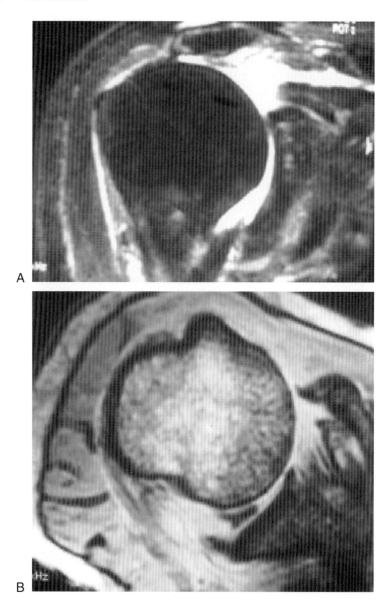

FIGURE 17.3. Imaging studies of anterosuperior rotator cuff tear. (A) Superior migration due to supraspinatus tear. (B) Anterior subluxation and dislocated biceps tendon with subscapularis failure.

17.2. Arthroscopic Evaluation

The arthroscopic examination is a systematic approach to evaluation of the articular structures, tissues concealed within the biceps pulley system, the bursal aspect of the rotator cuff, and surrounding bone restraints to anterior and superior translation (Table 17.1). This information, combined with the clinical and imaging findings, allows physicians to have the most complete picture prior to deciding on repair. The evaluation includes an examination under anesthesia, articular exam, bursal exam, and a dynamic exam.

The examination under anesthesia is designed to understand range of motion and to test translation of the humerus. Patients with excessive external rotation may be found to have subscapularis detachment. Anterior, inferior, and posterior load-and-shift is often normal, because the inferior capsular system is normal. In young patients with a suspicious instability event, this study reduces the concern of a typical capsule labrum detachment.

The patient is placed in either the lateral decubitus or beach chair position. Protective supports are used against dependent areas adjacent to the table. Supports for the axillae, head, and neck are important to avoid potential neurological traction injuries. Additional tape or supportive belts can be used to secure the torso. When lateral decubitus is chosen, the arm is placed in gentle traction of 10 to 12 pounds positioned with the arm abducted 30°. Access to anterior, lateral, and posterior portals is important to complete the evaluation and repair.

The posterior viewing portal is placed 2 cm distal to the angle of the acromion and spine of the scapula. After joint irrigation, an anterior portal is placed in the rotator interval, inferior to the acromion and biceps. The diagnosis begins through the posterior portal. The biceps tendon is visualized and probed. As the tendon is pulled into the joint, the quality of the tendon can be assessed, as well as the capsular restraints. The biceps tendon can be drawn superiorly and inferiorly to examine the hidden portions of the pulley system.

The subscapularis evaluation begins with the exposed portion of the superior tendon. As the shoulder is internally rotated, the attachment to the lesser tuberosity is exposed. Tears may include the articular

TABLE 17.1. Arthroscopic Diagnostic Checklist.

Posterior viewing portal
Biceps tendon
Biceps pulley
Subscapularis attachment
Supraspinatus insertion
Bursoscopy

superior third of the tendon, the entire subscapularis tendon, and the inferior border of the biceps pulley restraints. A grasping instrument allows re-approximation of the tendon to the tuberosity to judge proper anatomy and tension. A suture hook can be placed through the anterior portal and a monofilament suture introduced through the superior portion of the retracted tendon for tendon manipulation and to provide a landmark when visualizing from the bursal viewing portals.

The supraspinatus is visualized along the superior quadrant and adjacent superior labrum. The scope should be placed in the anterior portal to allow further visualization of tears that extend posteriorly. Use the posterior portal as a reference to visualize infraspinatus tear extension. Position the scope in the anterior and inferior pouch, confirm capsule ligament integrity, and visualize the subscapularis and lesser tuberosity with gentle internal rotation.

Remove the scope and place it in the subacromial space through the posterior portal. A portal 3 cm lateral to the anterior acromion allows access to this area with a shaver to remove superficial bursal tissue. The bursae should be peeled back to visualize the most posterior aspect of the tear. As the scope is advanced, the greater tuberosity can be visualized, biceps tendon groove, and interval. The scope can be placed in the lateral portal, and further bursectomy can be performed anteriorly beneath the subacromial arch and behind the coracoid. If the subscapularis or biceps tendon has migrated inferiorly, create a second anterior portal lateral to the coracoid and visualize from the anterior superior portal and debride from the inferior portal. The monofilament sutures will provide a useful landmark to the superior border of the subscapularis. Use a gentle grasping instrument to mobilize tendons, and plan repair of the large crescent tear.

The acromion, distal clavicle, and coracoid may compromise the working space for instruments. Decompression of the articular side of these structures may be helpful. A systematic approach of tendon evaluation, tissue mobilization, and planned reattachment is important to avoid swelling from a prolonged procedure. If a decompression is anticipated, surgeons should avoid complete detachment of the coracoacromial ligament. Small portions of bone can be removed without significant bone resection. A modified decompression will allow easy surgical access to the rotator cuff (Figure 17.4). If a more formidable resection is felt to be needed, this can be completed at the end of the repair.

17.3. Surgical Technique

Surgeons must become proficient in a number of approaches to be able to treat anterosuperior rotator cuff tears. They include articular-sided repairs,

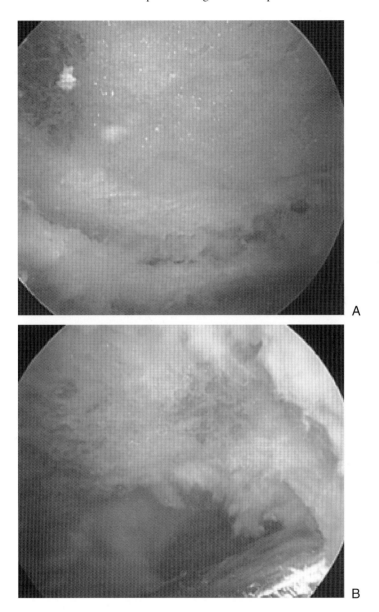

FIGURE 17.4. Modified subacromial decompression. Anterior soft tissue structures are not detached or excised with acromioplasty. (A) posterior view, (B) lateral view.

bursal-sided repairs, combination repairs, as well as repairs for biceps instability and tears (Table 17.2).

Articular repairs are most commonly performed on superior border subscapularis detachment, partial articular-sided tear avulsion (PASTA) tears, and biceps pulley lesions. The scope is positioned in the posterior portal. The biceps is probed to confirm proper position with the groove. If there is subluxation of the biceps over the anterior edge of the groove, you need to decide whether it can be safely repositioned or if tenotomy or tenodesis should be considered. The majority of patients will have a more predictable outcome with a tenodesis, particularly if they are middle-aged or older.

Many tears can be approached with an articular-side subscapularis repair and a bursal-side supraspinatus repair (Figure 17.5). It is important to recognize capsular detachments, including the coracohumeral ligament. This is best visualized from the bursal view. Suture anchor placement can be posterior and anterior to the biceps tendon.

Rotate the upper humerus to visualize the exposed lesser tuberosity. A shaver or burr can be used to gently remove devitalized tissue via the anterior portal. A percutaneous needle can be directed from medially into the prepared footprint. A double-loaded Super Revo® anchor (Linvatec, Largo, FL) can be inserted percutaneously into the superior border of the lesser tuberosity. This coincides with the inferior border of the biceps groove. After anchor placement, a large cannula can be inserted in the anterior portal and a Spectrum® suture hook (Linvatec) or an ExpresSew (Smith & Nephew, Andover, MA) can pass sutures through full-thickness subscapularis tendon. Larger avulsions of the subscapularis are best performed with an open interval and the scope placed anteriorly to allow for inferior and superior anchors.

The PASTA supraspinatus repair is described elsewhere in this text (see Chapter 11). A percutaneous anchor can be placed adjacent to the articular

TABLE 17.2. Arthroscopic Repair Procedure.

Articular suture in subscapularis
Prepare lesser tuberosity
Percutaneous anchor
Subscapularis suture pass
Complete subscapularis repair
Introduce scope into posterior bursal portal
Decompression
Biceps decision: leave alone, tenotomy, or tenodesis
Percutaneous greater tuberosity anchor
Suture pass/retrieval
Incorporate biceps tendon (non–post suture)
Tie knots posterior to anterior

junction with the greater tuberosity. Sutures can be percutaneously placed through the supraspinatus and superior pulley. Sutures are retrieved with a suture shuttle (Linvatec) into a debrided subacromial space. The knots are tied on the bursal side of the tendon.

The bursal repair is a more common approach to larger, full-thickness tears. The bursal tissue is debrided, and a modified decompression is performed. Tears should be visualized from posterior, anterior, and lateral portals. It is often helpful to place a suture anchor into the middle of the tear pattern. Because these are often crescent-shaped tears, this provides a useful landmark to complete the repair posteriorly and anteriorly to this anchor. Avoid tying the knot, to reduce difficulty in making full-thickness suture passes on additional suture anchors.

In large retracted avulsions, the anterior quadrant is best approached with the scope in the anterosuperior portal or the lateral portal. Another alternative is to leave the scope in the posterior portal and to create a hole in the rotator interval. The arthroscope can visualize the articular surface and the bursal surface with small movements with the scope through the interval defect. Instrumentation can be used in the subcoracoid space, and suture retrieval and knot tying can be performed on the exterior of the tendon. Biceps tendon dislocation is not uncommon with large avulsions.

After completing the anterior repair, the scope is removed and placed in the subacromial space. Super Revo® suture anchors (Linvatec) can be placed through percutaneous techniques into the greater tuberosity. If tears extend posteriorly into the infraspinatus, margin convergent technique is used to reduce the hole size prior to anchor placement (Figure 17.6).

Biceps problems are common with anterosuperior tears.[5] Tendons that have tears and are subluxed are best treated with tenotomy or tenodesis. In most cases, a tenodesis can be performed with a suture anchor that is used to repair the cuff tear. If a tenodesis is anticipated, a monofilament suture is placed through the tendon prior to division along the superior labrum. Cutting a small portion of labrum will resist distal migration of the tendon. As suture anchors are placed for rotator cuff repair, the monofilament suture can be used as a shuttle to retrieve the non–post arm of the stitch.

There are a number of very young patients with this rotator cuff tear pattern. Currently, I have chosen to repair the pulley and not divide the biceps. Meticulous care with anchors on both sides of the pulley has allowed these athletes to retain the biceps (Figure 17.7). In these cases, the tendons look pristine. If the tendon has a small tear associated with subluxation, a tenodesis would be a better option.

If surgeons are not familiar with subscapularis repairs, a mini-open technique can be used to repair the subscapularis. Monofilament sutures are placed in the subscapularis, and possibly the biceps, and retrieved through the anterior portal. A decompression and arthroscopic repair is

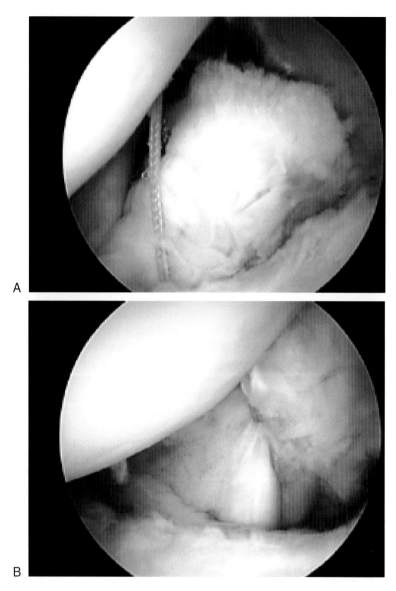

FIGURE 17.5. Combined approach for anterosuperior tear. (A) Articular view of superior border subscapularis tear with suture used to mobilize the lateral margin of the subscapularis tendon. (B) Suture anchor repair of subscapularis via articular view from posterior portal. (C) Surgical repair of subscapularis from articular approach and supraspinatus from bursal approach. (D) Completed supraspinatus bursal repair of supraspinatus tendon.

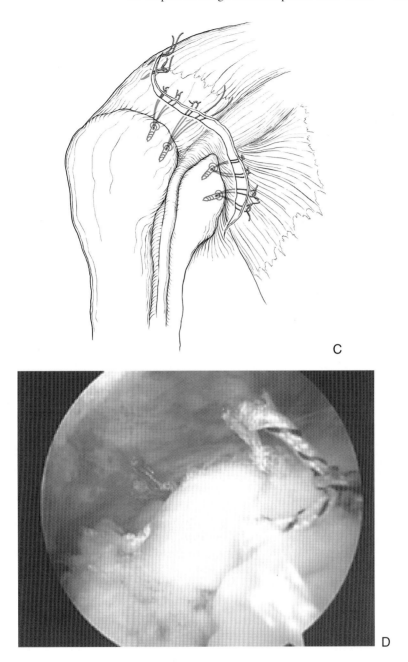

C

D

FIGURE 17.5. *Continued*

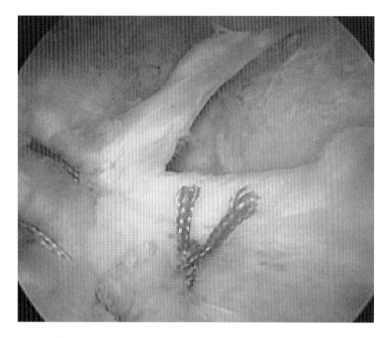

FIGURE 17.6. Posterior extension of tear treated with margin convergence.

performed on the supraspinatus tear. Knots are secured repairing the posterosuperior aspect of the tear. The arm is taken out of traction, and a deltopectoral incision is made. Remember, the anterior portal is superior to the incision, and this needs to extend toward the axillae. After enlarging the deltopectoral interval, the sutures are retrieved and the subscapularis is repaired, along with the biceps tenodesis.

Postoperatively, shoulders are immobilized in a small pillow sling. The shoulder has restricted external rotation to avoid subscapularis disruption. External rotation is generally allowed to 20°. After 4 to 5 weeks, supine passive flexion is allowed. Upright, active-assist flexion begins at 8 weeks. Strengthening exercises begin at 10 to 12 weeks. Return to activities should not be anticipated for 6 months. Young patients with acute tears may improve quickly and have an accelerated recovery pattern.

17.4. Results

There were 37 patients arthroscopically repaired with anterosuperior rotator cuff tears. Patient ages were between 15 and 75, with five patients being younger than 35 years old. Five patients had failed prior surgery, and five were referred from workmen's compensation.

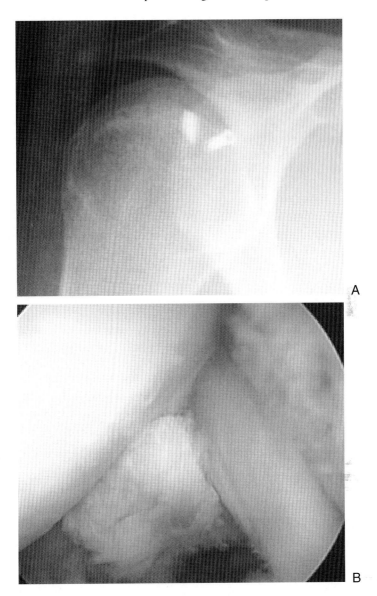

FIGURE 17.7. Biceps pulley repair in young patients. (A) Suture anchor repair of capsular ligaments comprising biceps pulley, anterior margin of supraspinatus, and superior margin of subscapularis. (B) Radiograph of anchor sewing pulley.

Biceps tendon ruptures were seen in 3 patients, and an additional 12 patients underwent surgical tenotomy (2), tenodesis (7), and stabilization (3). Stabilization was performed in three young patients (15, 17, and 19 years old) because their shoulders had biceps subluxation but no visible tears within the tendon. In this series, 41% of the patients had subluxed, partially torn, or ruptures of the long head of the biceps.

Subscapularis repairs were performed in all but one patient. Twenty-five of the patients required one or two anchors to repair the superior margin of the subscapularis (Figure 17.8). The other 11 required full tendon repair, inferiorly and superiorly, with two suture anchors. Infraspinatus tears were repaired in 10 of the shoulders, often with margin convergence and suture anchor techniques.

The surgical outcome is fairly early for most of these shoulders; repairs were performed from 2000 to 2005. Currently, there were 11 excellent, 22 good, 4 fair, and no poor results (Figure 17.9). Four of the five workmen's compensation cases returned to work at their previous jobs. Of the 28 employed patients or student athletes, all but two returned to employment and sport. Weakness was not uncommon. Five patients with pseudoparalysis improved, and one patient continued to be unable to flex above 100°. Internal rotation weakness was noted in many patients with chronic tears. These patients had positive belly press signs but often normal lift off tests.

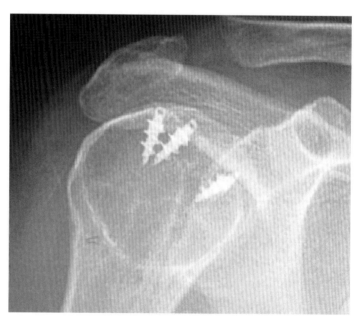

FIGURE 17.8. Postoperative X ray of suture anchors repairing supraspinatus and subscapularis.

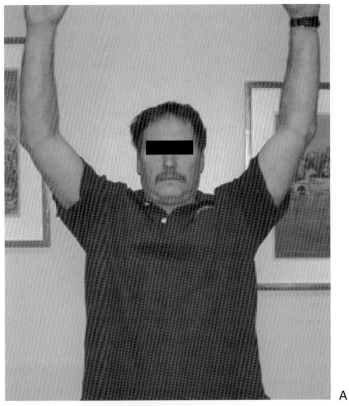

A

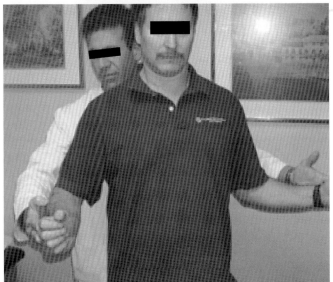

B

FIGURE 17.9. (A) Postoperative improvement in forward flexion 6 months following surgery. (B) Improved but continued weakness postoperatively in external rotation.

One patient had an irreparable subscapularis tendon avulsion and is considering a pectoralis transfer. He has returned to work and has been functioning well with his strength deficit. The University of California at Los Angeles (UCLA) range scores improved from 5 to 10 preoperatively to 27 to 31 postoperatively (35 is the maximum score).

17.5. Conclusions

Anterosuperior cuff tears are challenging to diagnose and treat. Arthroscopy has been a helpful instrument to visualize and treat articular pathology. Biceps tendon tears and subluxation can complicate management. Arthroscopic repair of anterosuperior cuff tears and treatment of biceps lesions have had promising results. Early intervention will limit muscular and tendon deterioration, improving cuff integrity and function.

17.5.1. Pearls

1. Arthroscopy is the best technique to visualize articular structures: superior subscapularis attachment, biceps tendon, biceps capsular pulley, and supraspinatus.

2. Subacromial decompression can be modified to avoid complete detachment of the coracoacromial ligament. Bone decompression is helpful to visualize, to utilize arthroscopic equipment, and to mobilize tendons.

3. Biceps tendon tears and subluxation are present in 41% of the cases. Young patients (<30 years old) are treated with repair of the pulley ligaments with an anchor securing capsular and tendinous structures along the pillars at the margin of the groove. Middle-aged and older patients should be treated with tenodesis or tenotomy.

4. Arthroscopic repair of the anterosuperior tear may combine articular techniques to repair the superior border of the subscapularis with bursal repair of the supraspinatus and infraspinatus.

5. Early recognition and repair can limit irreversible muscular atrophy and tendon deterioration.

References

1. Warner JJP, Higgins L, Parsons IM, Dowdy P. Diagnosis and treatment of anterosuperior rotator cuff tears. J Shoulder Elbow Surg 2001;10:37–46.
2. Sakurai G, Ozaki J, Tomita Y, Kondo T, Tamai S. Incomplete tears of the subscapularis tendon associated with tears of the supraspinatus tendon: cadaveric and clinical studies. J Shoulder Elbow Surg 1998;7:510–515.
3. Walch G, Nové-Josserand L, Levigne C, Renaud E. Complete ruptures of the supraspinatus tendon associated with "hidden lesions" of the rotator interval. J Shoulder Elbow Surg 1994;3:353–360.

4. Nové-Josserand L, Gerber C, Walch G. Lesions of the anterosuperior rotator cuff. In: Warner JJP, Iannotti JP, Gerber C, eds. Complex and revision problems in shoulder surgery. Philadelphia: Lippincott-Raven; 1997:165–176.
5. Bennett WF. Arthroscopic repair of anterosuperior (supraspinatus/subscapularis) rotator cuff tears: A prospective cohort with 2–4 year follow-up classification of biceps subluxation instability. Arthroscopy 2003;19:21–23.

18
Natural Extracellular Matrix Grafts for Rotator Cuff Repair

Joseph P. Iannotti, Michael J. DeFranco, Michael J. Codsi, Steven D. Maschke, and Kathleen A. Derwin

The results of open or arthroscopic repair of the rotator cuff vary widely in the literature.[1-15] The factors that have been shown to affect outcome relate to the technique of surgery,[3,9,16-18] the size of the tear,[9-11] the quality of the tissue and age of the patient,[10,11,15] the chronicity of the tear,[9-11,19,20] the degree of muscle atrophy, and the degree of tendon retraction.[9-11,20] In many cases, the size of the tear is correlated with the degree of tendon retraction, muscle atrophy, and loss of tissue quality. Postoperative care influences outcome and is dependent upon the length and type of protection in the first 6 weeks after surgery,[9,17,21] as well as the progression of the rehabilitation program from passive range of motion through active motion and resistance exercises. The larger and more chronic the tear, the more likely the patient will benefit from an abduction brace or pillow and a slower progression of the rehabilitation program.

Despite our understanding of the factors that affect surgical outcome, a high percentage of larger tears fail to heal after either open or arthroscopic repair.[5,9,14,22] Here, we must make a clear distinction between clinical and anatomical outcome. Historically, it was thought that good clinical outcomes could be achieved despite the persistence of a rotator cuff defect. Although many patients with persistent defects [as noted on magnetic resonance imaging (MRI), arthrography, or ultrasonography] have favorable clinical outcome when compared to their preoperative, patient-oriented, functional outcome scores, their objective (strength) and subjective (pain, functional activities and satisfaction) results are even better when the tear either partially or completely heals after surgery. Therefore, our goals for rotator cuff repair should include improvement in subjective scores and strength as well as a healed tendon. Hence, strategies to enhance the biological potential of the rotator cuff tendon to heal must be developed and investigated.

18.1. Biological Enhancement of Rotator Cuff Repair

Methods to enhance the biological potential of tendons to heal include the use of cell therapy, growth factors, gene delivery systems, and biological scaffolds.[23] A thorough review of each of these methods is beyond the scope of this chapter. However, each will be discussed briefly here.

Mesenchymal progenitor cells (MPCs) are known to differentiate into a variety of cell phenotypes and are essential for natural wound healing. Accordingly, autologous or allogeneic MPCs can be obtained from bone marrow, blood, or adipose tissue, and can be culture expanded and delivered to a tendon repair site to enhance healing. Animal studies using MPCs delivered in collagen gel or poly-lactide-*co*-glycolide acid (PLGA) scaffolds to patellar or Achilles tendon defects have demonstrated improvements in the mechanical properties of the repair tissue compared to natural repair.[24–27] Further, if MPC constructs are first mechanically conditioned in culture, such as allowing contracture around a suture,[27] the resulting improvement in repair biomechanics is even more substantial. In addition, cell therapy using autologous tenocytes was shown to enhance flexor tendon repair in an avian model.[28] Currently, cell therapy is used clinically for the effective treatment of skin wounds; however, its use has not been documented for rotator cuff (or any) tendon repair in humans to date.

A recent review article describes the roles of five growth factors that are known to be involved during tendon healing.[29] These include insulin-like growth factor-I (IGF-I), transforming growth factor beta (TGF-β), vascular endothelial growth factor (VEGF), platelet-derived growth factor (PDGF), and basic fibroblast growth factor (bFGF). All five are markedly upregulated following tendon injury and are active at multiple stages of the healing process. These molecules or members of their superfamilies [such as cartilage-derived morphogenetic protein-2 (CDMP2) or osteogenic protein-1 (OP-1), members of TGF-β superfamily], have been explored in animal models as therapeutic agents to increase the efficacy and efficiency of tendon and ligament healing. Results demonstrate that exogenous application of these growth factors into the wound site (either singly or in combination) can improve the efficacy and efficiency of tendon or ligament healing. The challenges that remain in using growth factor therapies include attaining specific and sustained delivery of growth factors to target cells and determining optimal spatial and temporal delivery strategies. In addition, we must better understand how growth factors work together with one another and other molecules in the repair site. Clearly, growth factor therapies will require rigorous investigation in preclinical and clinical trials before they could become practical for general clinical use.

Using gene therapy, it is possible to increase the cellular production of certain proteins (such as growth factors) that are important for tendon healing. The feasibility of gene transfer to normal and injured tendon and ligaments has been demonstrated in animal models.[30–35] Gene therapy

TABLE 18.1. Commercial Extracellular Matrices (ECMs) with Indication for Rotator Cuff Tendon Augmentation.

Product name	Manufacturer	Industrial source	Tissue type	Source	Chemically cross-linked
Restore® Orthobiologic Implant	DePuy Orthopaedics (Warsaw, IN)	DePuy Orthopaedics (Warsaw, IN)	Small Intestine Submucosa	Porcine	No
CuffPatch® Bioengineered Tissue Reinforcement	Organogenesis, Inc. (Canton, MA)	Arthrotek, Inc. (Warsaw, IN)	Small Intestine Submucosa	Porcine	Yes (carbodiimide)
GraftJacket® Regenerative Tissue Matrix	LifeCell Corporation (Branchburg, NJ)	Wright Medical Technology (Arlington, TN)	Dermis	Human	No
TissueMend® Soft Tissue Repair Matrix	TEI Biosciences, Inc. (Boston, MA)	Stryker Orthopaedics (Mahwah, NJ)	Dermis (fetal)	Bovine	No
Zimmer® Collagen Repair Patch	Tissue Science Laboratories, plc (Aldershot, Hampshire, UK)	Zimmer, Inc. (Warsaw, IN)	Dermis	Porcine	Yes (diisocyanate)

Source: Derwin K. Commercial extracellular matrix scaffolds for rotator cuff repair: biomechanical, biochemical, and cellular properties. J Bone Joint Surg 2006;88(12):2665–2672. Modified by permission from the Journal of Bone and Joint Surgery, Inc.

has shown promise in improving the function of healing ligaments.[36,37] Adenovirus-mediated gene transfer to human rotator cuff cells has been shown,[30] and genetically engineered, muscle-derived cells have been shown to differentiate toward a fibroblastic phenotype when injected into the supraspinatus tendon of nude mice.[38] Hence, gene delivery systems may potentially be useful in modulating the healing environment of the rotator cuff; however, considerable research is still required to understand and optimize this strategy for safe and efficacious clinical use.

Currently, the most common method to biologically enhance the healing of rotator cuff repair is the use of natural extracellular matrices (ECMs). Several ECMs have been marketed as patches to reinforce soft tissue repair during rotator cuff surgery (Table 18.1). These products include collagen-rich ECMs such as dermis (GraftJacket®, TissueMend™, Zimmer® Collagen Repair Patch) and small intestine submucosa (Restore®, CuffPatch™). Based upon sales reports, it is estimated that the annual use of these products in the United States alone numbers in the thousands. Although the use of biological scaffolds is becoming more popular, no human clinical trial has yet proven their efficacy in improving rotator cuff tendon healing. In fact, there is little retrospective data even describing the complications or adverse events associated with the use of these products.

The modification, characterization, use, and clinical investigation of natural ECMs for rotator cuff repair are rapidly evolving, and any attempt to provide a current report will no doubt be out of date before it is published. With that disclaimer in mind, this chapter will attempt to describe the current state of knowledge regarding natural ECMs, referencing the peer-reviewed literature (where is exists) as well as select unpublished data from national meetings and anecdotal clinical experience of orthopedic surgeons who have used these materials. We will attempt to identify the source of our information so that readers can make their own judgments regarding the level of evidence that may exist to support the data. The experience of the authors in the writing of this chapter includes the use of Restore® Orthobiologic Implant for repair augmentation in approximately 30 clinical cases, including 15 patients undergoing primary complete repair of chronic two tendon tears (supraspinatus and infraspinatus) that were enrolled in a prospective, randomized clinical trial. This study is currently in peer review for publication. Further, our laboratory is investigating the biological and material properties of several natural ECMs in both in vitro studies and preclinical animal models. Some of this data is presented herein.

18.2. Indications for Use of an Extracellular Matrix Graft

The use of ECMs for human tendon repair is supported largely by animal studies of acute tendon injury and repair. However, a lack of sound clinical data prevents us from defining the best indications for ECM products in a clinical setting. In the senior author's opinion (JPI), the role of an ECM graft is to provide augmentation of a repair that has a high chance of not healing but is otherwise optimal for surgery and postoperative rehabilitation. Specifically, we feel an ECM graft is indicated for chronic (longer than 3 months), medium-to-large tears and massive tears that are repairable. These types of tears fail to heal in 20% to 70% of cases.[5,9,22] Tears that are largely irreparable, with moderate-to-severe muscle atrophy are, in our view, not good candidates for this type of adjunct treatment. There may be some rationale for using an ECM graft when a large tear is almost completely repairable except for a small defect. We would not use an ECM graft to span a large, irreparable cuff defect because simply providing a soft tissue cap to the humeral head is not likely to reverse muscle atrophy or restore a functioning muscle–tendon unit.[9] Further, because primary repairs of small- and medium-sized acute cuff tears are likely to heal with proper surgical and postoperative care in 90% of cases, the use of ECM technology, which at this time has little clinical data to demonstrate efficacy and complications, is not justified.

18.3. Regulatory Aspects

Natural ECMs by definition are derived from human or animal tissues and are harvested, processed, sterilized, and marketed for clinical use. ECMs derived from animal tissues require U. S. Food and Drug Administration (FDA) approval. The FDA currently regulates these products through the device mechanism rather than the biological or drug mechanisms. When an ECM product is FDA approved as a device through a 510(k) application, the manufacturer needs only to demonstrate that the design and manufacture of the product are equivalent in safety and effectiveness to another device already approved in this device category. Demonstration of clinical efficacy in a preclinical or clinical trial is not required.

Table 18.1 lists the ECMs currently marketed for rotator cuff repair. In general, all of the animal-derived products have been FDA 510(k) approved "for reinforcement of the soft tissues, which are repaired by suture or suture anchors, during rotator cuff repair surgery." The FDA website provides an excellent resource to independently determine the intended use and 510(k) status and of any approved ECM product (http://www. accessdata.fda.gov/scripts/cdrh/cfdocs/cfpmn/pmn.cfm). Consistent with many other allograft products, GraftJacket® Regenerative Tissue Matrix is classified as human tissue for transplantation under 21 CFR, Part 1270. Under these regulations, no premarket review [510(k) or premarket approval (PMA)] is required. The specific and unique regulatory details for each product are described below.

18.4. Specific Product Information

18.4.1. Restore® Orthobiologic Implant

The Restore® Orthobiologic Implant is manufactured and marketed by DePuy Orthopaedics, a Johnson and Johnson Company (Warsaw, IN).

18.4.1.1. Product Description

The Restore® Orthobiologic Implant is a disc composed of 10 layers of porcine small intestine submucosa (SIS). SIS is a collagenous biomaterial consisting of the tunica submucosa of the small intestine. SIS is disinfected and after processing with peracetic acid and ethanol does not contain any viable cells. The SIS extracellular matrix contains predominately type I collagen, fibronectin, chondroitin sulfate, heparin, heparin sulfate, hyaluronan, and growth factors (such as FGF-2, TGF-β, VEGF).[39–42] To produce the Restore® Orthobiologic Implant, 10 individual SIS layers are laminated together under a vacuum press. The implant is terminally sterilized using electron beam radiation. The product is packaged dry with a shelf life of up to 1 year and requires rehydration prior to implantation.

Restore® is not artificially cross-linked and is approximately 0.8 to 1 mm thick.

18.4.1.2. FDA Regulatory Status and Indications [510(k) Approvals in 1998, 2000, 2003]

The Restore® Orthobiologic Implant is intended for use in general surgical procedures for reinforcement of soft tissue where weakness exists. The Restore® implant reinforces soft tissue and provides a resorbable scaffold that is replaced by the patient's own soft tissue. The device is also intended for use for reinforcement of the soft tissues, which are repaired by suture or suture anchors, during rotator cuff repair surgery. The use of Restore® is not limited to the supraspinatus tendon. The Restore® implant is not intended to replace normal body structure or provide the full mechanical strength to repair the rotator cuff. Sutures to repair the tear and suture or bone anchors to reattach the tissue to the bone provide mechanical strength for the rotator cuff repair.

18.4.2. CuffPatch® Bioengineered Tissue Reinforcement

CuffPatch® Bioengineered Tissue Reinforcement is developed and manufactured by Organogenesis, Inc. (Canton, MA) and marketed by Arthotek, Inc. (Warsaw, IN).

18.4.2.1. Product Description

CuffPatch® is an 8-layer, acellular, porcine SIS sheet. A nondetergent, nonenzymatic chemical cleaning protocol removes cells and cellular debris from SIS without damaging the native collagen structure. Following lamination of the individual SIS layers, the product is cross-linked with water-soluble carbodiimide. The implant is packaged hydrated and terminally sterilized using gamma radiation. CuffPatch® is approximately 0.6 mm thick. It has a shelf life of 2 years.

18.4.2.2. FDA Regulatory Status and Indications [510(k) Approved in 2004]

CuffPatch® is intended for reinforcement of soft tissues repaired by sutures or suture anchors, during tendon repair surgery including reinforcement of rotator cuff, patellar, Achilles, biceps, quadriceps, or other tendons. It is not intended to replace normal body structure or to provide the full mechanical strength to support tendon repair.

18.4.3. GraftJacket® Regenerative Tissue Matrix

GraftJacket® Regenerative Tissue Matrix is manufactured by LifeCell Corporation (Branchburg, NJ) and is distributed by Wright Medical

Technology (Arlington, TN) for the orthopaedic and podiatric markets. GraftJacket® is decellularized and freeze dried in the same manner as LifeCell's AlloDerm® product for abdominal wall repair. GraftJacket® is differentiated from AlloDerm® by the addition of several quality control testing procedures and requirements designed to ensure that the Graft-Jacket® material meets or exceeds minimum strength and consistency requirements for orthopedic applications.

18.4.3.1. Product Description

GraftJacket® is derived from human allograft skin that is processed using a patented technique to remove the epidermis, cells, and cell remnants. The remaining acellular, dermal layer is preserved by utilizing a proprietary freeze drying method that retains the native extracellular architecture and vascular channels. The matrix contains biochemical components including collagen, elastin, and proteoglycans and is not artificially cross-linked. It is packaged with a shelf life of up to 2 years and requires rehydration prior to use. The material is a single layer and is provided in a variety of thicknesses (0.5–2mm) and sizes for targeted surgical indications.

18.4.3.2. FDA Regulatory Status and Indications

Consistent with many other allograft products, GraftJacket® Regenerative Tissue Matrix is classified as human tissue for transplantation under 21 CFR, Part 1270. Under these regulations, no premarket review [510(k) or PMA] is required prior to distribution of the tissue. The product must meet requirements for Good Tissue Practices regarding donor screening and testing, as well as American Association of Tissue Banks (AATB) guidelines. GraftJacket® is marketed as a regenerative tissue matrix for soft tissue repair, including tendon and ligament reinforcement and wound repair. GraftJacket® is not recommended as a replacement of the patient's own tendon or ligament, but rather as an augmentation to primary suture repair.

18.4.4. Zimmer® Collagen Repair Patch

The Zimmer® Collagen Repair Patch is developed and manufactured by Tissue Science Laboratories, plc (Aldershot, Hampshire, UK) and is not substantively different than the Permacol™ Surgical Implant. It is distributed by Zimmer, Inc. (Warsaw, IN) for rotator cuff indications.

18.4.4.1. Product Description

The Zimmer® Collagen Repair Patch (ZCR) is an acellular sheet of cross-linked porcine dermis. Organic and enzymatic extractions are undertaken to remove fat, cellular material, and soluable proteins. The material is then cross-linked with diisocyanate and thus resistant to enzymatic degradation.

It is one layer and approximately 1.5 mm thick. It is packaged hydrated and terminally sterilized by gamma radiation. It has a shelf life of 3 years.

18.4.4.2. FDA Regulatory Status and Indications
[510(k) Approved in 2002]

Zimmer® Collagen Repair Patch is intended for use to reinforce soft tissues that are repaired by suture or suture anchors limited to the supraspinatus tendon during rotator cuff repair surgery.

18.4.5. TissueMend® Soft Tissue Repair Matrix

TissueMend® Soft Tissue Repair Matrix is developed and manufactured by TEI Biosciences, Inc. (Boston, MA) and marketed by Stryker Orthopaedics (Mahwah, NJ).

18.4.5.1. Product Description

TissueMend® is an acellular, nondenatured collagen membrane derived from fetal bovine dermis. It is not artificially cross-linked. The device is one layer and approximately 1 mm thick. TissueMend® is composed primarily of type I and type III collagen fibers. As a result of the patented production process, carbohydrate, lipid, and the fat cells are removed from the implant. It is lyophilized and packaged dry with a shelf life of 3 years.

18.4.5.2. FDA Regulatory Status and Indications
[510(k) Approved in 2002, 2003]

TissueMend® is intended for use as a soft tissue patch to repair and reinforce soft tissues where weakness exists. In addition, the device is intended to reinforce soft tissues that are repaired by suture or suture anchors, limited to the supraspinatus, during rotator cuff surgery.

18.5. Comparison of Extracellular Matrix Biomaterials

To date, there is no peer-reviewed literature comparing the physical or biological properties of these ECM biomaterials.

In a recent abstract, Fox and colleagues investigated the retention and infiltration of fibroblastlike synoviocytes into Restore®, GraftJacket®, CuffPatch®, and Permacol™ scaffolds.[43] Under nonloaded conditions, Restore® scaffolds had significantly higher cell infiltration than all other materials, and only cells in Restore® scaffolds were associated with new collagen formation.

In another recent abstract, Cook and colleagues reported on the viability and retention of various cell types seeded onto Restore®, GraftJacket®, CuffPatch®, Permacol™, and TissueMend® scaffolds, as well as the in vivo tissue healing and regeneration using these materials in a rat abdominal wall model.[44] The SIS biomaterials (Restore® and CuffPatch®) were consistently superior to other biomaterials in terms of cell retention, cell infiltration, new tissue formation, integration, and resorption. The dermis biomaterials (GraftJacket®, Permacol™, and TissueMend®) did not undergo significant resorption during 12 weeks implantation and were associated with little to no new tissue formation or integration. Overall, Restore® was reported to have superior cell integration characteristics in vitro, was replaced with regenerative tissue most rapidly in vivo and scored the highest in all subjective evaluations on ease of use. The differences noted among these materials could be related to tissue source/species, biomaterial processing, bioactive factors present, porosity and/or three-dimensional architecture.

In our laboratory, we have been investigating the biomechanical properties of these biomaterials. In a recent abstract, test strips, 4 mm wide by 30 mm in gage length, were tested from different lots of Restore®, Graft-Jacket®, CuffPatch®, and TissueMend®.[45] All samples were subjected to a uniaxial tension test to failure at 10 mm/min while submerged in saline maintained at 37°C. All ECMs required 10% to 30% stretch before they begin to carry significant load. However, if stretched enough, each material demonstrated a stiff, linear region, and an appreciable breaking strength. In the strain range of ~5%, these materials have a very low modulus relative to tendon. Maximum properties of ECMs were realized at 30% to 80% strain but remain one order of magnitude less than tendon.

These mechanical data suggest that these ECMs would not offer significant functional support as a load-sharing augmentation devices for tendon repair. If used as a primary graft to connect tendon to bone, these materials would stretch appreciably under the associated muscle and joint loads. While prestretching at implantation may improve their functional contribution, for tendon repair these ECMs may offer more of a biological advantage than a functional one. It should be noted that the suture retention properties of these materials cannot be inferred by this type of strip testing. However, suture retention will further impact the comparative biomechanical stiffness and strength of any graft augmentation procedure.

18.6. Studies in Peer-Reviewed Literature

Here, we review both the peer-reviewed literature as well as scientific presentations presented in abstract form. We have made a clear distinction in the text as to the source of the material cited. Keep in mind that information available in abstracts may be preliminary or incomplete. We have chosen to include these, however, because in some cases abstracts represent the only available data on these products.

18.6.1. Preclinical (Animal) Studies

18.6.1.1. Restore® Orthobiologic Implant

There are several animal studies in the peer-reviewed, published literature on the use of porcine SIS devices (single- and multilayer) in a tendon, ligament, or meniscus applications.[46–57] These studies support the use of an SIS device, such as the Restore® Orthobiologic Implant, to enhance the repair of musculoskeletal tissues. SIS appears to promote cell migration into the wound site and is associated with rapid angiogenesis, graft resorption, and constructive remodeling. SIS grafts are resorbed by 3 months after implantation.[48,58,59] While an acute inflammatory response occurs with SIS implantation,[60] little to no evidence of chronic inflammation or encapsulation has been observed.[47,51,56,60] The immune response is consistent with graft resorption and remodeling rather than rejection.[60] Further, SIS has been shown to resist infection.[61]

The histomorphometric appearance of SIS regenerated tissues appears similar to specific tissue it was intended to repair.[47,51,53] Biomechanically, the properties of SIS regenerated tendon and ligament are equal to or greater than control repairs (autogenous, without SIS) but remain less than those of normal tissue up to 6 months postoperatively.[47,51,56] Long-term assessments (greater than 1 year) have not been done in these animal models. In general, SIS grafting has not resulted in the formation of peripheral adhesions,[48,51] however, when used as a full-length intrasynovial tendon graft, ubiquitous adhesion to the digital sheath, together with impaired digital function, was observed.[52]

One animal study has specifically investigated the use of SIS for rotator cuff repair.[51] A 10-ply implant was used as an interpositional graft to replace a 2-cm segment of the infraspinatus tendon in a canine model. As a control, the contralateral tendon was elevated from its boney insertion and immediately reattached. Dogs were allowed free cage activity postoperatively. At 3 and 6 months there was no difference in the histological appearance or failure load between the SIS and control repaired tendons. No evidence of foreign body or immune-mediated reactions or peripheral adhesions was observed. Tissue remodeling consistent with a tendon phenotype (oriented, collagenous matrix) and a normal appearing tendon–bone insertion were observed in both groups at 6 months. These data suggest that acute tendon repair with SIS performs as well as natural tendon healing in this animal model. However, the failure strength of both repair types remained significantly less than native (uninjured) tendon at 6 months. In the authors' opinion, the surgical technique and postoperative care in this animal model make it difficult to predict from these data the efficacy of this material for clinical use.

In a recent abstract, acute supraspinatus tendon repair using a 10-layer SIS graft performed biomechanically as well as natural healing in the rat model.[62] In the chronic tendon repair (rat) model, SIS grafts were smaller in cross section than native tendon repairs but had similar material properties.[62] The authors suggest that the decreased tendon area with an SIS graft could allow for improved tendon glide under the acromial arch compared to the native tendon repair.

18.6.1.2. GraftJacket® Regenerative Tissue Matrix

To date, there are no peer-reviewed preclinical studies on the use of Graft-Jacket® for any tendon or rotator cuff repair.

In a recent abstract, Adams and colleagues reported on the use of Graft-Jacket® as an interpositional graft for infraspinatus tendon repair in the canine rotator cuff model.[63] No evidence of infection or rejection was noted with this graft material. Native cell infiltration was observed. At 6 weeks, 3 months, and 6 months, there was no significant difference in the ultimate failure stress between the GraftJacket® and autologous tendon graft repairs.

Three preclinical models were used to evaluate GraftJacket® as a scaffold for periosteum regeneration. The combined studies provided preliminary evidence that the dermal membrane material allowed cellular repopulation, revascularization, and bone defect restoration.[64]

18.6.1.3. Zimmer® Collagen Repair Patch

To date, there are no peer-reviewed preclinical studies on the use of Zimmer® Collagen Repair Patch (or Permacol™) for any tendon or rotator cuff repair.

Recently, the host response to the Permacol™ biomaterial was reported.[65] Permacol™ was implanted subcutaneously in the rat model over a 20-week period and compared histologically to two other porcine biomaterials (SIS and glycerol treated, ethylene oxide sterilized dermis). Implants were scored on the degree of acute inflammation, chronic inflammation, fibrosis, stromal response, vascularity, and percentage collagen. Permacol™ was reported to be well tolerated as a subcutaneous implant, with only a minor chronic inflammatory response remaining after 20 weeks. There was some evidence of collagen degradation during this period, and vascular ingrowth into Permacol™ was limited.

18.6.1.4. CuffPatch® Bioengineered Tissue Reinforcement

To date there are no peer-reviewed preclinical studies on the use of Cuff-Patch® for any tendon or rotator cuff repair.

18.6.1.5. TissueMend® Soft Tissue Repair Matrix

To date there are no peer-reviewed preclinical studies on the use of TissueMend® for any tendon or rotator cuff repair.

18.6.2. Surgical Technique

There are insufficient data at this time to recommend the best surgical methods and the most appropriate postoperative rehabilitation protocols for any of these ECM products for rotator cuff repair.

We believe that the role of the ECM is to both provide modest mechanical augmentation of a repair as well as a scaffold for host cell infiltration. As a scaffold, the ECM allows mechanical signals to be transmitted to cells, signals that are essential to drive their differentiation toward a tendon phenotype. Although the precise magnitude and mode of these mechanical signals are not known, it is likely that they may be influenced by surgical technique and the postoperative rehabilitation. Therefore, it seems advisable to secure the ECM graft to both the tendon and bone under tension. This means that the ECM graft should be first secured at one edge, stretched until taut, and then sutured along the opposite edge. It can be inferred that the material should extend from healthy, intact tendon tissue to its bony insertion site, and it should be closely applied to the native tissue to allow host cell infiltration and avoid gaps.

In the senior author's (JPI) practice, the Restore® Orthobiologic Implant has been applied after repair of chronic, large to massive rotator cuff tears by standard, open techniques. The tendon is first debrided of all devitalized and mechanically unsound tissue, judged by qualitative macroscopic criteria. Next, the tendon is mobilized to the maximum extent possible by all necessary means. The tendon is repaired to bone (#2 FiberWire®, Arthrex, Naples, FL) using a Modified Mason–Allen suture configuration and to tendon (#2 FiberWire®) using simple suture technique, achieving complete or near complete closure of the cuff tear with the arm in 0° of abduction in the plane of the scapula. The Restore® graft is then rehydrated in saline for approximately 15 min (range, 10–30 min) and then cut to the approximate the size of the tear. The graft should cover the entire anterior–posterior extent of the original tear site. It is sutured to the tendon, as far medially as can be achieved, to the intact tendons from the most anterior to the most posterior of the repaired tendons and to the greater tuberosity using a second set of trans-osseous sutures. We use multiple simple 2.0 nonabsorbable sutures for the Restore® graft (Figure 18.1).

To date, the senior author (JPI) has not used ECM grafts for arthroscopic cuff repair. Arthroscopic repair is used routinely as the preferred method of treatment for all tears with no or mild muscle atrophy and no more than 2.5 cm tendon retraction in tears up to 4 cm. In these cases, our rate of tendon healing (85%) and excellent clinical results (95% good to

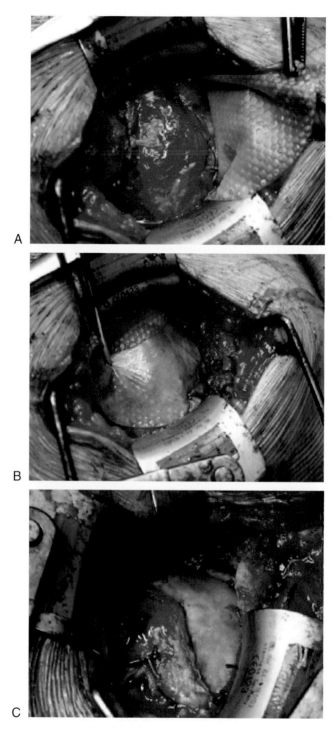

FIGURE 18.1. Intraoperative photographs of a study patient receiving a Restore® patch. The cuff was completely repairable. (A) The Restore® patch was first sewn to the medial aspect of the tendon. (B) The patch was then stretched over the repair to the greater tuberosity and (C) then sewn to the greater tuberosity.

excellent) do not in our view justify the use of ECM grafts at this point in time. Tears that do not have these characteristics are preferentially treated by open repair when preoperative imaging studies support a tear configuration that is likely to be repairable. In these circumstances, an ECM graft patch is considered if the patient is enrolled in a study protocol. We know that ECM grafts are used by others during arthroscopic repair, but we do not feel comfortable commenting on the surgical methods used as this falls outside of our own experience.

Our preferred postoperative protocol for large or massive tears treated by open techniques where an ECM patch could be indicated is placement in an abduction brace (Don Joy SCOI brace in 20° of abduction) for 4 weeks after surgery. The brace is removed daily for dressing, washing, meals, and daily passive supine range of motion exercises. The brace should be worn at all other times for 4 weeks, and we expect it to be worn at least 20 h of each day.

18.6.3. Clinical (Human) Studies

18.6.3.1. Restore® Orthobiologic Implant

Limited clinical data on the use of The Restore® Orthobiologic Implant has been published in the peer-reviewed literature. In one series, 11 consecutive patients underwent open repair of large and massive rotator cuff tears augmented with the Restore® Implant.[66] All patients underwent an MRI exam 6 months postoperatively, and only 1 of the 11 repairs remained intact. American Shoulder and Elbow Surgeons (ASES) scores were worse in five patients, which lead the authors to conclude that the use of Restore® Implant to reinforce large and massive cuff repairs is ineffective.

In a recent abstract, Rivenburgh and Davidson reported results of a randomized trial comparing Restore® augmentation of mini-open rotator cuff repairs to no augmentation in a group of 43 patients.[67] The size of the tears was not reported. After a minimum 1 year follow-up, the mean Constant score for the Restore group was 70.1 and for the control group was 64.5 ($p = 0.24$). The mean SST score for the Restore group was 10.1 and for the control group was 8.3 ($p = 0.19$). Although an anatomical analysis by MRI or ultrasound was not performed postoperatively to assess the integrity of the repairs and the results presented did not reach statistically significant levels, the authors concluded that the Restore® patch improved their results.

The senior author (JPI) undertook a prospective, randomized clinical trial at The Cleveland Clinic Foundation to study the efficacy of the Restore® Orthobiologic Implant in the treatment of reparable, two-tendon, chronic rotator cuff tears (large and massive).[68] The surgery and postoperative rehabilitation was as described above except a sling was used postoperatively instead of an abduction brace. Thirty patients were randomized to receive a standard, open repair with or without Restore® augmentation. All other parameters of care were identical between the two groups. Patients were evaluated by subjective outcome questionnaire and by post-operative MR arthrogram a minimum of 1 year after surgery. Based upon the preoperative MRI, 9 patients had large tears and 21 patients had massive tears (Figure 18.2). After adjusting for tear size, repairs without Restore® augmentation were 7% more likely to heal than repairs augmented with Restore® ($p = 0.07$). The median (interquartile range) postoperative shoulder score for the Restore® group was 83 (70–92) of 100 points and for the control group was 91 (81–99), $p = 0.08$. Healing of the cuff defect was strongly correlated with patient clinical scores regardless of whether Restore® was used. The postoperative shoulder total scores for the healed repairs was significantly greater than for the failed repairs [96 (83–98) vs. 81 (74–91), respectively, $p = 0.007$]. The preoperative to postoperative percentage change in the patient satisfaction score for the healed repairs was 400% (267%–450%) and for the failed repairs was 50% (0%–350%), which was statistically significant ($p = 0.04$).

This outcome study demonstrated that for large and massive chronic cuff tears, Restore® augmentation did not improve the likelihood of tendon healing or increase clinical outcome scores. We believe that in this patient population, poor tendon quality or high tissue tension secondary to severe muscle atrophy precipitated early failure (within the first 4 weeks) of the tendon repair. If the mechanical environment did not allow for maintenance of an intact repair in the early postoperative period, any potential, biological benefit of using Restore® would not be realized. It is possible that use of an ECM graft with these larger chronic tears could be advantageous with a slower rehabilitation protocol and/or use of an abduction brace in the early postoperative period.

18.6.3.1.1. Complications

Malcarney and colleagues reported the results of 25 patients who underwent repair of the rotator cuff with Restore® augmentation.[69] Four patients (16%) developed an inflammatory reaction that required operative debridement. No bacteria were present in the cultures from these patients, leading the authors to conclude that the Restore® Implant incites a nonspecific inflammatory reaction that may cause breakdown of the rotator cuff repair.

Zheng and colleagues observed noninfectious edema and severe pain in patients after they received Restore® during tendon repair, and as a result they examined the Restore® Implant more closely.[70] Their histological data suggested the presence of nuclear material as well as mast cell granules, and molecular methods confirmed the presence of porcine DNA material. Subcutaneous implantation into mice and rabbits demonstrated that Restore® caused an inflammatory reaction characterized by massive

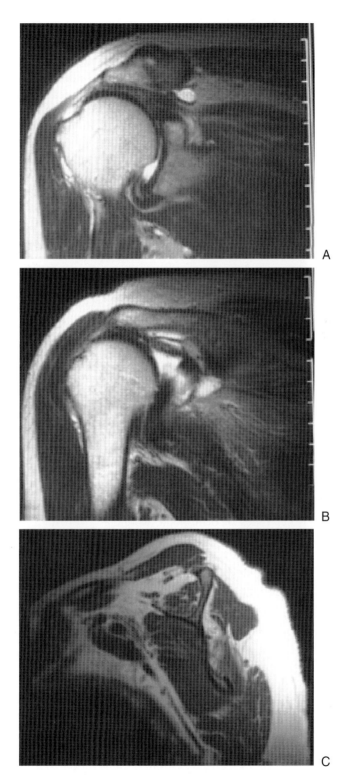

FIGURE 18.2. Preoperative MRI showing a massive rotator cuff tear of (A) the supraspinatus and (B) the infraspinatus tendons with (C) moderate-to-severe muscle atrophy of the supraspinatus and infraspinatus.

lymphocyte infiltration. Their results demonstrate that Restore®, as it is currently manufactured, is not a fully free of nuclear material and cellular debris. This may explain the nonspecific inflammatory reactions found in their patients after rotator cuff augmentation with Restore®, a finding consistent with the previously reported acute inflammatory response to SIS.[60]

Using the Restore® Implant in our clinical trial, a sterile inflammatory reaction was seen in 3 of 15 patients within the first few weeks after surgery. There was no patient in the study with a known history of allergy to pork or pork products. In all three cases, there were no signs of infection. In two of the three patients, the tear did not heal, and the third patient had partial healing on postoperative MR arthrogram. All three patients had an excellent clinical result with shoulder scores above 85 points. In the senior author's total clinical experience with the Restore® Implant (approximately 30 cases), this type of sterile inflammatory reaction has been observed in five patients for an overall incidence of approximately 15% of cases.

18.6.3.2. GraftJacket® Regenerative Tissue Matrix

There are no peer-reviewed clinical series on the use of GraftJacket® for rotator cuff repair.

There is a published case report of GraftJacket® augmentation of a gastrocnemius recession repair of a chronic Achilles tendon rupture in a 64-year-old female.[71] GraftJacket® allowed for adequate repair without a tendon transfer or a free tendon graft. The patient had early return to activity and good plantar flexion strength postoperatively.

GraftJacket® has been shown to be effective is management of major lower extremity diabetic foot ulcers, suggesting that this tissue matrix is applicable to other types of orthopedic wounds.[72–74] Further, there is an extensive literature on the use of acellular dermal grafts (e.g., AlloDerm®) for plastic reconstructive, burn, and dental applications.

18.6.3.3. Zimmer® Collagen Repair Patch

Permacol™ has been used clinically to reinforce soft tissues in a variety of non-orthopedic applications, including urogynelogical and plastic and reconstructive surgery.[75] To date, there are no peer-reviewed clinical studies on the use of the Zimmer® Collagen Repair Patch (or Permacol™) for any tendon or rotator cuff repair.

18.6.3.3.1. Complications

Interposition of Permacol™ grafts was shown to be detrimental to the results of trapeziectomy.[76] Twenty-six hands in 26 adults with osteoarthrosis of the thumb trapeziometacarpal joint were randomized to undergo either trapeziectomy alone (control) or with the interposition of porcine dermal collagen xenograft (Permacol™). The study was terminated prematurely because of apparent reactions to the implants in 6 of 13 patients. The Permacol™ group required more frequent review on clinical grounds and were discharged later after surgery. Three of the implants have been removed, and histology revealed foreign body reactions in all. There was no difference in thumb movement or power after surgery between the two groups. However, improved grip strength was observed and improved function was reported only in the control group. Permacol™ patients reported greater pain and were less satisfied with their operations than control patients.

18.6.3.4. CuffPatch® Bioengineered Tissue Reinforcement

To date there are no peer-reviewed clinical studies on the use of CuffPatch® for any tendon or rotator cuff repair.

18.6.3.5. TissueMend® Soft Tissue Repair Matrix

To date there are no peer-reviewed clinical studies on the use of Tissue-Mend® for any tendon or rotator cuff repair.

18.7. Conclusions

The authors firmly believe that the use of natural ECMs holds great promise for our ability to enhance and accelerate the healing of rotator cuff tendon repair. There are now several products on the market for general use, and it is the responsibility of our profession, the government, and industry to perform careful clinical trials and postmarketing surveillance to define the efficacy, proper indications, and methods of application of each of these products. This is a daunting task given the lack of consensus on basic issues such as optimal repair technique and postoperative care for the routine case as well as how best to measure outcomes. The track record for our profession in performing careful clinical trials does not suggest that many of these studies will be done in the near term. It is critical that this track record change as orthopedic surgeons continue to explore the use of many biological products being developed to enhance healing of bone and soft tissue.

There is still much to be learned about natural ECMs. We cannot engineer optimal repair strategies using these materials until we better understand their mechanism of action. As more knowledge is gained through basic science and preclinical animal studies, modification of ECM products may further enhance and improve their benefit for the human condition. For example, fabricating ECMs in parallel with other materials may increase their mechanical advantage. Natural ECMs could be modified prior to implantation to add growth factors, or seeded with autologous stem cells or tenocytes. Cell-seeded ECM grafts could be preconditioned in bioreactors to improve both their mechanical and biological properties.

Finally, our most challenging clinical cases are those patients with large, chronic, rotator cuff tears and poor strength and function. Surgical treatment of these types of tears is no longer a simple issue of tendon repair. The associated muscle is atrophied and infiltrated with fat. Repair and healing of the tendon alone may not reverse these muscle changes. Much has been done recently to characterize the muscle changes, but little effort has been directed toward uncovering the mechanisms or strategies for treating the muscle disease. Improving outcomes for our most challenging rotator cuff cases requires our attention to understanding and treating the entire musculo-tendinous unit.

References

1. Adamson GJ, Tibone JE. Ten-year assessment of primary rotator cuff repairs. J Shoulder Elbow Surg 1993;2:57–63.
2. Bigliani LU, Cordasco FA, Mcflveen SJ, Musso ES. Operative treatment of massive rotator cuff tears: long-term results. J Shoulder Elbow Surg 1992;1: 120–130.
3. Cordasco FA, Bigliani LU. The rotator cuff. Large and massive tears. Technique of open repair [review]. Orthop Clin North Am 1997;28:179–193.
4. Ellman H, Hanker G, Bayer M. Repair of the rotator cuff. End-result study of factors influencing reconstruction. J Bone Joint Surg Am 1986;68: 1136–1144.
5. Galatz LM, Ball CM, Teefey SA, Middleton WD, Yamaguchi K. The outcome and repair integrity of completely arthroscopically repaired large and massive rotator cuff tears. J Bone Joint Surg Am 2004;86:219–224.
6. Galatz LM, Griggs S, Cameron BD, Iannotti JP. Prospective longitudinal analysis of postoperative shoulder function: a ten-year follow-up study of full-thickness rotator cuff tears. J Bone Joint Surg Am 2001;83:1052–1056.
7. Gartsman GM, Khan M, Hammerman SM. Arthroscopic repair of full-thickness tears of the rotator cuff. J Bone Joint Surg Am 1998;80:832–840.
8. Gartsman GM, O'Connor DP. Arthroscopic rotator cuff repair with and without arthroscopic subacromial decompression: a prospective, randomized study of one-year outcomes. J Shoulder Elbow Surg 2004;13:424–426.
9. Gerber C, Fuchs B, Hodler J. The results of repair of massive tears of the rotator cuff. J Bone Joint Surg Am 2000;82:505–515.
10. Iannotti JP. Full thickness rotator cuff tears: factors affecting surgical outcome. J Am Acad Orthop Surg 1994;2:87–95.
11. Iannotti JP, Bernot MP, Kuhlman JR, Kelley MJ, Williams GR. Postoperative assessment of shoulder function: a prospective study of full-thickness rotator cuff tears. J Shoulder Elbow Surg 1996;5:449–457.
12. Jones CK, Savoie FH III. Arthroscopic repair of large and massive rotator cuff tears [review]. Arthroscopy 2003;19:564–571.

13. Murray TF Jr, Lajtai G, Mileski RM, Snyder SJ. Arthroscopic repair of medium to large full-thickness rotator cuff tears: outcome at 2- to 6-year follow-up. J Shoulder Elbow Surg 2002;11:19–24.

14. Rokito AS, Cuomo F, Gallagher MA, Zuckerman JD. Long-term functional outcome of repair of large and massive chronic tears of the rotator cuff. J Bone Joint Surg Am 1999;81:991–997.

15. Romeo AA, Hang DW, Bach BR Jr, Shott S. Repair of full thickness rotator cuff tears. Gender, age, and other factors affecting outcome. Clin Orthop 1999; 367:243–255.

16. Flatow EL, Kelkar R, Raimondo RA. Active and passive restraints against superior humeral translation: the contributions of the rotator cuff, the biceps tendon, and the coracoacromial arch. J Shoulder Elbow Surg 1996;5:S111.

17. Gerber C, Schneeberger AG, Beck M, Schlegel U. Mechanical strength of repairs of the rotator cuff. J Bone Joint Surg Br 1994;76:371–380.

18. Goldberg BA, Lippitt SB, Matsen FA III. Improvement in comfort and function after cuff repair without acromioplasty [review]. Clin Orthop 2001; 390:142–150.

19. Bassett RW, Cofield RH. Acute tears of the rotator cuff. The timing of surgical repair. Clin Orthop 1983;175:18–24.

20. Goutallier D, Postel JM, Bernageau J, Lavau L, Voisin MC. Fatty muscle degeneration in cuff ruptures. Pre- and postoperative evaluation by CT scan. Clin Orthop 1994;304:78–83.

21. Hersche O, Gerber C. Passive tension in the supraspinatus musculotendinous unit after long-standing rupture of its tendon: a preliminary report. J Shoulder Elbow Surg 1998;7:393–396.

22. Harryman DT, Mack LA, Wang KY, et al. Repairs of the rotator cuff. Correlation of functional results with integrity of the cuff. J Bone Joint Surg Am 1991;73:982–989.

23. DeFranco MJ, Derwin K, Iannotti JP. New therapies in tendon reconstruction [review]. J Am Acad Orthop Surg 2004;12:298–304.

24. Awad HA, Boivin GP, Dressler MR, et al. Repair of patellar tendon injuries using a cell-collagen composite. J Orthop Res 2003;21:420–431.

25. Awad HA, Butler DL, Boivin GP, et al. Autologous mesenchymal stem cell-mediated repair of tendon. Tissue Eng 1999;5:267–277.

26. Ouyang HW, Goh JC, Thambyah A, Teoh SH, Lee EH. Knitted poly-lactide-co-glycolide scaffold loaded with bone marrow stromal cells in repair and regeneration of rabbit Achilles tendon. Tissue Eng 2003;9:431–439.

27. Young RG, Butler DL, Weber W, et al. Use of mesenchymal stem cells in a collagen matrix for Achilles tendon repair. J Orthop Res 1998;16:406–413.

28. Cao Y, Liu Y, Liu W, et al. Bridging tendon defects using autologous tenocyte engineered tendon in a hen model. Plast Reconstr Surg 2002;110: 1280–1289.

29. Molloy T, Wang Y, Murrell G. The roles of growth factors in tendon and ligament healing [review]. Sports Med 2003;33:381–394.

30. Dai Q, Manfield L, Wang Y, Murrell GA. Adenovirus-mediated gene transfer to healing tendon–enhanced efficiency using a gelatin sponge. J Orthop Res 2003;21:604–609.

31. Gerich TG, Kang R, Fu FH, Robbins PD, Evans CH. Gene transfer to the patellar tendon. Knee Surg Sports Traumatol Arthrosc 1997;5:118–123.

32. Hildebrand KA, Deie M, Allen CR, et al. Early expression of marker genes in the rabbit medial collateral and anterior cruciate ligaments: the use of different viral vectors and the effects of injury. J Orthop Res 1999;17:37–42.
33. Lou J, Manske PR, Aoki M, Joyce ME. Adenovirus-mediated gene transfer into tendon and tendon sheath. J Orthop Res 1996;14:513–517.
34. Nakamura N, Shino K, Natsuume T, et al. Early biological effect of in vivo gene transfer of platelet-derived growth factor (PDGF)-B into healing patellar ligament. Gene Ther 1998;5:1165–1170.
35. Natsu-ume T, Nakamura N, Shino K, et al. Temporal and spatial expression of transforming growth factor-beta in the healing patellar ligament of the rat. J Orthop Res 1997;15:837–843.
36. Hildebrand KA, Woo SL, Smith DW, et al. The effects of platelet-derived growth factor-BB on healing of the rabbit medial collateral ligament. An in vivo study. Am J Sports Med 1998;26:549–554.
37. Nakamura N, Hart DA, Boorman RS, et al. Decorin antisense gene therapy improves functional healing of early rabbit ligament scar with enhanced collagen fibrillogenesis in vivo. J Orthop Res 2000;18:517–523.
38. Pelinkovic D, Lee JY, Engelhardt M, et al. Muscle cell-mediated gene delivery to the rotator cuff. Tissue Eng 2003;9:143–151.
39. Hodde JP, Badylak SF, Brightman AO, Voytik-Harbin SL. Glycosaminoglycan content of small intestinal submucosa: a bioscaffold for tissue replacement. Tissue Eng 1996;2:209–217.
40. Hodde JP, Record RD, Liang HA, Badylak SF. Vascular endothelial growth factor in porcine-derived extracellular matrix. Endothelium 2001;8:11–24.
41. McPherson TB, Badylak SF. Characterization of fibronectin derived from porcine small intestine submucosa. Tissue Eng 1998;4:75–83.
42. Voytik-Harbin SL, Brightman AO, Kraine MR, Waisner B, Badylak SF. Identification of extractable growth factors from small intestinal submucosa. J Cell Biochem 1997;67:478–491.
43. Fox DB, Kuroki K, Cockrell M, Cook JL. Comparison of collagen scaffolds for in vitro tissue engineering using synoviocytes and dynamic compressive load. Trans Orthop Res Soc 2005;30:1716.
44. Cook JL, Kuroki K, Fox DB. In vitro and in vivo comparison of five biomaterials used for orthopaedic soft tissue augmentation. Trans Orthop Res Soc 2005;30:982.
45. Baker AR, DeFranco MJ, Iannotti JP, Derwin KA. Commercial ECMs for rotator cuff tendon repair or reinforcement. Proc Int Soc Ligaments Tendons 2005;5:15.
46. Aiken SW, Badylak SF, Toombs JP, et al. Small intestinal submucosa as an intra-aricular ligamentous graft material: a pilot study in dogs. Vet Comp Orthop Traumatol 1994;36–40.
47. Badylak S, Arnoczky S, Plouhar P, et al. Naturally occurring extracellular matrix as a scaffold for musculoskeletal repair. Clin Orthop 1999;367(suppl):S333–S343.
48. Badylak SF, Tullius R, Kokini K, et al. The use of xenogeneic small intestinal submucosa as a biomaterial for Achilles tendon repair in a dog model. J Biomed Mater Res 1995;29:977–985.
49. Cook JL, Tomlinson JL, Arnoczky SP, et al. Kinetic study of the replacement of porcine small intestinal submucosa grafts and the regeneration of meniscal-

like tissue in large avascular meniscal defects in dogs. Tissue Eng 2001;7: 321–334.

50. Cook JL, Tomlinson JL, Kreeger JM, Cook CR. Induction of meniscal regeneration in dogs using a novel biomaterial. Am J Sports Med 1999;27: 658–665.

51. Dejardin LM, Arnoczky SP, Ewers BJ, Haut RC, Clarke RB. Tissue-engineered rotator cuff tendon using porcine small intestine submucosa. Histologic and mechanical evaluation in dogs. Am J Sports Med 2001;29: 175–184.

52. Derwin K, Androjna C, Spencer E, et al. Porcine small intestine submucosa as a flexor tendon graft. Clin Orthop 2004;423:245–252.

53. Gastel JA, Muirhead WR, Lifrak JT, et al. Meniscal tissue regeneration using a collagenous biomaterial derived from porcine small intestine submucosa. Arthroscopy 2001;17:151–159.

54. Gu Y, Dai K. Substitution of porcine small intestinal submucosa for rabbit Achilles tendon, an experimental study. Chung-Hua i Hsueh Tsa Chih 2002; 82:1279–1282.

55. Ledet EH, Carl AL, DiRisio DJ, et al. A pilot study to evaluate the effectiveness of small intestinal submucosa used to repair spinal ligaments in the goat. Spine J 2002;2:188–196.

56. Musahl V, Abramowitch SD, Gilbert TW, et al. The use of porcine small intestinal submucosa to enhance the healing of the medial collateral ligament — a functional tissue engineering study in rabbits. J Orthop Res 2004;22: 214–220.

57. Welch JA, Montgomery RD, Lenz SD, Plouhar P, Shelton WR. Evaluation of small-intestinal submucosa implants for repair of meniscal defects in dogs. Am J Vet Res 2002;63:427–431.

58. Badylak SF, Kropp B, McPherson T, Liang H, Snyder PW. Small intestinal submucosa: a rapidly resorbed bioscaffold for augmentation cystoplasty in a dog model. Tissue Eng 1998;4:379–387.

59. Record RD, Hillegonds D, Simmons C, et al. In vivo degradation of 14C-labeled small intestinal submucosa (SIS) when used for urinary bladder repair. Biomaterials 2001;22:2653–2659.

60. Allman AJ, McPherson TB, Badylak SF, et al. Xenogeneic extracellular matrix grafts elicit a TH2-restricted immune response. Transplantation 2001;71: 1631–1640.

61. Badylak SF, Wu CC, Bible M, McPherson E. Host protection against deliberate bacterial contamination of an extracellular matrix bioscaffold versus Dacron mesh in a dog model of orthopedic soft tissue repair. J Biomed Mater Res B Appl Biomater 2003;67:648–654.

62. Perry SM, Van Kleunen JP, Gimbel JA, et al. Use of small intestine submucosa in an acute and chronic rotator cuff tear rat model. Trans Orthop Res Soc 2005;30:719.

63. Adams JE, Zobitz ME, Reach JS, et al. Rotator cuff repair using an acellular dermal matrix graft: an in vivo canine study. Trans Orthop Res Soc 2005; 30:1733.

64. Beniker D, McQuillan D, Livesey S, et al. The use of acellular dermal matrix as a scaffold for periosteum replacement. Orthopedics 26(suppl 5): s591–s596.

65. Macleod TM, Williams G, Sanders R, Green CJ. Histological evaluation of Permacol as a subcutaneous implant over a 20-week period in the rat model. Br J Plast Surg 2005;58:518–532.
66. Sclamberg SG, Tibone JE, Itamura JM, Kasraeian S. Six-month magnetic resonance imaging follow-up of large and massive rotator cuff repairs reinforced with porcine small intestinal submucosa. J Shoulder Elbow Surg 2004; 13:538–541.
67. Rivenburgh D, Davidson PA. A prospective, randomized evaluation of the Restore Soft Tissue Implant in rotator cuff repair. Trans AAOS Annual Meeting 2005;P270.
68. Iannotti JP, Codsi MJ, Kwon YW, Derwin K, Ciccone J, Brems JJ. Porcine small intestine submucosa augmentation of surgical repair of chronic two-tendon rotator cuff tears. A randomized, controlled trial. J Bone Joint Surg Am 2006;88:1238–1244.
69. Malcarney HL, Bonar F, Murrell GA. Early inflammatory reaction after rotator cuff repair with a porcine small intestine submucosal implant: a report of 4 cases. Am J Sports Med 2005;33:907–911.
70. Zheng MH, Chen J, Kirilak Y, et al. Porcine small intestine submucosa (SIS) is not an acellular collagenous matrix and contains porcine DNA: possible implications in human implantation. J Biomed Mater Res B Appl Biomater 2005;73:61–67.
71. Lee MS. GraftJacket augmentation of chronic Achilles tendon ruptures. Orthopedics 2004;27(suppl 1):s151–153.
72. Brigido SA. The use of an acellular dermal regenerative tissue matrix in the treatment of lower extremity wounds: a prospective 16-week pilot study. Int Would J 2006;3:181–187
73. Brigido SA, Boc SF, Lopez RC. Effective management of major lower extremity wounds using an acellular regenerative tissue matrix: a pilot study. Orthopedics 27(suppl 1):s145–149.
74. Harper C. Permacol: clinical experience with a new biomaterial. Hosp Med 2001;62:90–95.
75. Belcher HJ, Zic R. Adverse effect of porcine collagen interposition after trapeziectomy: a comparative study. J Hand Surg [Am] 2001;26:159–164.
76. Belcher HJ, Zic R. Adverse effect of porcine collagen interposition after trapeziectomy: a comparative study. J Hand Surg [Br] 2001;26:159–164.

19
Biceps Tenotomy: Alternative When Treating the Irreparable Cuff Tear

E. Peter Sabonghy, T. Bradley Edwards, and Gilles Walch

Massive rotator cuff tears are a common cause of shoulder pain and dysfunction. A tear can be determined to be irreparable based on the quality of tendon tissue, quality of the rotator cuff musculature (high-grade fatty infiltration is a poor prognostic indicator for attempted repair), static or advanced humeral head superior migration or subluxation, and the presence of a noncompliant or poorly motivated patient. Pathology of the rotator cuff represents the most common cause of biceps tendon disease and can be classified by the type of underlying lesion.[1,2]

Large tears of the rotator cuff, including disruption of the supraspinatus, infraspinatus, and rotator interval, invariably lead to some degree of long head of the biceps tendon instability and progressive pathology. Once the infraspinatus is disrupted, this allows proximal migration of the humeral head, entrapping the biceps tendon between the humeral head and coracoacromial arch, and resulting in mechanical pain with elevation of the arm.

The observation that spontaneous rupture of the biceps tendon provided pain relief in the face of massive rotator cuff tear led to the development of arthroscopic biceps tenotomy as a treatment option for the irreparable cuff tear.[3] Concomitant acromioplasty is not performed in cases of irreparable rotator cuff tear as this risks anterior superior escape of the humeral head.[4]

19.1. Indications and Contraindications for Treatment

Treatment options for irreparable cuff tears include nonoperative interventions and surgical treatment. Nonoperative interventions can include rest, anti-inflammatory medications, physiotherapy, and corticosteroid injection.[5,6] Nonoperative treatment is most effective in patients with primary biceps tendonitis (tenosynovitis). After a macroscopic structural change in the biceps tendon has occurred, the usefulness of nonoperative interventions is usually limited to providing transitory relief.

Surgical indications for rotator cuff debridement and biceps tenotomy include failure of nonoperative measures, large tear size not amenable to repair, high-grade fatty infiltration of the rotator cuff musculature, and poor patient motivation for compliance with postoperative rehabilitation regimens following rotator cuff repair.[3]

The contraindications to biceps tenotomy would include low-demand elderly patients who are poor surgical candidates, patients with a stiff shoulder, and patients who find the possibility of developing a cosmetic deformity of the arm unacceptable. In the latter case, we recommend a biceps tenodesis.

19.2. Preoperative Planning

Patients with irreparable rotator cuff tears proceeding to arthroscopic debridement are candidates for a biceps procedure. Our treatment of choice for these patients is biceps tenotomy. In our experience, debridement is not effective at eliminating symptoms and recentering of dislocated or subluxated biceps has not yielded acceptable results.[2]

The decision to perform biceps tenotomy versus biceps tenodesis is based on multiple factors. The main advantage of tenodesis over tenotomy is cosmetic, though improved pain relief with tenotomy has been suggested by some authors.[7] In our experience, pain relief has been comparable with both procedures. When considering biceps tenotomy, we preoperatively educate the patient about the possibility of developing a cosmetic deformity of the arm (Popeye muscle), which in our experience occurs in about half of patients.[3]

19.3. Surgical Procedure

19.3.1. Positioning and Setup

Although arthroscopic biceps tenotomy can be performed in the lateral decubitus, we prefer the modified beach chair position. We utilize an operating table that allows removal of a panel just posterior to the shoulder to provide easy accessibility.

19.3.2. Instrumentation

The recommended instrumentation includes a 30° arthroscope, arthroscopic cannulas, arthroscopic scissors, arthroscopic shaver, and an arthroscopic electrocautery or an arthroscopic soft tissue ablator.

19.3.3. Surgical Technique

Through a standard posterior arthroscopic portal, a routine glenohumeral diagnostic arthroscopy is performed. This includes assessment of the subscapularis tendon, the biceps tendon, the glenoid labrum, the glenoid articular surface, the humeral articular surface, and the superior, middle, and inferior glenohumeral ligaments.

The stabilizing ligamentous pulley of the biceps consists of the confluence of the superior glenohumeral ligament and the coracohumeral ligament with fibrous contributions from the subscapularis and supraspinatus tendons.[8] In the vast majority of cases, lesions of the bicipital pulley will predominately involve the medial aspect. Flexing the arm to approximately 60° facilitates visualization of the ligamentous pulley and bicipital groove when looking through the posterior arthroscopic portal. A standard 30° arthroscope can be positioned anterior within the glenohumeral joint and used to "look around the corner" of the humeral head to evaluate for lesions of the biceps tendon, ligamentous pulley, and subscapularis insertion (Figure 19.1). Variable amounts of internal rotation and/or use of a 70° arthroscope may further facilitate visualization of these structures. Additionally, too lateral placement of the anterior glenohumeral arthroscopic operating portal canula can hinder visualization of these structures.[9]

Tenotomy is performed through a lateral arthroscopic portal in the patient with a full-thickness rotator cuff tear or an anterior glenohumeral portal if the rotator cuff is intact or only partially torn. If the intra-articular portion of the biceps tendon and associated structures appear normal, a blunt probe is used to pull the extra-articular portion of the biceps into the glenohumeral joint allowing visual inspection for macroscopic structural changes (Figure 19.2).[9]

The biceps tendon is then released from its insertion on the superior glenoid labrum using arthroscopic scissors, an arthroscopic electrocautery, or an arthroscopic soft tissue ablator (Figure 19.3). The arm and elbow are then extended ensuring retraction of the biceps tendon out of the glenohumeral joint. Any residual biceps tendon stump is removed with the arthroscopic shaver or tissue ablator. The entrance to the bicipital groove is visualized arthroscopically after tenotomy to further confirm adequate tendon retraction.

19.4. Postoperative Management

No immobilization is needed; however, we advise patients that heavy manual labor or activity, specifically eccentric-type biceps muscle contractions, should be avoided for 6 to 12 weeks following the procedure to allow scarring of the tendon in the bicipital groove, which minimizes the chance for cosmetic deformity.

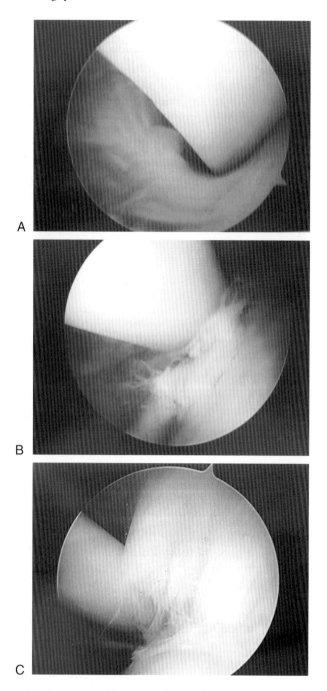

FIGURE 19.1. (A) A normal biceps tendon and ligamentous pulley visualized arthroscopically from the posterior portal while "looking around the corner." (B) Lesion of the medial aspect of the ligamentous pulley. (C) Articular-sided, partial-thickness tear of the supraspinatus tendon extending into the lateral aspect of the ligamentous pulley.

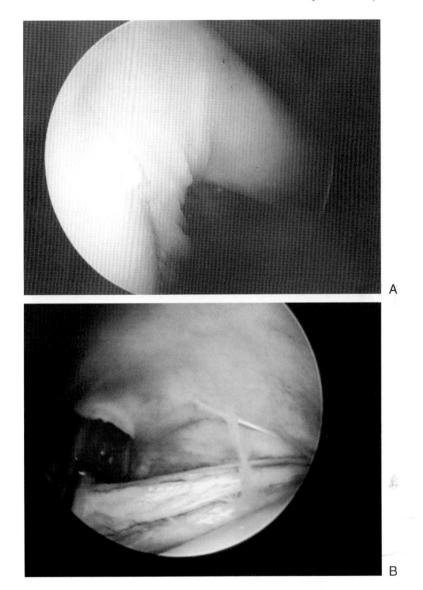

A

B

FIGURE 19.2. (A) A biceps tendon that appears normal during initial inspection. (B) When the tendon is pulled into the joint using a blunt probe, deep surface hemorrhage and fraying becomes apparent.

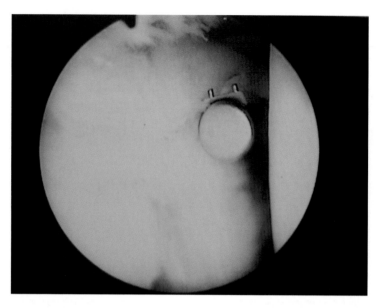

FIGURE 19.3. Release of the biceps tendon from its superior labral insertion with a soft tissue ablator.

19.5. Results

Most of our experience with biceps tenotomy has been in the treatment of massive, irreparable rotator cuff tears in older patients (>55 years). In this scenario, arthroscopic biceps tenotomy has proven very successful in providing pain relief and restoring some function by virtue of providing pain relief.[3,10] In 307 patients undergoing biceps tenotomy for the treatment of a full-thickness rotator cuff tear, the mean Constant score improved from 48 points preoperatively to a mean of 68 points postoperatively.[3] Eighty-seven percent of patients were satisfied with the operative outcome. Less than 3% of patients underwent another operation during the average 57-month follow-up period. No acute postoperative superior migration of the humeral head was noted after biceps tenotomy for irreparable rotator cuff tear; however, the natural radiographic arthritic progression that occurs in patients with longstanding rotator cuff tears was not altered.

19.6. Complications

Complications specific to this technique are rare. Postoperative stiffness was noted with the greatest frequency (4.9%) and resolved by a mean of 9 months postoperatively without further surgery.[3] We do not consider the change in contour in the arm that infrequently occurs in these patients to be a complication, but we do preoperatively educate every tenotomy patient, letting them know that this change in contour is a possible outcome of the procedure.

References

1. Walch G, Nové-Josserand L, Boileau P, et al. Subluxations and dislocations of the tendon of the long head of the biceps. J Shoulder Elbow Surg 1998;7: 100–108.
2. Habermeyer P, Walch G. The biceps tendon and rotator cuff disease. In: Burkhead WZ, ed. Rotator cuff disorders. Baltimore: Williams and Wilkins; 1996:142–159.
3. Walch G, Edwards TB, Boulahia A, et al. Arthroscopic tenotomy of the long head of the biceps in the treatment of rotator cuff tears: clinical and radiographic results of 307 cases. J Shoulder Elbow Surg 2005;14:238–246.
4. Gartsman GM. Arthroscopic acromioplasty for lesions of the rotator cuff. J Bone Joint Surg 1990;72:169–180.
5. Burkhead WZ Jr, Arcand MA, Zeman C, et al. The biceps tendon. In: Rockwood CA, Matsen FA, eds. The shoulder, 2nd ed. Philadelphia: Saunders; 1998:1009–1063.
6. Edwards TB. Treatment of chronic proximal biceps tendonitis: classification and nonoperative management. Paper presented at: 28th Annual Meeting of the American Orthopaedic Society for Sports Medicine, Orlando, FL, June 30–July 3, 2002.
7. Yamaguchi K. Disorders of the biceps tendon. Paper presented at: 28th Annual Meeting of the American Orthopaedic Society for Sports Medicine, Orlando, FL, June 30–July 3, 2002.
8. Bennett WF. Subscapularis, medial, and lateral head coracohumeral ligament insertion anatomy: arthroscopic appearance and incidence of "hidden" rotator interval lesions. Arthroscopy 2001;17:173–180.
9. Bennett WF. Visualization of the anatomy of the rotator interval and bicipital sheath. Arthroscopy 2001;17:107–111.
10. Walch G, Madonia G, Puzzi I, et al. Arthroscopic tenotomy of the long head of the biceps in rotator cuff ruptures. In: Gazielly DF, Gleyze P, Thomas T, eds. The cuff. Paris: Elsevier; 1997:350–355.

20
Biceps Soft Tissue Tenodesis

Alessandro Castagna, Raffaele Garofalo, Marco Conti, and Victor M. Naula

Surgical treatment options for long head biceps (LHB) tendon disorders varies between preservation of tendon to tenotomy or tenodesis. Optimal management is debated among orthopaedic surgeons. This discussion lies in the fact that there is great controversy existing in literature on the possible functional role of LHB and on its influence on shoulder function.[1] In fact, based on scientific evidence, different authors believe that the LHB tendon plays a key role as humeral head depressor, and as a secondary anterior stabilizer.[2–4] LHB seems to reach its maximal efficacy in abduction and external rotation (throwing position) giving torsional rigidity to the shoulder.[1,5,6] This stabilizer role seems to become most important when the primary shoulder stabilizer such as capsule-ligamentous complex or dynamic stabilizer such as rotator cuff are injured. On the other hand, some authors consider LHB tendon as a structure without any function.[1,7,8] In surgical decision making, the balance between the supposed functional role of LHB and the type LHB tendon pathology responsible for shoulder pain should be taken into account.[1] Numerous authors have recommended tenotomy in cases of symptomatic tendinopathy, partial or full thickness tears, subluxation or dislocation of LHB tendon with pulley lesion, isolated or associated with rotator cuff tear.[7,9,10] Nevertheless, if we think about a possible functional role of LHB in shoulder biomechanics, and in particular about a secondary stabilizing effect, a simple tenotomy can be considered a critical approach.[3,11] In situations in which the LHB tendon is unstable or in presence of chronic degeneration and incomplete tear causing shoulder pain, tenodesis has been advocated to preserve tendon function.[5,11,12] In this chapter we will review functional anatomy of LHB tendon, its pathological conditions responsible for shoulder pain, and will describe and discuss the rationale of soft tissue LHB tenodesis technique.

Sections of this chapter are adapted from Castagna A, Conti M, Mouhsine E, et al. Arthroscopic biceps tendon tenodesis: the anchorage technical note. Knee Surgery, Sports Traumatology, Arthroscopy 2006;14(6):581–585 with permission from Springer.

20.1. Functional Anatomy of the Long Head of Biceps Tendon

The LHB has a variable origin from both the supraglenoid tuberosity and the superior portion of the glenoid labrum.[13] Vangsness,[14] in a cadaveric study, has found four types of biceps attachment to the labrum: type I is all posterior (22%); type II is mostly posterior with a small amount anterior (33%); type III is equally anterior and posterior (37%); and type IV is all anterior (8%). The route of the tendon is an oblique one from the superior rim of the humeral head, down through the rotator cuff interval, toward the intertubercular groove, which can be explained by the fact that during the ninth week of gestation, the elbow undergoes dorsal rotation. This rotation translates at the level of the humerus in an average retroversion of 35° and hence induces the biceps to cross the articulation in an oblique fashion with a corresponding angle, rather than proceed in a linear fashion, as is the case in quadrupeds.[15] Such a delicate process of development, if threatened by critical conditions, can give rise to the onset of abnormalities and alterations to the anatomical structures and, hence, LHB diseases.

Anatomically speaking, even though the bicipital tendon is intraarticular, it lies in an extrasynovial space. In reality, the synovial sheath reflects on itself, ending as a blind pouch completely enveloping the tendon within the bicipital groove. The most critical anatomical area is the insertion of the tendon in the bicipital groove. In this area, formed by the lateral border of the lesser tuberosity and the medial border of the greater tuberosity, the supraspinatus and subscapularis tendon, the coracohumeral ligament, and the superior glenohumeral ligament play an important role; with the transverse ligament, they form the static–dynamic bonds that keep the LHB in its groove. The shape of the groove has been indicated as the cause of some bicipital tendon diseases.[16] A flattened groove is linked to instability and subluxation of the LHB; a narrow groove, together with an osteophyte, is associated with tendonitis and tendon rupture. It is very likely that some of these anatomical variations concerning the groove are in reality secondary to the disease of the LHB.

The precise biomechanical function of the LHB at the level of the shoulder remains under debate. According to some literature on the subject, the biceps is considered a weak flexor muscle of the shoulder. However, some reports suggest that the LHB functions as a static depressor of the head, preventing migration of the same against the acromion. Electrical stimulation of the LHB during arthroscopy visualization showed a glenohumeral compression.[17] Other studies[6,18] revealed that it acts like a muscle that contributes to shoulder anterior stability during throwing motion. Itoi[19] observed the stabilizing function of the LHB and reported a decreased anterior, posterior, and superior displacement of the humeral head with loading of the tendon. In a study simulating superior labral tears, Pagnani[20] found that the biceps acts as a significant shoulder stabilizer that can reduce strain on the inferior glenohumeral ligament.[4]

The role of the humeral head as static–dynamic depressor seems to become most important in the presence of rotator cuff tear,[21] which is confirmed by the flattening and hypertrophy of LHB tendon found in this setting. Interestingly, rotator cuff diseases (tendinitis, tears) represent the most common cause of secondary LHB tendon abnormalities. Recent developments in the field of research have better re-evaluated the role of LHB tendon in rotator cuff diseases, with important therapeutic consequences.[22] On the basis of its position, the LHB tendon can operate like a superior belt of the humeral head and functions as a depressor of the same. Providing the tendon is positioned normally within its groove, the humeral head is able to glide on the tendon and the glenoid surface. However, when the rotator cuff is torn and the LHB subluxated medially, this depressor action becomes compromised.[23] Proprioceptive roles for the LHB tendon remain to be studied.

20.2. Classification of Pathological Findings

The spectrum of chronic disorders involving LHB tendon can be divided into degenerative, inflammatory, overuse, and tendon instability. We differentiated the arthroscopic findings of the LHB into morphological and functional parameters, which were then further divided into six subtypes:

1. Normal LHB tendon with an intact synovial sheath.
2. Hyperemic LHB in the intra-articular portion, without signs of tendinosis.
3. Hyperemic LHB with the tendon imprinting on the anterior–superior humeral head cartilage, evidence of weakening of the synovial sheath at the entrance of the bicipital groove.
4. Flattened and enlarged LHB showing anatomo-arthroscopic signs of medial subluxation. Humeral chondropathy. Evidence of weakening and macroscopic degeneration of the synovial sheath.
5. Medial dislocation of the tendon with pathological adhesions involving the subscapularis.
6. Prerupture of the LHB, macroscopic signs of tendon degeneration visible as partial tears from fraying of the tendon accompanied by laceration and widespread weakening of the synovial sheath.

The anatomo-pathological situations described above can be associated with various degrees of the rotator cuff lesion, hence creating an unspecified number of anatomo-arthroscopic associations.

20.3. Surgical Procedure

20.3.1. Positioning and Setup

Once the patient has been brought into the operating room, anesthesia is administered in the form of an interscalene regional block. Patient position is dependent on the surgeon's preference. We prefer use the lateral decubitus position. The anatomical profiles of the osseous structures are drawn on the skin to identify the spine of scapula, the acromion, the coracoid process, and the coracoacromial ligament.

20.3.2. Diagnostic Arthroscopy

A standard posterior portal is created. A 30° arthroscope is introduced into the glenohumeral joint through it. A pressure-sensing fluid pump is used with a medium level of fluid flow and the pressure setting at 35 to 40 mm Hg. Anterior mid-glenoid portal is established with a taper-tipped guide rod inserted in the cannula of the scope. A thorough diagnostic arthroscopy examination is performed by positioning the arthroscope in both the anterior and posterior portals. In particular, the LHB tendon is carefully evaluated to assess any tenosynovitis, degeneration, tears, or prerupture and to evaluate stability in the bicipital groove. LHB tendon pathology is often in the intertubercular groove portion. To visualize this segment of the LHB, a probe is brought in through the anterior portal and positioned above the tendon to pull it into the joint. The remainder of the glenohumeral inspection identifies any other intra-articular pathology. In particular, the rotator cuff is assessed to evaluate concomitant disorders. An injury to the subscapularis tendon requires a thorough evaluation of biceps stability. Commonly, the disruption of the superior lateral edge of the subscapularis from its insertion point on the lesser tuberosity will result in the loss of the normal restraint of the LHB to medial translation. The associated rotator cuff tears are evaluated in terms of size, and the retraction and mobility of the edges of the lesion are estimated.

20.3.3. Anterosuperior Bursectomy

Once intra-articular diagnostic arthroscopy performed, the arthroscope, still in the posterior portal, is removed from the joint and reoriented under the acromion into the subacromial bursa. The anteromedial cannula is reoriented into the anterosuperior bursa (lateral to the coracoacromial ligament). In the case of partial rotator cuff lesions, an intra-articular and subacromial evaluation is performed, and a bursectomy and debridement of the subacromial space as necessary is carried out with a motorized shaver. This step is very important in order to facilitate the following knotting procedure for LHB soft tissue tenodesis.

20.3.4. Surgical Technique

If a tenodesis is planned, after completion of subacromial space decompression, the arthroscopic equipment is transferred to the intra-articular space. Any degenerative changes of the LHB tendon are debrided [Figure 20.1(A,B)]. An 18-gauge spinal needle equipped with stilet is introduced through the skin in the location of the lateral deltoid immediately adjacent to the anterior–lateral corner of the acromion. The spinal needle is then visualized under arthroscopic visualization as it penetrates through the rotator cuff. The route of the spinal needle within the rotator cuff is influenced by the pattern of the cuff lesion. In the presence of a partial lesion, the needle will pass through the supraspinatus in the anterior, pre-insertion area. In the case of full-thickness lesions, however, the morphology and width of the tendinous gap are determining factors. If the complete rupture is found to be retracted, a useful technique is that of exerting traction on the edge of the tendon with a clamp to facilitate the passage through the cuff tendon. At this point, the tip of the needle is oriented towards the base of the bicipital tendon approximately 1 cm away from its glenoid origin [Figure 20.2(A)]. The best orientation of the needle is as much as possible perpendicular to the long axis of LHB tendon. Once the spinal needle pierces the LHB tendon, the shuttle relay is introduced into the needle and manually driven until it appears within the joint. A grasping clamp introduced through anterior portal allows the surgeon to extract the shuttle relay and then to retract the spinal needle without damaging the nylon sheath [Figure 20.2(B)].

After removing the needle, a #2 braided, nonabsorbable polyester suture (Ethibond Excel Ethicon, Somerviller NJ) is loaded in the eyelet of the shuttle, taking care to avoid acute angles and subsequent damage to the surrounding tissues. In this way, the suture is carefully drawn through the rotator cuff and the LHB tendon until its exit from the anterior cannula [Figure 20.2(C)]. At this point, one limb of the suture protrudes from the skin adjacent to the acromion; the other limb exits from the anterior cannula and, during its route, traverses the lateral deltoid, the rotator cuff, and the LHB tendon. At this moment, the shuttle relay is released, after which the same steps are repeated, taking care to position the needle at least 0.5 cm from the first needle route to guarantee adequate resistance of the tissues at the moment of suturing [Figure 20.3(A)]. During the second route, the shuttle is retrieved and the eyelet pulled out of the anterior portal. The end of suture limb that was pulled and protrudes through the anterior cannula is promptly tied to the eyelet of the shuttle and then pulled back through the anterior cannula and through the biceps tendon to be recuperated out of the skin [Figure 20.3(B)]. At this point, both suture limbs protrude from the skin just lateral to the acromion and envelope the LHB tendon and the rotator cuff in a U shape. A bipolar electrocautery (VAPR, Mitek, Westwood MA) is introduced through the anterior cannula to release the LHB close its base while a mild tension force is

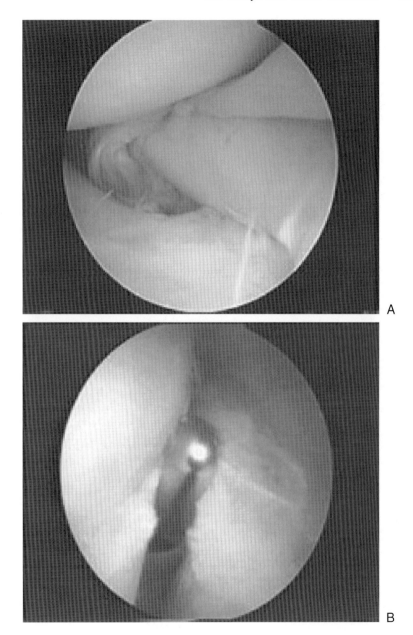

FIGURE 20.1. (A) Arthroscopic view of a right shoulder showing synovitis on the undersurface of rotator cuff. Partial rotator cuff tear associated with a LHB tendon partial tear (fraying). (B) Motorized shaver introduced through anterior portal debrides degenerative tissue.

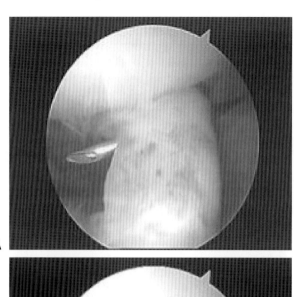

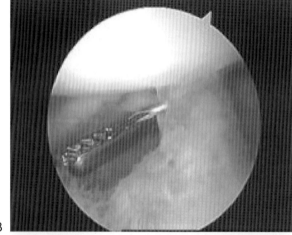

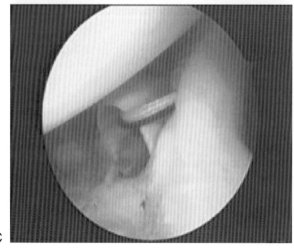

A

B

C

FIGURE 20.2. (A) Arthroscopic view of the first spinal needle transfixing the LHB tendon. (B) Shuttle relay driven through the spinal needle, pulled out by a grasping clamp introduced through anterior portal (C) a #2, braided, non-absorbable polyester suture loaded in the eyelet of the shuttle is pulled through the anterior cannula and out of the anterior region of shoulder.

FIGURE 20.3. (A)
Arthroscopic view of
a second spinal needle
with shuttle relay,
transfixing the LHB
tendon more proximal
than the first spinal
needle passage. (B)
The limb of suture
tied to the eyelet of
the shuttle is pulled
back through the
anterior cannula,
through the biceps
tendon to be
recaptured out of the
skin. (C) The two
limbs of the suture
are held by an
assistant and the LHB
is released close its
base with a bipolar
electrocautery
introduced through
the anterior cannula.

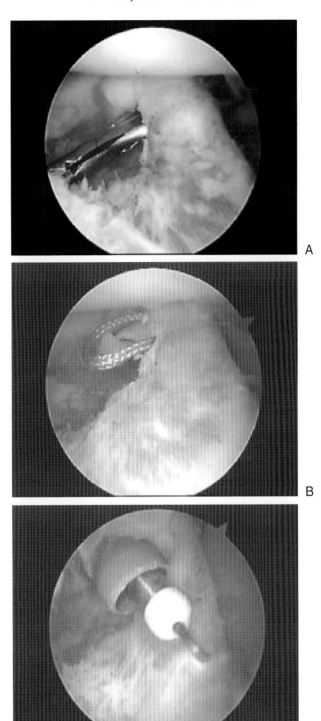

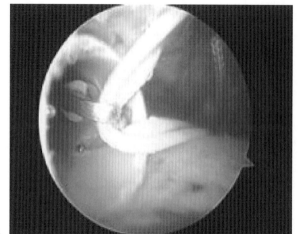

A

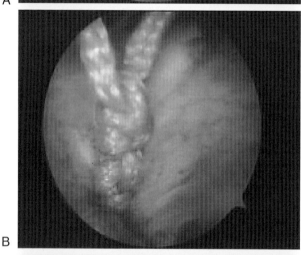

B

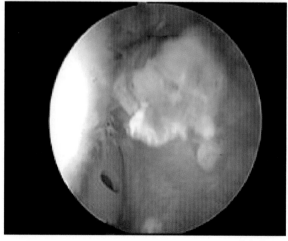

C

FIGURE 20.4. (A) Arthroscopic view of subacromial space showing the sutures that are extracted through the anterior cannula using a grabber. (B) The sutures are tied using a knot pusher, securing the LHB tendon to the rotator cuff. (C) Final aspect of soft tissue tenodesis.

applied on the sutures to protect them from potential damage and also to facilitate the release of the tendon [Figure 20.3(C)]. The residual stump of the LHB tendon is debrided to a stable margin. After bicipital release, the suture protruding from the skin is taut to evaluate the final effect that can be obtained with the knotting procedure.

At this point, the arm position is changed to approximately 20° of abduction to open the subacromial space. The arthroscope is now inserted through the posterior portal into the subacromial space, and a further arthroscopic examination is performed. Once the sutures are well visualized, they are extracted through the anterior cannula using a grabber and tied [Figure 20.4(A)]. The knot can be a sliding one (we prefer the SMC knot specifically for this procedure), or nonsliding one, like the Revo knot, according to the degree of friction produced by the soft tissues [Figure 20.4(B)]. In order to promote adequate gliding and contact between the two tendon surfaces, we prefer to choose the posterior limb as the post [Figure 20.4(C)]. Once the knot has been tied, the operation is completed in accordance with the specific clinical situation present. Treatment consists of acromioplasty, tendon-to-bone repair, partial side-to-side repair, or a combination of the three. In partial side-to-side repair for massive rotator cuff tears, the bicipital tendon stump can effectively be used as additional tissue when the tendinous gap is very wide or the quality of the tissues is found to be poor (Figure 20.5).

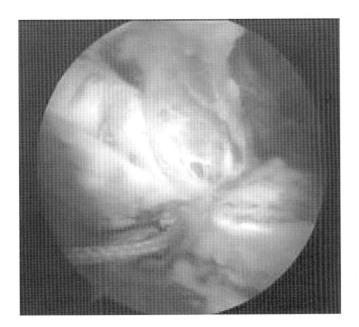

FIGURE 20.5. Arthroscopic view of bicipital tendon stump including a patch in a partial side-to-side repair for massive rotator cuff tears.

20.4. Postoperative Management

Rehabilitation is typically dictated by the procedures that have been performed in conjunction with the biceps tenodesis (i.e., rotator cuff repair).
If an isolated arthroscopic biceps soft tissue tenodesis is performed, the
patient is immediately started on passive pendulum exercises and active
wrist and hand range of motion exercises. At 1 week after surgery, gentle
passive elbow and shoulder range of motion are begun in all planes under
the guidance of a therapist. To avoid presence of anterior shoulder pain
after this technique active flexion of elbow should be restricted for 6 weeks
to protect the healing time period for tenodesis. Active extension of the
elbow is allowed. The sling is used for 4 weeks. After 6 to 8 weeks, active
range of motion exercises and gentle strengthening of the shoulder and
elbow are commenced. Unrestricted use of extremity is allowed 4 to 6
months after surgery.

20.5. Conclusions

Treatment of LHB tendon pathology has become an area of renewed
interest and debate among orthopedic surgeons in recent years. Tenotomy
and tenodesis of the LHB are undoubtedly the most favored surgical
techniques now.[1] Recently, anatomical and biomechanical studies have
reconsidered previous theories of the functional role of the LHB
tendon in glenohumeral stability and humeral head depression.[2–5,19]
Characterization of the role of LHB tendon is important to arrive at a
consensus about the need for biceps preservation. We now know that the
painful shoulder caused by diseases of the LHB that is left undiagnosed
and consequently untreated during surgery performed for other reasons,
such as subacromial decompression for chronic rotator cuff tendonitis
or tear, can be a common cause of persistent pain and shoulder
malfunction.[7]

   A possible explanation of this shoulder pain could be the close, anatomopathologic links among the LHB, the acromial arch, and rotator cuff
disease. The sheath of the biceps tendon is an extension of the synovial
lining of the glenohumeral joint and is intimately related to the rotator cuff,
so any inflammatory process affecting one of the structures can also potentially affect the other.[24] However, it is not always easy to identify lesions
involving the LHB by arthroscope because these lesions are macroscopically evident in only about 50% of the cases.[6] Nevertheless, arthroscopy
remains the most specific and sensitive method of evaluation of the various
pathological conditions of the LHB, and when pathological findings of
LHB tendon, such as hyperaemic LHB tendon associated to weakening of

the synovial sheath, are found, we think that the LHB tendon should be surgically addressed.

Recent reports[5,7] suggest a higher percentage of success in relation to tenodesis, about 80% to 90%, both for open surgery and arthroscopy. The arthroscopic procedures reduce the morbidity of surgery, with less soft tissue dissection. One controversy related to tenodesis is related to the site where it is performed. Some authors maintain that the site for tenodesis should not be in the bicipital groove. In fact, the groove may be part of the LHB tendon pathology,[16] so tenodesis within the groove may not relieve the symptoms. Biceps soft tissue tenodesis obviates this problem. This type of tenodesis can represent an additional option especially in cases of rotator cuff tears with associated LHB tendon disorders requiring treatment. The objective is to obtain a triple, biomechanical effect.[25] The first of these biomechanical effects that we try to promote through the procedure of transposition is the elimination of the deviation and oblique angle that occurs as the LHB completes its intra-articular course prior to reaching the bicipital groove. Tenodesis of the LHB to the rotator cuff can also ensure continual dynamic action of the tendon that depresses the head and impedes lateral translation [Figure 20.6(A,B)]. Furthermore, this technique can be extremely useful in the presence of large ruptures of the rotator cuff with muscle retraction. In these cases, infraspinatus tenodesis allows the infraspinatus to shift in an anterior direction, thus facilitating the practice of side-to-side suturing and anchorage to the bone. The bicipital tendon

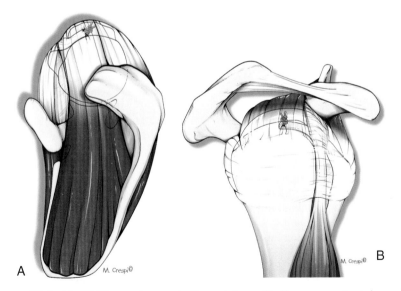

FIGURE 20.6. (A, B) The anchorage to the rotator cuff allows a constant dynamic action of the tendon that depresses the head and impedes lateral translation.

stump can effectively be used as additional tissue when the tendinous gap is very wide.

This surgical technique has a short learning curve and is quick, safe, and reproducible with low cost (one spinal needle and one suture). It represents an all-arthroscopic, inexpensive technique that causes minimal trauma. The most common complication, observed in less than 3% of patients, is failed biological fixation that manifests as subsidence of the tenodesis and consequent descent of the tendon with evident aesthetic deformity. This is a very low percentage considering that it is the expected final outcome of a simple tenotomy.

References

1. Ball C, Galatz LM, Yamaguchi K. Tenodesis or tenotomy of the biceps tendon: why and when do it. Techniques Shoulder Elbow Surg 2001;2:140–152.
2. Neer CS. Anterior acromioplasty for the chronic impingement syndrome in the shoulder. A preliminary report. J Bone Joint Surg Am 1972;54:41–50.
3. Pagnani MJ, Deng XH, Warren RF, Torzilli PA, O'Brien SJ. Role of the long head of the biceps brachii in glenohumeral stability: a biomechanical study in cadavers. J Shoulder Elbow Surg 1996;5:255–262.
4. Rodosky MW, Harner CD, Fu FH. The role of the long head of the biceps muscle and superior glenoid labrum in anterior stability of shoulder. Am J Sports Med 1994;22:121–130.
5. Berlemann U, Bayley I. Tenodesis of the long head of biceps brachii in the painful shoulder: improving results in the long term. J Shoulder Elbow Surg 1995;4:429–435.
6. Murthi AM, Vasburgh CL, Neviaser TJ. The incidence of pathologic changes of the long head of the biceps tendon. J Shoulder Elbow Surg 2000;9:382–385.
7. Gill TJ, McIrvin E, Scott MD, Hawkins RJ. Results of biceps tenotomy for treatment of pathology of the long head of the biceps brachii. J Shoulder Elbow Surg 2001;10:247–249.
8. Lippmann RK. Bicipital synovitis. N Y State J Med 1944;90:2235–2241.
9. Barber A, Byrd T, Wolf E, Burkhart S. Point counterpoint: how would you treat the partially torn biceps tendon? Arthroscopy 2001;17:636–639.
10. Edwards T, Walch G. Biceps tendonitis: classification and treatment with tenotomy. Oper Tech Sports Med 2003;11:2–5.
11. Becker DA, Cofield RH. Tenodesis of the long head of the biceps brachii for chronic bicipital tendinitis. J Bone Joint Surg Am 1989;3:376–381.
12. Boileau P, Krishnan S, Coste J, Walch G. Arthroscopic biceps tenodesis: a new technique using bioabsorbable interference screw fixation. Arthroscopy 2002;18:1002–1012.
13. Habermeyer P, Schmidt-Wiethoff R, Lehmann M. [Diagnosis and therapy of shoulder instability]. Wien Med Wochenschr 1996;146:149–154.
14. Vangsness CT Jr, Jorgenson SS, Watson T, et al. The origin of the long head of biceps from the scapula and glenoid labrum: an anatomical study of 100 shoulders. J Bone Joint Surg Br 1994;76:951–954.

15. Rockwood CA, Matsen FA, eds. The shoulder. Philadelphia: Saunders; 1998.
16. Pfahler M, Branner S, Refiar HJ. The role of the bicipital groove in tendinopathy of the long biceps tendon. J Shoulder Elbow Surg 1999;8:419–424.
17. Andrews JR, Carson WG Jr, McLeod WD. Glenoid labrum tears related to the long head of the biceps. Am J Sports Med 1985;13:337–341.
18. Gowan ID, Jobe FW, Tibone J, Perry J, Moynes DR. A comparative electromyographic analysis of the shoulder during pitching. Professional versus amateur pitcher. Am J Sports Med 1987;15:586–590.
19. Itoi E, Kuechle DK, Newman SR, et al. Stabilising function of the biceps in stable and unstable shoulders. J Bone Joint Surg Br 1993;75:546–550.
20. Pagnani Deng XH, Warren RF, et al. Effect of lesions of the superior portion of the glenoid labrum on glenohumeral translation. J Bone Joint Surg Am 1995;77:1003–1010.
21. Rowe CR. The shoulder. New York: Churchill Livingstone; 1998:145.
22. Sethi N, Wright R, Yamaguchi K. Disorders of the long head of the biceps tendon. J Shoulder Elbow Surg 1999;8:644–654.
23. Walch G, Novè-Josserand L, Boileau P, Levigne C. Subluxations and dislocations of the tendon of the long head of the biceps. J Shoulder Elbow Surg 1998;7:100–108.
24. Neviaser TJ. The role of the biceps tendon in the impingement syndrome. Orthop Clin North Am 1987;18:383–386.
25. Castagna A, Mouhsine E, Conti M, Vinci E, Borroni M, Giardella A, Garofalo R. Arthroscopic biceps tendon tenodesis: the anchorage technical note. Knee Surg Sports Traumatol Arthrosc 2006 Jun; 14(6):581–585. Epub 2005 Dec 23.

21
Biceps Tenodesis with Interference Screw

Pascal Boileau and Christopher R. Chuinard

The tendon of the long head of the biceps (LHB) is a frequent source of pain in the shoulder and is subject to numerous pathologies.[1-3] Treatment of pathology of the LHB involves resection of the intra-articular portion with a simple tenotomy or a tenodesis. Tenodesis of the LHB, with or without a rotator cuff repair, is an intervention known to reliably and effectively reduce the pain.[4,5] We were not satisfied with the results obtained with other techniques. Because of our experience with the use of interference screw for surgery of the anterior cruciate ligament (ACL), we developed a technique for tenodesis of the biceps utilizing a bioresorbable interference screw.[6,7]

21.1. Indications and Contraindications

The conditions affecting the LHB tendon are numerous: tenosynovitis, delamination, prerupture, subluxation, frank dislocation, or incarceration of the tendon in the groove (the "hourglass" biceps). Lesions of the biceps tendon can be seen with or without rotator cuff lesions. Tenotomy or tenodesis of the biceps is indicated in any of the following circumstances:

1. In massive, irreparable rotator cuff tears with accompanying pathology of the biceps tendon;
2. In arthroscopic rotator cuff repair when there is concomitant biceps pathology;
3. In cases of isolated biceps pathology and an intact rotator cuff, particularly when young athletes present with tenosynovitis, subluxation, prerupture, or a superior labral anterior posterior (SLAP) lesion; and
4. In cases of failed cuff repair with the biceps pulley in place but pathological or the tendon fixed in a manner that affects the normal kinematics of the shoulder.

The sole contraindication, ultimately, is the presence of a biceps without pathology, but it would be rare to find a healthy biceps in a patient older than 50 who has a rotator cuff tear![8] Tenodesis is preferable to tenotomy in active patients; it avoids the retraction of the muscle, possible cramping during physical activities with the arm, and loss of supination strength.[9]

21.2. Preoperative Planning

Patients often complain of pain in the anterior region of the shoulder with occasional distal radiation along the anterior aspect of the upper arm and forearm. However, these symptoms are often concomitant with impingement symptoms, such as overhead activity pain and night pain. Speed's test is often positive; tenderness with palpation of the bicipital groove (approximately 2 cm distal to the anterolateral border of the acromion with the arm in slight internal rotation) is often present. Tenderness with passive external rotation of the arm, as the examiner is palpating the bicipital groove, is also a common sign, as the pathological biceps is "rolled" under the examiner's fingers. Often patients will localize a point of maximum discomfort at the level of the superior portion of the bicipital groove. Radiographic examination should include a standard roentenographic series (anterior–posterior X rays in neutral, internal, and external rotation, an axillary view, and a scapular Y-view/supraspinatus outlet view), to rule in or out any associated abnormalities. Osteophytes around the bicipital groove can also be identified and indicate bicipital pathology. Specialized imaging studies [magnetic resonance imaging (MRI) with gadolinium, arthrographic computerized tomography (artho-CT), and/or ultrasound imaging] can assist in preoperatively diagnosing pathology of the biceps tendon. Magnetic resonance imaging, in particular, is useful to assess both the position of the biceps and possible intra-tendinous pathology.

We have recently described a new pathological entity of the LHB that cannot be detected without dynamic exploration of the shoulder and is, perhaps, a cause of failure of simple tenotomy: the entrapped LHB (the "hourglass" biceps). Hypertrophy of the intra-articular portion of the biceps creates a situation in which the tendon becomes incarcerated in the glenohumeral joint during elevation of the arm because the enlarged portion is unable to glide through the groove.[10] The hourglass biceps is the origin of pain and blockage of motion of the shoulder [Figure 21.1(A,B)]; the diagnosis is suspected when the pain is localized to the anterior aspect of the shoulder and there is accompanying loss of the last 20° or 30° of elevation (forward flexion) or abduction in the recumbent position [Figure 21.2(A)]. The limitation of motion persists with passive range of motion under anesthesia (the hourglass test) [Figure 21.2(B–D)]. The treatment consists of both resection of the intra-articular portion of the tendon and tenodesis; this restores normal elevation of the shoulder. The hourglass biceps is often associated with medial subluxation of the

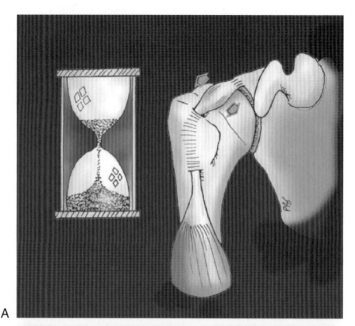

A

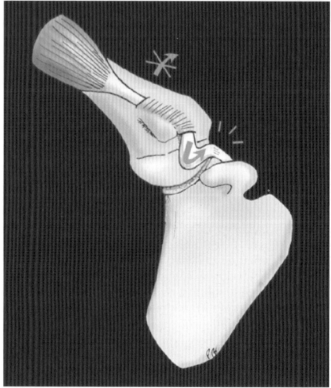

B

FIGURE 21.1. (A) Entrapment of the biceps in the glenohumeral joint during elevation of the arm because of hypertrophy of the tendon (the "hourglass" biceps);
(B) functional representation. (From Boileau P, Ahrens PM, Hatzidakis AM.
Entrapment of the long head of the biceps tendon: the hourglass biceps — a cause
of pain and locking of the shoulder. J Shoulder Elbow Surg 2004;13(3):249–257.
Adapted with permission from the Journal of Shoulder and Elbow Surgery Board
of Trustees.)

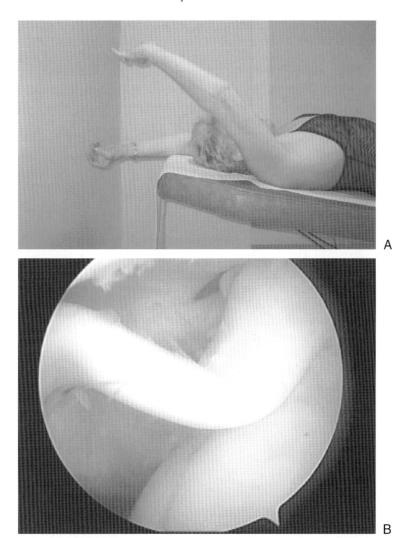

FIGURE 21.2. Shoulder pain and loss of 20° to 30° of passive elevation (A) because of squeezing of the biceps between the glenoid and humeral head; arthroscopic view at the beginning of humeral elevation shows that the tendon does not slide into the groove (B). (From Boileau P, Ahrens PM, Hatzidakis AM. Entrapment of the long head of the biceps tendon: the hourglass biceps — a cause of pain and locking of the shoulder. J Shoulder Elbow Surg 2004;13(3):249–257. Reprinted with permission from the Journal of Shoulder and Elbow Surgery Board of Trustees.)

tendon by dilatation of the orifice to the bicepital groove and cleavage of the upper border of the subscapularis tendon.

Another cause of entrapment of the tendon is inclusion of the LHB in cuff repair, the "accordion biceps" (i.e., when sutures are placed between the supraspinatus and the subscapularis), or tenodesis at the entrance to the groove without detachment from the supraglenoid tubercle.[11] Again, the normal physiology of the shoulder is perturbed because the tendon of the LHB is unable to pass freely through the bicipital groove with elevation of the arm. The tendon folds back upon itself and becomes entrapped in the glenohumeral articulation. It is, therefore, incumbent on the surgeon to perform a dynamic arthroscopic examination of the shoulder to evaluate for instability or entrapment of the LHB.

An exquisitely thin, friable tendon that is almost completely ruptured represents the potential limitation to arthroscopic tenodesis with interference screw. When this is the case, it is easier to perform a simple arthroscopic tenotomy or to convert to an open tenodesis. The choice between tenotomy and tenodesis depends not only on surgical preference but also on technical expertise.

21.3. Surgical Procedure

The principle of the technique is to first exteriorize the tendon through an anterior portal, then fold it on itself for 20mm or 25mm. Next, a bone tunnel is prepared approximately 5 to 10mm from the summit of the bicipital groove. The tendon is then fixated in the groove with a bioresorbable interference screw (Figure 21.3). Recently, interference screw fixation has been shown to have double the load to failure for biceps tenodesis than

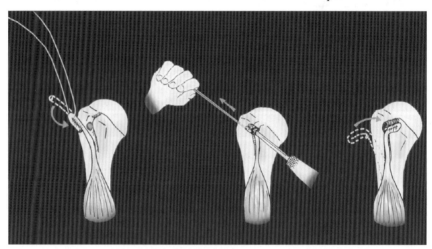

FIGURE 21.3. Schematic of the procedure. (Adapted from Boileau P, et al. Entrapment of the long head of the biceps tendon: the hourglass biceps — a cause of pain and locking of the shoulder. J Shoulder Elbow Surg 2004;13(3):249–257 with permission from The Journal of Shoulder and Elbow Surgery Board of Trustees and from Boileau P, et al. Arthroscopic biceps tenodesis: a new technique using bioabsorbable interference screw fixation. Arthroscopy 2002;18(9):1002–1012 with permission from the Arthroscopy Association of North America.)

suture anchor fixation.[11] Doubling the biceps tendon has at least three advantages: (1) it reinforces the strength of the tendon, which is not damaged by the interference screw; (2) it prevents a possible sliding of the tendon after screw insertion ("stop-block" effect); and (3) it allows an optimal tensioning of the biceps muscle.

21.3.1. Position and Setup

While it is possible to perform the procedure in the lateral decubitus position, we prefer the 30° beach chair position without traction, because this offers the surgeon greater freedom and better control of the rotation of the shoulder and flexion of the elbow. The arm is placed on a U support (a Trillat knee holder, Orleans, France); the position of the support is at the level of the epicondyles and should hold the arm parallel to the floor (about 45° of shoulder flexion) in about 30° of abduction when the elbow if fully extended (remember to account for the drapes when positioning the vertical height of the U support). Alternatively, a commercially available articulated arm holder can be used. We do not routinely use traction during shoulder arthroscopy, but gentle, manual traction is possible in this position if needed. The forearm is placed in neutral or slight internal rotation; the hand can be placed against the operative Mayo stand for support. This position relaxes the deltoid and allows the space needed to work anteriorly, providing the optimum exposure to the bicipital groove. One must understand that the work is not done in the subacromial space; rather, it is an anterior region of the subdeltoid bursa.

21.3.2. Portals

It is necessary to have two working portals in addition to the standard posterior portal: an anterior–medial (AM) portal and an anterior–lateral (AL) portal. The AM is the "work horse," and the AL is the "eye" on the bicipital groove (Figure 21.4). The two anterior portals are located about two fingerbreadths distal to the anterior border of the acromion and are separated by about two fingerbreadths, forming a triangle with the anterior edge of the acromion (of course, "two fingerbreadths" is a general guideline).

21.3.3. Instrumentation

Standard arthroscopic equipment is employed: a 30° scope, shaver (Smith & Nephew Endoscopy, Andover, MA), arthroscopic meniscal tip bovie, VAPR probe (Depuy Mitek, Westwood, MA), Tenoscrew® (Phusis, Tornier, Stafford, TX), Beath needle and ACL reamers and sizers, and a disposable cannula for the working instruments (CLEAR-TRAC COMPLETE Cannula System, Smith & Nephew Endoscopy). An optional targeting device is available (Shoulder Guide, Future Medical Systems, Glen Burnie, MD). A spinal needle will be required to transfix the biceps tendon after

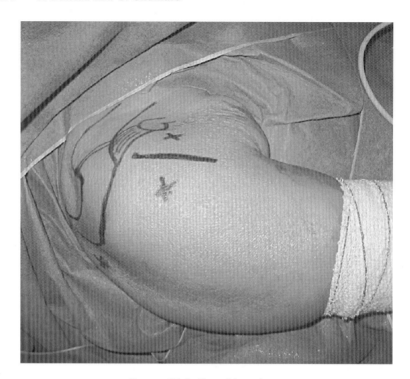

FIGURE 21.4. Portal locations.

tenotomy, and a vascular clamp is extremely helpful to allow for appropriate exteriorization of the biceps tendon without damaging the structure of the tendon itself. Sutures required will be a large nonabsorbable suture (#5 Ethibond, Ethicon, Inc., a Johnson and Johnson Company, or #7 Flexidene, Braun, Germany), a smaller absorbable suture (usually #0 or #1 Vicryl, Ethicon, Inc., a Johnson and Johnson Company), and a guiding suture (usually #1 PDS Ethicon, Inc., a Johnson and Johnson Company).

21.3.4. Surgical Technique

21.3.4.1. Step 1: Tenotomy of the Long Head of the Biceps

The glenohumeral joint is explored though the standard posterior viewing portal. The AM is realized through an inside-out technique just above the tendon of the subscapularis, lateral to the coracoid process and the coracohumeral ligament. An arthroscopic cannula is then placed over the trochar as it is passed from posterior to anterior. The rotator cuff is explored, and pathology of the biceps is confirmed: tenosynovitis, subluxation (medial or lateral), dislocation, hypertrophy (hourglass biceps), delamination, or prerupture. It is of paramount importance to probe the tendon with a crochet hook through the anterior portal and to perform the flexion maneuver with the elbow extended to evaluate its mobility (Figure 21.2). The

LHB is transfixed at the entrance of the groove with a spinal needle; this facilitates locating the gutter during the anterior bursoscopy and prevents retraction of the tendon after tenotomy. Arthroscopic scissors or the electrocautery are used to tenotomize the LHB at the supraglenoid tubercle.

21.3.4.2. Step 2: Anterior Subdeltoid Bursectomy and Transhumeral Ligament Release

The arthroscope is removed from the joint, and the AL is established two fingers lateral to the AM in the horizontal plane and two fingers inferior to the anterior border of the acromion in the vertical plane. Now, the AL becomes the viewing portal and the AM is the working portal until completion of the tenodesis. The cannula in the AM is withdrawn from the GH joint and is directed anteriorly and laterally to the subdeltoid bursa. A shaver or Depuy Mitek VAPR is used to perform the bursectomy up to the transfixing needle. The bicipital groove is identified. The overlying transverse humeral ligament is opened from distal to proximal with the bovie, taking care to avoid contact with the tendon itself. The tendon is then grasped (Figure 21.5) and mobilized from both the joint and the groove with the aid of the probe and elbow extension.

21.3.4.3. Step 3: Exteriorization and Preparation of the Biceps

The LHB is grabbed at the most proximal part with graspers placed through the AM. Removal from the exposed groove is facilitated by extension of the elbow. The cannula is temporarily withdrawn from the

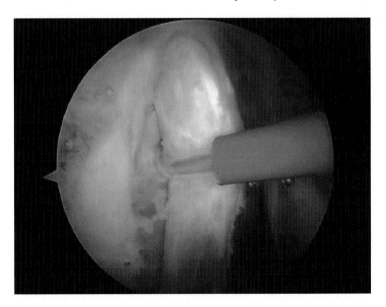

FIGURE 21.5. Staying medial to the ascending vessels located on the lateral border of the bicipital groove.

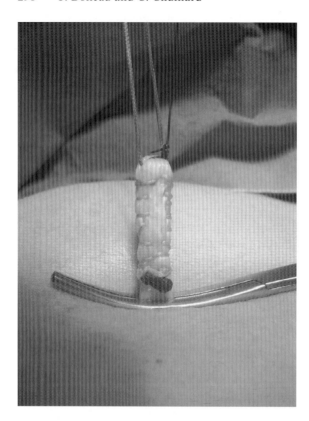

FIGURE 21.6. The prepared tendon with PDS Ariadne guide suture and indelible mark to show the end of the tendon and the orientation.

AM; the LHB is delivered from the portal. The elbow is then flexed and traction is applied to the tendon in order to obtain approximately 5 to 6 cm of length. A vascular clamp is pushed against the surface of the skin and secured around the tendon to hold it in place.

At this stage, if the tendon is hypertrophied or widened through the degenerative process, the tendon is trimmed with a scalpel to normalize its size to the remainder of the tendon. The tendon is then doubled over both a traction suture (#1 Ethibond) and a guide suture (the Ariadne stitch) for the interference screw (#1 PDS). The tendon is then sutured to itself with a braided resorbable suture (#3 Dexon or Vicryl) in a whipstitch fashion for about 25 mm (its doubled length). The PDS is tied at the tip in a simple fashion; this serves two purposes: it secures the guide stitch and tapers the tip of the tendon for insertion (Figure 21.6). Mark the end of the tendon with a sterile marker to visually confirm that the tendon is seated to the depth of the tunnel. The diameter of the tendon is measured (ACL sizing guides can be used for this step); this measurement determines the diameter of the bone tunnel (7–8 mm is ideal). The cannula is reintroduced through the AM, but the tendon remains exterior, "parked" outside of the cannula.

21.3.4.4. Step 4: Reaming the Humeral Socket

The bicipital groove is debrided with a shaver (Smith & Nephew Endoscopy) and/or VAPR (Depuy Mitek), and a synovectomy is done around the tendon. Take care to avoid the ascending vessels on either side of the groove. The point of entry for the bone tunnel should be approximately 5 to 10 mm from the summit of the groove to prevent contact with the coracoacromial (CA) arch (transverse white fibers in the floor of the tunnel provide a visual reference for the approximate location).

An awl is used to make a pilot hole in the floor of the groove and to prevent drill point slippage. A guide pin is drilled perpendicular to the humerus and parallel to the lateral border of the acromion; the target is the posterior portal. The surgeon places a finger over the posterior portal so that once the pin perforates the posterior cortex, it can be withdrawn through the posterior portal without injuring the muscle or skin. A 7-mm or 8-mm reamer is placed over the guide pin, and the humerus is reamed to a depth of 25 mm under visual control. The guide pin and reamer are removed, and the orifice to the bone tunnel is smoothed with a shaver and VAPR to bevel the edges for passage of the tendon into the bone socket (Figure 21.7).

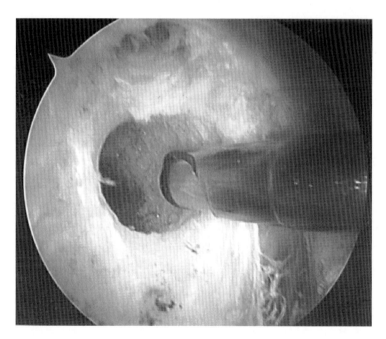

FIGURE 21.7. The entry of the humeral socket is smoothed using a shaver to avoid damage of the tendon. (From Boileau P, Krishnan SG, Coste J-S et al. Arthroscopic biceps tenodesis: a new technique using bioabsorbable interference screw fixation. Arthroscopy 2002;18(9):1002–1012. Reprinted with permission from the Arthroscopy Association of North America.)

21.3.4.5. Step 5: Passage of the Beath Needle

The sutures are retrieved into the cannula with a grasper in retrograde fashion prior to drilling the needle through the humerus; this avoids incarceration of deltoid fibers. To centralize the needle in the socket, we temporarily place the needle inside a reamer that is one size smaller than the prepared tunnel and introduce this through the cannula into the socket; the reamer is then withdrawn. The needle is then driven through the humerus and out of the posterior portal. Alternatively, the shoulder guide can be used (Figure 21.8). The two limbs of the traction suture (Ethibond) are placed in the eyelet of the needle. As the needle is pulled through the humerus, the traction suture of tendon is delivered into the bone tunnel. The guide suture (Ariadne suture) remains secured outside of the AM for placement of the screw. With the elbow in flexion, the tendon is drawn into the tunnel under arthroscopic control; the blue mark on the LHB should sit flush to slightly recessed in the tunnel.

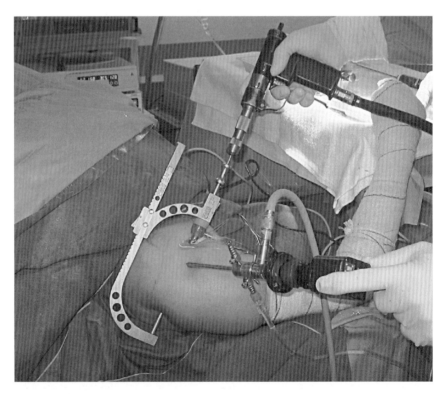

FIGURE 21.8. A Beath pin is centered in the humeral socket and is drilled until it exits the bone and the skin through the posterior portal.

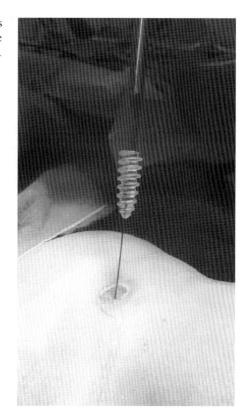

FIGURE 21.9. The traction sutures pull the tendon into the tunnel while the Ariadne stitch guides the screw.

21.3.4.6. Step 6: Fixation with the Interference Screw

The working cannula is again removed from the AM; traction is applied to the traction sutures, which are now out off the posterior portal. An interference screw (Tenoscrew®, Phusis, Tornier) is then placed over the Ariadne guide suture (PDS), which is out of the AM, while gentle traction is applied to this suture. The tendon is pulled into the tunnel by means of the traction sutures (Figure 21.9). An 8.5-mm screw is used for an 8-mm tunnel. The screw is placed along the superior aspect of the tendon and is tightened until it is level or slightly recessed with the tunnel (Figure 21.10). The elbow should be in extension during screw placement to avoid excessive tension on the tendon. The guide suture is cut with arthroscopic scissors; one limb of the traction suture is cut, and it is pulled through the posterior portal. As a variation, a tendon "fork" can be used to push the tendon to the base of the tunnel; the screw is then placed over the fork. This obviates the transhumeral drilling. With the probe, the surgeon should verify that the tendon is taut when the elbow is extended and slack when the elbow is flexed.

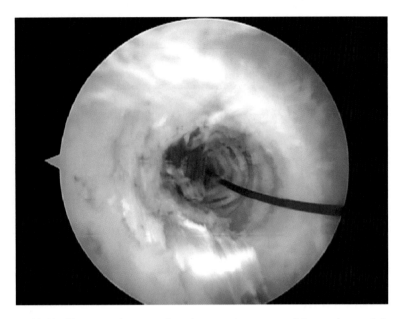

FIGURE 21.10. The screw is secured on the superior aspect of the tendon and should be flush to slightly recessed. The tendon should be taut when the elbow is extended, to preserve the strength and contour of the muscle.

21.4. Postoperative Management

No immobilization is needed postoperatively; only a sling for comfort is used for 1 or 2 weeks. Active and passive motion is allowed as tolerated. Resisted elbow flexion and supination, as well as return to sport, are allowed at 6 weeks.

21.5. Results and Complications

Review of the initial 43 cases performed between 1997 and 1999 with a minimum of 2-year clinical follow-up showed encouraging results that led us to adopt this technique.[7] Average age was 63 years (range, 25–78 years). Average preoperative Constant score was 43 points (range, 13–60 points) with an improvement to 79 postoperatively (range, 59–89 points). The strength, measured with a spring balance, was 90% of the contralateral extremity (Figure 21.11). The shape and contour of the biceps was preserved in all but two of the cases (95%).

21.5.1. Failure of Fixation with Retreat of the Tendon and Retraction of the Muscle

For the interference screw technique, failure of fixation is usually a result of a technical error. The primary error is to not double the tendon on itself; doubling the tendon allows the tissue to be reinforced when it is of poor quality and prevents slipping past the interference screw. Furthermore, it does not change the tension of the muscle. Another error is to use a screw of inadequate diameter; the fixation is best when the screw is of a greater diameter than the tunnel (i.e., an 8.5-mm screw for an 8-mm tunnel). Another technical error is to place the tunnel too low (at the level of the diaphysis) where there is a scant amount of cancellous bone. Finally, not all screws are created equally; the Tenoscrew® was specifically designed for this application and has nonaggressive threads and a tapering diameter.

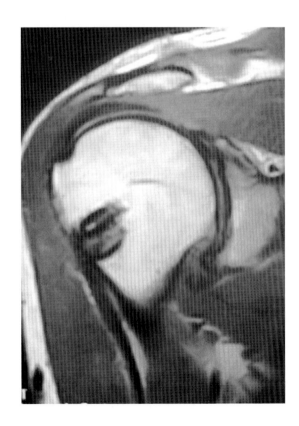

FIGURE 21.11. An MRI demonstrating healing.

21.5.2. Incarceration of Deltoid Fibers with the Tenodesis

This complication can occur if you do not take care when you pass the needle through the shoulder and re-introduce the tendon into the shoulder (Step 5). A simple trick is to replace the traction sutures in the cannula in a retrograde fashion prior to pulling the pin through the humerus.

21.5.3. Pain at the Level of the Bicipital Groove

Residual, anterior shoulder pain after tenodesis of the LHB, in our experience, has two potential causes: (1) overly aggressive shaving that extended into the deltoid muscle and (2) excessive tension on the LHB. Because of this, doubling the tendon and placement 10 mm from the top of the groove presents another advantage: it maintains both the tension and the shape of the muscle if you extend the elbow when tightening the screw. Finally, our studies have shown that the incidence of anterior shoulder pain is the same for both tenodesis with an interference screw and tenotomy. A certain number will have unexplainable rest pain, but recently it has been shown that the LHB is surrounded by a network of nerve fibers along its length, especially near its insertion.[12] Therefore, we felt that the synovectomy is an important associated step.

21.5.4. Nerve Injury

We have yet to see a neurological complication. The axillary nerve is not in danger during preparation of the humeral tunnel, provided one drills strictly perpendicular to the long axis of the humerus and parallel to the lateral border of the acromion and the target is palpated through the posterior portal. By following this protocol, the transhumeral pin always springs from the posterior portal. The axillary nerve passes 3 to 5 cm below the posterior border of the acromion far from the exit of the pin. We have made a guide specifically to facilitate placement of the pin that can be used at surgeon's discretion (Shoulder Guide, Future Medical Systems).

21.6. Conclusions

The LHB tendon is a major source of shoulder pain and dysfunction, altering the normal kinematics. Its agency in failed cuff repair has been underestimated. While a tenotomy can relieve pain, there is the possibility of cosmetic deformity (the Popeye sign), cramping with activity, and decreased supination strength. Arthroscopic biceps tenodesis with an interference screw is a safe, reliable, reproducible procedure that gives excellent clinical and cosmetic results. This procedure has become a routine part of our practice since 1998. It provides a stronger fixation than other methods of tenodesis (suture or suture and anchors). We do not kill the biceps; rather, arthroscopic tenodesis with an interference screw transfers the insertion so that its function is preserved while removing the pathological portion.

References

1. Burkhead WZ Jr. The biceps tendon. In: Rockwood CA Jr. and Matsen III FA, eds. The shoulder, 2nd ed. Philadelphia: Saunders; 1990:791–836.
2. Walch G, Nové-Josserand L, Boileau P, Lévigne C. Subluxations and dislocations of the tendon of the long head of the biceps. J Shoulder Elbow Surg 1998; 72:100–108.
3. Murthy AM, Vasburg CL, Neviaser TJ. The incidence of pathologic changes of the long head of the biceps tendon. J Shoulder Elbow Surg 2000;9:382–385.
4. Dines D, Warren RF, Inglis AE. Surgical treatment of lesions of the long head of the biceps. Clin Orthop 1982;164:165–174.
5. Berleman U, Bayley I. Tenodesis of the long head of the biceps brachii in the painful shoulder: improving the results in the long term. J Shoulder Elbow Surg 1995;4:429–435.
6. Boileau P, Krishnan SG, Walch G. Arthroscopic biceps tenodesis: a new technique using bioabsorbable screw fixation. Tech Shoulder Elbow Surg 2000; 2:153–164.
7. Boileau P, Krishnan SG, Coste JS, Walch G. Arthroscopic biceps tenodesis: a new technique using bioabsorbable screw fixation. Arthroscopy 2002;9: 1002–1012.
8. Boileau P, Walch G. So-called "isolated" supraspinatus tears: a plea for systematic opening of the rotator interval. In: Gazielly D, Gleyze P, Thomas T, eds. The cuff. Paris: Elsevier; 1997:320–323.
9. Osbahr DC, Diamond AB, Speer KP. The cosmetic appearance of the biceps muscle after long head tenotomy versus tenodesis. Arthroscopy 2002;18: 483–487.
10. Boileau P, Ahrens PM, Hatzidakis AM. Entrapment of the long head of the biceps tendon: the hourglass biceps — a cause of pain and locking of the shoulder. J Shoulder Elbow Surg 2004;13:249–257.
11. Richards DP, Burkhart SS. A biomechanical analysis of two biceps tenodesis fixation techniques. Arthroscopy 2005;21:861–866.
12. Alpantaki K, McLaughlin D, Kargogeos D, Hadjipavlou A, Kontakis G. Sympathetic and sensory neural elelments in the tendon of the long head of the biceps. J Bone Joint Surg Am 2005;87:1580–1583.

22
Biceps Subpectoral Mini-Open Tenodesis

Stephen C. Weber, Jeffrey I. Kauffman, and Deanna L. Higgins

The biceps has been recognized as an important pain generator in the shoulder.[1-8] Becker and Cofield disparaged the results of isolated biceps tenodesis[9]; however, in retrospect, most of these patients probably had impingement unaddressed by their tenodesis. Neer's concerns about resection of the biceps aggravating impingement problems by removing one restraint to superior migration of the humeral head seconded this negative assessment of biceps tenodesis.[10] With the advent of arthroscopy, more accurate assessment of pathology of the glenohumeral joint in general and the biceps in particular became possible. Sethi and colleagues did a thorough review of the pathology and treatment of biceps tendon problems, describing four potential sources of pain originating from the biceps tendon: (1) instability of the biceps tendon; (2) inflammation of the biceps tendon with rotator cuff disease; (3) isolated biceps tenosynovitis; and (4) traumatic injuries to include partial or complete tearing of the biceps tendon.[11]

Treatment options have traditionally centered on tenodesis. While generally deemed effective, tenodesis done through a deltoid splitting or deltopectoral approach carries significant morbidity, especially if a coexistent glenohumeral arthrotomy is required to address the intra-articular pathology.[1-7] Arthroscopic resection of associated biceps and labral damage was an initial step in decreasing morbidity related to this procedure.[12] Several surgeons have noted that spontaneous rupture of the biceps was associated with minimal strength loss from 10%[13] to 21% in supination,[14] suggesting that repair of complete ruptures might not be indicated. Walch and colleagues[15] also noted this and popularized tenotomy rather than tenodesis due to the marked decrease in perioperative morbidity. Subsequently, Gill and colleagues,[16] Osbahr and coworkers,[17] and Speer[18] also noted that autotenodesis occurred in a high proportion of patients with tenotomy. Gill and colleagues[16] noted less morbidity and greater patient satisfaction with tenotomy than tenodesis. More recent articles noted that the reported high rates of autotenodesis with tenotomy were not reproduced in subsequent studies,[19] though a small but disturbing number of patients develop cramping in the muscle belly with tenotomy.

To avoid these problems, techniques of arthroscopic biceps tenotomy were developed.[20–23] All of these techniques can be technically difficult. If it is the surgeon's desire to correct concomitant shoulder pathology arthroscopically, arthroscopic biceps tenodesis can be difficult due to limited operating time secondary to swelling incurred from the prior procedures. Transhumeral drilling, required with interference screw techniques,[20,23] put the axillary nerve at risk and place a large, bioabsorbable implant at the tenodesis site, which has led to resorptive inflammatory changes and pain when used in other areas of the body. The technique of Gross and colleagues applied arthroscopic tenolysis for isolated biceps tenosynovitis[24] as another means of avoiding tenotomy, but this was applicable only to the category of isolated bicipital tenosynovitis and has raised concerns about creating biceps instability. None of the arthroscopic techniques allow for treatment of a complete biceps rupture, as the tendon is retracted distal to the bicipital groove and not accessible arthroscopically.

Dr. Richard Caspari developed a technique of a subpectoral approach to the biceps, originally for use in his arthroscopic Gallie procedure in the early 1980s, and taught this to the senior author in 1986 (SW; R. B. Caspari, personal communication, 1986). The senior author first published this technique in 1993,[25] showing good results and predictable short-term outcome. In view of the proliferation of complex and expensive techniques for arthroscopic biceps tenodesis over the last decade, it seemed of interest to revisit this simple technique to see if the outcomes might compare with these more challenging, expensive techniques.

22.1. Indications and Contraindications

Subpectoral biceps tenodesis can be used for any disease of the biceps for which tenodesis is appropriate, for both intra-articular and extra-articular problems. Relative contraindications would be those lower demand patients in whom biceps rupture could be tolerated, and those patients with intra-articular biceps lesions where it would be the surgeon's preference to correct the pathology with a pure arthroscopic technique.

22.2. Preoperative Planning

Equipment needs are minimal. Small Hohman retractors serve well to expose the tenodesis site. Normally, any intra-articular and subacromial work to be done is performed first; at a minimum, the stump of the ruptured biceps is removed, along with correction of any labral damage. If this work is performed beach chair, the patient need not be repositioned. If done lateral, the arm will be taken out of traction and externally rotated, but the patient left otherwise lateral. Radiographic control is not necessary.

22.3. Surgical Procedure

22.3.1. Position and Setup

All patients in this series had a diagnostic arthroscopy in the lateral decubutis position with the arm in lateral traction.

22.3.2. Instrumentation

Standard arthroscopic instruments are necessary. As noted, small Hohman retractors are all that is needed for exposure. Tenodesis was accomplished in this series with an A.O./A.S.I.F. screw and washer, and so large-fragment A.O./A.S.I.F. instrumentation is necessary. Other surgeons have preferred different techniques of fixation, and so different instrumentation would be needed depending on the fixation technique desired.

22.3.3. Surgical Technique

With the patient in lateral or beach chair position, intra-articular pathology should be corrected arthroscopically as required. If the biceps is partially torn, the tendon is tagged using a #0 PDS suture through an 18-gauge spinal needle. The tendon is then tenotomized using electrocautery and allowed to retract. If completely torn, damage to the superior labrum and the biceps stump is resected, with labral damage repaired as indicated. Any other intra-articular pathology is corrected at this time. Attention is then focused on the subacromial space. An arthroscopic acromioplasty is then performed as indicated, followed by repair of any rotator cuff pathology. If soft tissue swelling is modest at this point, attention can then be directed to the open portion of the procedure.

With the patient left lateral decubutis, the arm is taken out of traction and externally rotated and abducted. A 2-cm incision is then made in the mid-axillary line in the axillary fold, at the inferior border of the pectoralis major (Figure 22.1). Blunt dissection was then carried under the pectoralis

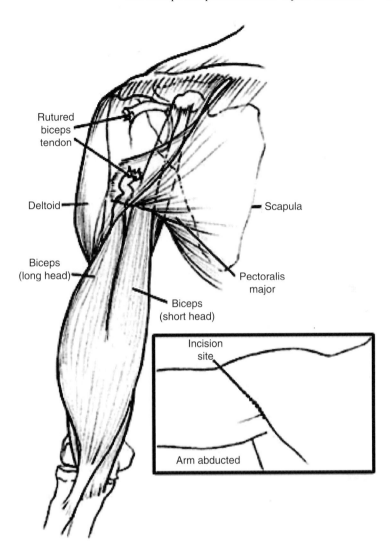

Rutured
biceps
tendon

Deltoid

Scapula

Biceps
(long head)

Pectoralis
major

Biceps
(short head)

Incision
site

Arm abducted

FIGURE 22.1. Anatomy of approach and skin incision for subpectoral approach. (Reprinted from Wiley et al., Arthroscopic assisted mini-open biceps tenodesis: surgical technique. Arthroscopy 2004;20:445–446 with permission from the Arthroscopy Association of North America.)

major (Figure 22.2), utilizing the interval between the pectoralis major and the conjoined tendon. This interval places the neurovascular structures on the medial side of the conjoined tendon and is thus safe. The tendon stump is identified deep to the pectoralis major, in the distal aspect of the bicipital groove, and then is pulled from the wound and tagged with a permanent

310   S.C. Weber et al.

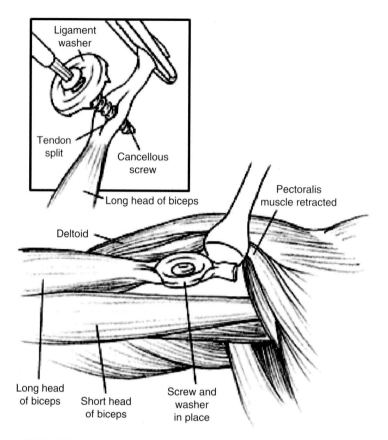

FIGURE 22.2. Schematic of completed exposure for subpectoral biceps tenodesis. (Reprinted from Wiley et al., Arthroscopic assisted mini-open biceps tenodesis: surgical technique. Arthroscopy 2004;20:445–446 with permission from the Arthroscopy Association of North America.)

suture (Figure 22.3). The bicipital groove is then subperiosteally stripped with an elevator. Fixation is then done according to the preference of the surgeon. In our series, all patients had the tendon fixed with a unicortical large fragment A.O./A.S.I.F. screw and spiked ligament washer. A unicortical, 3.5-mm drill hole is made, and tapped. Bicortical drilling is to be avoided to limit injury to the axillary nerve, which at this level lies posterior on the humerus. The biceps tendon is then split parallel to its fibers and fixed in place using a unicortical, large-fragment A.O./A.S.I.F. screw and spiked washer (Figure 22.4). Motion is then checked; restoration of normal cosmesis of the biceps is confirmed, and full extension of the elbow is documented. Overtensioning of the biceps is to be avoided, and full extension of the elbow should be possible at surgery. If restoration of biceps conformation is confirmed, the wound is closed with subcutaneous and subcuticular closure and steristrips.

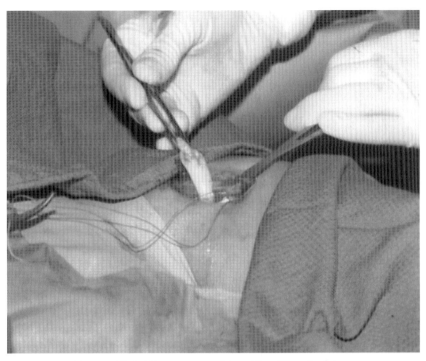

FIGURE 22.3. Biceps exposed in mid-axillary incision.

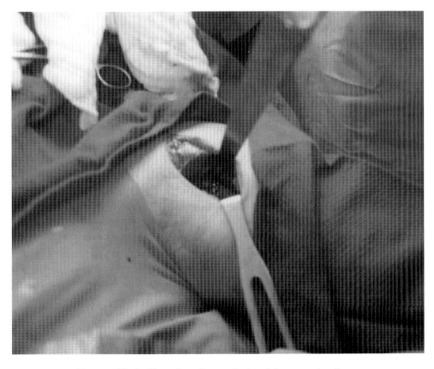

FIGURE 22.4. Completed tenodesis with screw in place.

22.4. Postoperative Management

All patients were treated on an outpatient basis. The arm is maintained in a sling for 6 weeks. Pendulum exercises with the elbow bent are done the day of surgery. Passive shoulder motion is started at the first week. Full elbow extension is avoided for 3 weeks. At 6 weeks, active shoulder motion is started, and elbow flexion exercises are started with light therabands. More vigorous resistance exercises, and return to unrestricted manual labors is not permitted for 3 months.

22.5. Results and Complications

All procedures over a 10-year period were retrospectively reviewed. All surgeries were performed by the senior author (SW), using the technique described.[25] Data were retrospectively reviewed by the two other authors (JF and DH). University of California at Los Angeles (UCLA) and sample shoulder test (SST) scores were obtained. Data was analyzed using Student's t test using an Excel spreadsheet.

Forty-three patients were identified as undergoing subpectoral biceps tenodesis during the course of the study from 1991 to 2000. Patient demographics are shown in Table 22.1. Most of the patients had associated diagnoses, as shown in Table 22.2. The condition of the biceps is shown in Table 22.3. Preoperative UCLA scores averaged 18.93, and SST scores averaged 3.21. Eleven of 44 patients had a preoperative magnetic resonance imaging (MRI), with four scans correctly diagnosing a biceps rupture (34%). With the exception of one superficial infection, no complications occurred; specifically no deep infections, neurological injuries, stiffness, bleeding, or postoperative deformity occurred. One patient, a workers' compensation patient, perceived that his hardware was painful postoperatively, it was removed without mitigation of his postoperative pain. Postoperative UCLA scores improved to 32.37 and SST scores to 10.25 ($p < 0.01$; Figure 22.5). In the workers' compensation population, mean UCLA scores averaged 32.55, not significantly different from the non-workers' compensation population. No patient lost range of motion at the elbow. Range of motion of the shoulder is shown in Figure 22.6. Shoulder motion at follow-up averaged 164.02° of flexion and 72.73° degrees of external rotation.

The concept of the biceps as a pain generator has waxed and waned over the last four decades. Improvements in diagnostic imaging and arthroscopy

TABLE 22.1. Patient Demographics for Biceps Tenodesis.

Age (years)	49.54
Right/left	29/15
Male/female	40/4
Workers' compensation/other	19/25

Source: Data from Weber SC, (25).

TABLE 22.2. Associated Diagnoses for Study Patients.

Partial rotator cuff tear	8
Complete rotator cuff tear	9
Impingement	17
SLAP lesion	1
Other	5
None	4

Source: Data from Weber SC, (25).

TABLE 22.3. Condition of the Biceps Tendon at Surgery.

Diagnosis	*n*
Partial rupture	10
Subluxed	4
Complete rupture	30

Source: Data from Weber SC, (25).

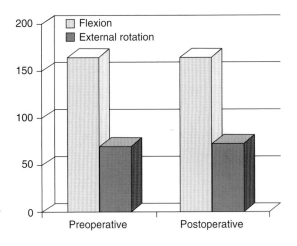

FIGURE 22.5. Pre- and postoperative range of motion. (Data from Weber SC, (25).)

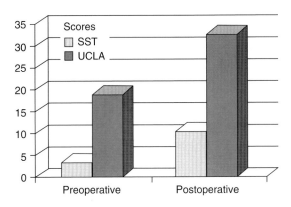

FIGURE 22.6. Pre- and postoperative UCLA and SST scores. (Data from Weber SC, (25).)

have reaffirmed the biceps as a significant cause of pain in the shoulder. Now that the biceps is recognized as a pain generator, treatment of biceps pathology is required for a successful surgical outcome.

Open tenodesis can be expected to manage all forms of biceps problems. The morbidity is the issue, with at least one comparative study showing a significant increase in morbidity and inferior outcome with tenodesis over tenotomy.[16] Most of the time, open tenodesis will require a separate incision and surgical approach from open treatment of other pathology, further increasing patient morbidity.

Tenotomy, as suggested by Walch[15] and others, obviates many of these concerns, and good results can be anticipated. While autotenodesis does occur, it is not universal, and results in at least modest weakness and deformity when it does not. More recent review of this technique shows disturbingly high levels of cosmetic deformity and residual biceps crampy pain.[19] In these authors' opinion, successful biceps tenodesis is rarely practical more than a month after spontaneous rupture or tenotomy, as the tendon atrophies and reattachment become impractical. For the rare patient with a painful, deformed biceps post-tenotomy, late correction of the unwanted deformity is not possible. Despite any surgeon's best efforts in both diagnostic acumen and preoperative informed consent, biceps pathology can sometimes be recognized only intraoperatively. In the unconsented patient, this presents the surgeon with the dilemma of treating the patient with tenotomy and possibly dealing with significant unconsented biceps deformity postoperatively.

Arthroscopic tenodesis does allow the surgeon the possibility of tenodesis without the morbidity of a second surgical exposure. Arthroscopic interference screw techniques have been championed by Boileau and colleagues[20] and others[23] but raise concerns about transhumeral drilling, and become especially difficult in a shoulder already swollen from other arthroscopic procedures. In addition to requiring purchase of a large set of instruments, the implants and required individual implants and tools are considerably more expensive (Table 22.4) and approach most physicians' surgical billing. These costs become especially relevant for the physician in the physician-owned surgery center.

Gartsman and colleagues[22] described tenodesing the tendon using suture anchors. This technique is especially applicable when the rotator cuff is torn, allowing easier visualization and fixation of the torn biceps through

TABLE 22.4. Cost of Implants for Different Techniques.

	Vendor price	Hospital markup	Vendor price	Hospital markup	Total
Biotenodesis screw	Screw = $195	$828	Passing wire = $95	$403	$1231
A.O./A.S.I.F. screw	$11.50	$35	Washer = $15	$45	$80

Source: Data from Weber SC, (25).

the cuff tear. Bursal side identification of the biceps with an intact cuff can be challenging, however, as it requires incision of the intact tissue over the bicipital sheath. All these techniques require significant operating time. If the surgeon is already confronted with a rotator cuff tear, labral tear, or other combination of pathology, arthroscopic tenodesis may simply not be practical for any but the most gifted surgeons. The technique developed by Castagna and colleagues[21] is a simple, soft tissue technique for biceps tenotomy. This technique allows fixation to the intact cuff and transverse ligament tissues with sutures. Castagna reported only one failure with this technique. All of these techniques permit tenodesis only if the biceps is not completely ruptured and retracted.

The technique of subpectoral tenodesis can be used for all of the described problems. Even a retracted ruptured tendon can be retrieved from the small axillary incision. Ruptures diagnosed late can be explored with little morbidity and tenodesed if adequate tissue is still available. Subpectoral tenodesis can be carried out in the presence of reasonable post-arthroscopic swelling without difficulty, allowing multiple arthroscopic procedures to be performed without compromising the subsequent fixation of the biceps. Results shown here would appear to be comparable to those obtained by interference screw fixation.[20,23] Bioabsorbable interference screws are not always benign, with these screws lasting up to 2.5 years with occasional serious synovitis associated with their resorption.[26–28] The suture anchor technique of Gartsman and colleagues[22] was described in a technique article, and no results were given. Subpectoral tenodesis is almost certainly much easier for the less experienced arthroscopist to perform. The cost as described is significantly less than other arthroscopic techniques. Snyder[29] has used our approach with similar success, labeling it the "Caspari–Weber" or "CW Subpectoralis Approach." He preferred a keyhole tenodesis to screw fixation; in fact, the approach is amenable to any fixation technique desired once the bicipital groove is visualized. The main problem with the subpectoral approach is the fact that it does require a small incision. Despite the low morbidity, it is the authors' current preference to perform the biceps tenodesis arthroscopically using suture anchors through an associated cuff tear when present and, using the soft tissue technique of Castagna when the cuff is intact, reserving subpectoral tenodesis for the patient with a complete rupture of the biceps.

22.6. Conclusions

Subpectoral biceps tenodesis, described in 1993, continues to be a safe, easy, and effective means of addressing biceps pathology. The subcutaneous nature of the approach through a 2-cm incision offers minimal morbidity and can be easily done as an outpatient procedure. Results of this predictable, simple procedure compare favorably with newer, more complex techniques of tenodesis.

References

1. Crenshaw AH, Kilgores WE. Surgical treatment of bicipital tenosynovitis J Bone Joint Surg Am 1966;48:1496.
2. DePalma AF, Callery GE. Bicipital tenosynovitis. Clin Orthop 1954;3: 69–84.
3. Froimson AI, Oh I. Keyhole tenodesis of the biceps origin at the shoulder. Clin Orthop 1975;112:245.
4. Gilcreest EL. Dislocation and elongation of the long head of the biceps brachii. Ann Surg 1936;104:118.
5. Hitchcock HH, Bechtol CO. Painful shoulder: observations on the role of the tendon of the long head of the biceps brachii in its causation. J Bone Joint Surg Am 1948;30A:263.
6. Post M. The shoulder. Surgical and nonsurgical management. Philadelphia: Lea and Febinger; 1988.
7. Soto-Hall R, Stroot JH. Treatment of ruptures of the long head of biceps brachii. Am J Orthop 1960;2:192.
8. Murthi AM, Vosburgh CL, Neviaser TJ. The incidence of pathologic changes of the long head of the biceps tendon. J Shoulder Elbow Surg 2000;9:382–385.
9. Becker DA, Cofield RH. Tenodesis of the long head of the biceps brachii for chronic bicipital tendonitis: long term results. J Bone Joint Surg Am 1989;71: 376–381.
10. Neer CS. Shoulder reconstruction. Philadelphia: Saunders; 1990.
11. Sethi N, Wright R, Yamaguchi K. Disorders of the long head of the biceps tendon. J Shoulder Elbow Surg 1999;8:644–654.
12. Burkhart SS, Fox DL. SLAP lesions in association with complete tears of the long head of the biceps tendon: a report of two cases. Arthroscopy 1992;8: 31–35.
13. Warren RF. Lesions of the long head of the biceps tendon. Inst Course Lect 1985;34:204–209.
14. Mariani EM, Cofield RH, Askew U, et al. Rupture of the tendon of the long head of the bieps brachii. Surgical versus nonsurgical treatment. Clin Orthop 1988;228:233–239.
15. Walch G, Nove-Josserand L, Boileau P, et al. Subluxation and dislocations of the tendon of the long head of the biceps. J Shoulder Elbow Surg 1998;7: 100–108.
16. Gill TJ, McIrvin E, Mair SD, et al. Results of biceps tenotomy for treatment of pathology of the long head of the biceps brachii. J Shoulder Elbow Surg 2001;10:247–249.
17. Osbahr DC, Diamond AB, Speer KP. The cosmetic appearance of the biceps muscle after long-head biceps tenotomy versus tenodesis. Arthroscopy 2002; 18:483–487.
18. Speer KP. Arthroscopic long head biceps tenotomy results in autotenodesis in patients with refractive bicipital pain. Arthroscopy 1999;15:543.

19. Cameron ML. The incidence of "popeye" deformity and muscle weakness following biceps tenotomy for recalcitrant biceps tendonitis. Annual Meeting Proceedings, AAOS 2003;442.
20. Boileau P, Krishnan SG, Coste JS, et al. Arthroscopic biceps tenodesis: a new technique using bioabsorbable interference screw fixation. Arthroscopy 2002; 18:1002–1012.
21. Castagna A, Sacchi G, D'Ortona A, et al. Rottura del capo lungo del bicipite, lesioni SLAP e conflitto suuperio-interno: trattamento chirurgico. G It Ort Trauma 2002;28(supp I):644–652.
22. Gartsman GM, Hammerman SM. Arthroscopic biceps tenodesis: operative technique. Arthroscopy 2000;16:550–552.
23. Klepps S, Hazrati Y, Flatow EL. Arthroscopic biceps tenodesis. Arthroscopy 2002;18:1040–1045.
24. Ruotolo C, Nottage WM, Flatow EL, et al. Controversial topics in shoulder arthroscopy. Arthroscopy 2002;18(suppl):65–75.
25. Weber SC. Arthroscopic "mini-open" technique in the treatment of ruptures of the long head of the biceps. Arthroscopy 1993;9:365.
26. Burkart A, Imhoff AB, Roscher E. Foreign-body reaction to the bioabsorbable suretac device. Arthroscopy 2000;16:91–95.
27. Martinek V, Niklaus FF. Tibial and pretibial cyst formation after anterior cruciate ligament reconstruction with bioabsorbable interference screw fixation. Arthroscopy 1999;15:317–320.
28. Martinek V, Seil R, Lattermann C, et al. The fate of poly-L-lactic acid interference screw after anterior cruciate ligament reconstruction. Arthroscopy 2001;17:73–76.
29. Snyder S. Treatment of biceps pathology using the CW tenodesis technique. San Diego Shoulder Arthroscopy Course, San Diego, California 2000.

23
Endoscopic Release of Suprascapular Nerve Entrapment at the Suprascapular Notch

Laurent Lafosse and Tony Kochhar

A problem that has recently been recognized as a potential etiology of shoulder pain and weakness is suprascapular nerve entrapment. This was first described by Thompson and Koppel in 1959.[1,2] As rotator cuff pathology is much more common, this problem was often overlooked and diagnosis was delayed. Other authors have recognized contributing causes including anomalous transverse ligament,[3,4] ganglion,[5,6,7,8] abnormal bone morphology,[9,10] sporting activities,[11,12,13] and large rotator cuff tears with retraction.[14,15,16]

Surgical decompression is indicated for those patients with chronic shoulder pain that has been refractory to nonoperative management and the diagnosis has been confirmed by electrodiagnostic studies.[17] Open surgical decompression has been reported as a reliable method of treatment.[18] For those cases associated with rotator cuff ruptures, margin convergence and reattachment of the tendon may treat the problem.[16] Some patients may benefit from procedures that combine nerve decompression.

Open decompression is performed through a superior incision beginning at the acromioclavicular joint and extending posteriorly. The trapezius muscle can be split or elevated from its insertion to expose the supraspinatus muscle. Along the anterior margin of the fossa the edge of the scapular is the origin of the medial edge of the ligament. This area of exposure can be difficult to visualize for a number of reasons. First, the space between the spine of the scapula and the clavicle is narrow. The

Sections of this chapter are adapted from Lafosse L, Tomasi A. Technique for endoscopic release of suprascapular nerve entrapment at the suprascapular notch. Techniques in Shoulder and Elbow Surgery 2006 Mar; 7(1):1–6. Reprinted with permission.

318

notch is deep and often is vascular, making visualization tricky. As techniques continue to evolve to treat rotator cuff problems, a new endoscopic method for decompression of the suprascapular nerve at the notch is presented.

23.1. Anatomy

The suprascapular nerve originates from the upper trunk of the brachial plexus (C5, C6 roots). The nerve passes deep to the trapezius muscle and through the suprascapular notch under the superior transverse ligament (STL; see Figure 23.1). Superficial to this, the suprascapular artery travels over the ligament. The nerve divides into the medial and lateral branches just before it passes under the STL. The medial branch supplies the supraspinatus while the lateral branch descends around the lateral margin of the scapular spine at the spinoglenoid ligament (SGL) and splits into several terminal branches which supply the infraspinatus.

The STL is attached to the scapula at the edge of the supraspinatus fossa and attaches laterally to the coracoid. If the arthroscope is visualizing

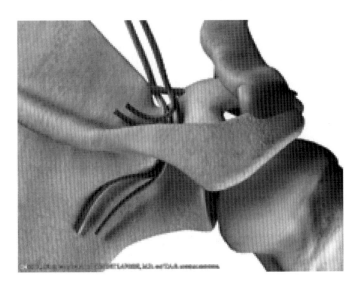

FIGURE 23.1. Artery going above and suprascapular nerve going under STL. (Reprinted with permission from Lafosse L, Tomasi A. Technique for endoscopic release of suprascapular nerve entrapment at the suprascapular notch. Techniques in Shoulder and Elbow Surgery 2006 Mar; 7(1):1–6.)

from the lateral portal, the coracoacromial ligament is the most lateral vertically-oriented structure. This is followed by trapezoid and conoid portions of the coracoclavicular ligaments, then medial to the STL. The nerve travels below the ligament and the artery traverses above the ligament.

23.2. Etiology

Suprascapular neuropathy can result from a single traumatic injury, repetitive traction events, as well as external compression from an abnormal transverse ligament, bone anatomy, or mass effect (i.e., a ganglia). The nerve can be placed under tension with the shoulder retracted and the head rotated in the opposite direction.

A large rotator cuff tear, particularly a posterosuperior rupture, may result in nerve injury due to traction on the nerve from the medial pull from the infraspinatus. It should also be noted that cuff repair with reduction of a chronic tear may pull on the nerve fixed by adhesions under the superior transverse ligament (STL). As the nerve has limited excursion under the STL and its supraspinatus attachment is very close to the suprascapular notch, muscle mobilization may affect the nerve conduction. The STL may become ossified with age or following trauma, and the suprascapular notch may become narrowed, thus increasing the risk of a nerve entrapment.

23.3. Diagnosis

Entrapment of the nerve at the suprascapular notch rarely causes pain, with most patients presenting with shoulder weakness. Physical examination usually reveals atrophy of both the infraspinatus and supraspinatus and weakness in abduction and external rotation compared to the other shoulder. Magnetic Resonance Imaging and/or Arthrogram Compute Tomography (CT) Scan confirm the integrity of the cuff, presence of a ganglion cyst at the suprascapular notch, or possible bony anomalies.

MRI will also demonstrate muscle atrophy of the cuff, without associated fatty degeneration. Fatty degeneration has been linked to chronic cuff tear independent of a neurologic problem. The diagnosis is made by electromyogram (EMG) which shows two characteristic features: reduction of the nerve conduction velocity by longer latency of the muscle following nerve stimulation at the Erb spot and reduced amplitude of muscle contraction due to chronic nerve entrapment and muscle atrophy.

In cases of cuff rupture, reattachment of the tendon to its insertion may treat the neuropathy, but releasing the nerve to allow better freedom may permit better function. When the rotator cuff is torn, we performed an EMG for all cases of retracted supraspinatus tear. A significant number of positive nerve injuries were detected, especially when associated with an infraspinatus tear. In addition, we have performed EMG for all patients with persistent pain and weakness following rotator cuff repair (RCR) and have noticed major SSN entrapment in a number of these cases even when the cuff repair was intact.

23.4. Indications

Surgical decompression is indicated in patients with chronic shoulder pain and weakness refractory to conservative treatment. The diagnosis is confirmed with electrodiagnostic testing. Symptoms are usually present for six months, although certain high-demand individuals may require early intervention if no improvement is demonstrated with a nonoperative approach.

23.5. Surgical Technique[17]

The patient can be positioned in the beach-chair position or lateral decubitus and surgery is performed under a general anesthetic with a supplementary interscalene block. To aid visualization (beach-chair), distraction of the humerus in flexion is done by applying longitudinal traction (Figure 23.2). The surgical field is prepared and draped as per other arthroscopic shoulder procedures.

Three portals are used to perform this surgery [Figures 23.3(A,B)]. In addition to the classic posterior portal and the lateral portal for the subacromial space, we utilize the superior SSN portal. This is a new portal which is created between the clavicle and the scapular spine, and is located approximately 7 cm medial to the lateral border of the acromion and 2 cm medial to the Neviaser portal. This third portal is created under arthroscopic visualization using an outside-in technique. A spinal needle is placed perpendicular to the suprascapular fossa. It passes through the trapezius muscle in a perpendicular orientation toward the suprascapular notch along the anterior border of the supraspinatus. Warner et al.[15] demonstrated that the suprascapular notch is 4.5 cm

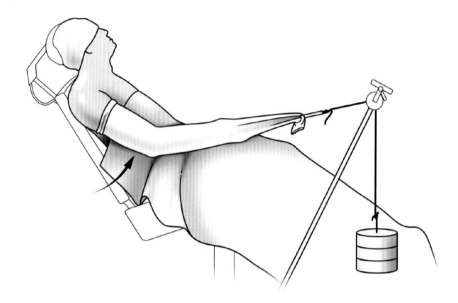

FIGURE 23.2. Beach-chair position and weight traction. (Reprinted with permission from Lafosse L, Tomasi A. Technique for endoscopic release of suprascapular nerve entrapment at the suprascapular notch. Techniques in Shoulder and Elbow Surgery 2006 Mar; 7(1):1–6.)

(±0.5 cm) from the posterolateral acromion. It should be remembered that the spinal accessory nerve passes along the medial border of the scapula; however, is located medial to the N. suprascapularis and is a safe distance.

The instrumentation to be used includes a standard shaver and burr to aid in the debridement of the subacromial space and bursa. We also find it very useful to use a radiofrequency device (Side-effect VAPR, Mitek; Norwood, MA) for the dissection and approach to the notch. A standard diagnostic arthroscopy is performed to assess the glenohumeral joint, followed by an inspection of the subacromial space, with the arthroscope being moved from the posterior portal to the lateral portal. Debridement is performed to remove the bursa and allow access towards the suprascapular notch. Instrumentation (VAPR and shaver) is used through the posterior portal. However, to decrease the swelling before the suprascapular notch area, the nerve dissection and release is performed before any decompression, acromioclavicular joint removal, or cuff repair.

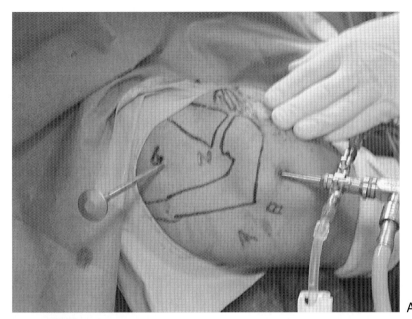

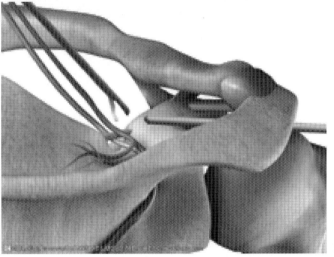

FIGURE 23.3. (A) Portals on a right shoulder: the normal posterior soft spot portal, the lateral portal as for acromioplasty and the new SSN-portal (suprascapularis nerve portal). (B) Portals and instrument positioning: viewing by the lateral portal, all other devices are passed through the SSN-portal. (Reprinted with permission from Lafosse L, Tomasi A. Technique for endoscopic release of suprascapular nerve entrapment at the suprascapular notch. Techniques in Shoulder and Elbow Surgery 2006 Mar; 7(1):1–6.)

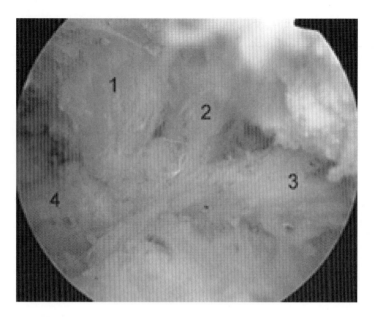

FIGURE 23.4. Right shoulder, lateral view: conoid (1) and trapezoid (2) coracocla-vicular ligaments, coracoacromial ligament (3), and STL (4). (Reprinted with permission from Lafosse L, Tomasi A. Technique for endoscopic release of supra-scapular nerve entrapment at the suprascapular notch. Techniques in Shoulder and Elbow Surgery 2006 Mar; 7(1):1–6.)

The dissection continues medially until we identify the base of the coracoid and the origin of the coracoclavicular ligaments (conoid and trapezoid). Visualizing the medial border of the attachment of these ligaments on the posterior part of the coracoid process, the lateral inser-tion of the superior transverse scapular ligament can be palpated above the scapular notch (Figure 23.4). By using the third SSN portal for instrumentation, dissection towards the notch is performed using a smooth trocar by carefully spreading the fat (Figure 23.5). To assist in the dissection, we recommend using a shaver or a radiofrequency device. However, care must be taken when using these devices so as to keep them always above the supraspinatus muscle and behind the base of the conoid ligament attachment at the coracoid. This will allow a safe distance lateral to the suprascapular artery to avoid injury to the neu-rovascular structures. Following adequate dissection, the suprascapular artery can clearly be seen coursing over the superior transverse liga-ment (STL), and the SSN can be identified underneath the ligament (Figure 23.6).

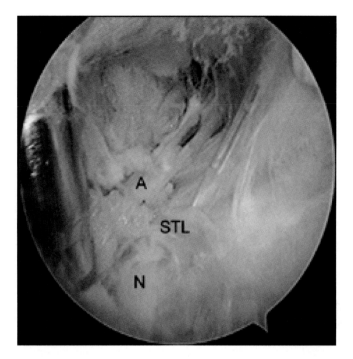

FIGURE 23.5. Suprascapular artery (A) crossing the superior transverse ligament (STL); right shoulder, lateral view. The device is inserted via the SSN portal.

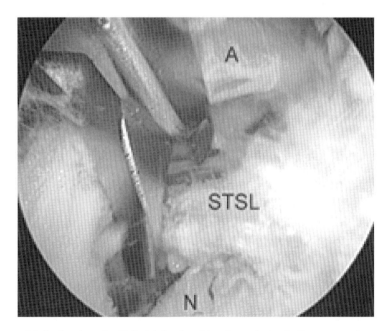

FIGURE 23.6. Cutting the STL (right shoulder, lateral view). Suprascapular artery (A), suprascapular nerve (N). The device is inserted by the SSN-portal. (Reprinted with permission from Lafosse L, Tomasi A. Technique for endoscopic release of suprascapular nerve entrapment at the suprascapular notch. Techniques in Shoulder and Elbow Surgery 2006 Mar; 7(1):1–6.)

Once the STL has been exposed, the nerve is located running under it, and its status and the degree of compression is assessed. A smooth trocar is introduced through an additional portal (Neviaser portal) and passed under the ligament and lateral to the nerve to protect it from the arthroscopic scissors. The nerve can be pushed downward and away from the ligament using a probe. With the nerve under visualization at all times, the STL is then sectioned [Figure 23.7(A,B)]. The SSN is then carefully probed and mobilized with the trocar to assess it and to ensure that compression is eliminated within the suprascapular notch. If there is any residual compression from the bony notch, a notch decompression is performed with a burr [Figure 23.8(A,B)]. The nerve is gently displaced and protected, while the notch is widened.

23.6. Postoperative Management

Patients should be monitored postoperatively due to general anesthesia and can be discharged from hospital on the day of surgery, especially if an interscalene block has been administered. The patient should wear a sling for the first two to three days to minimize postoperative pain. Active motion is allowed on Day 1, and activities of daily living can be started, dependent upon patient status. Pendulum exercises are allowed early on if pain is present. We recommend that the patient should attend an outpatient appointment for first follow-up at four weeks and then after six months. An EMG test should be performed on the next presentation to compare with the preoperative findings and to assess recovery of neural function.

23.7. Results

Eighteen patients underwent endoscopic SSN release between January 2003 and December 2004. Patients were evaluated pre and postoperatively, clinically and with electrodiagnostic studies.[17] The muscle strength was evaluated by a 0- to 5-point scale (5 indicates normal force). Supraspinatus force is measured with Jobe test, and the infraspinatus force with external rotation in neutral position. EMG nerve testing confirmed compression of the SSN at the scapular notch before surgery and was repeated six months after surgery to evaluate the result. All patients with SSN entrapment associated

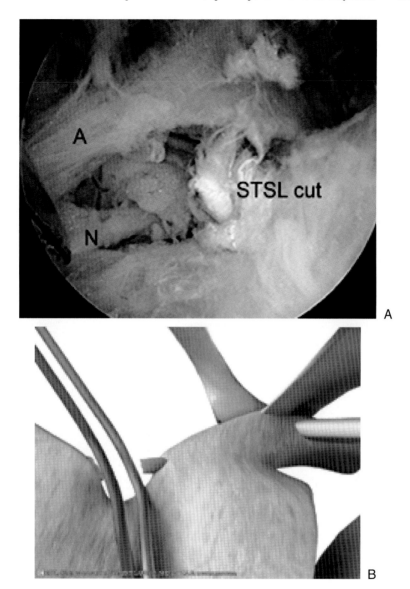

FIGURE 23.7. (A) Cut STL with suprascapular nerve (N) and artery (A) (right shoulder, lateral view). (B) Schema of the endoscopic view in (A): cut STSL with the suprascapular nerve and artery (right shoulder, lateral view). (Reprinted with permission from Lafosse L, Tomasi A. Technique for endoscopic release of suprascapular nerve entrapment at the suprascapular notch. Techniques in Shoulder and Elbow Surgery 2006 Mar; 7(1):1–6.)

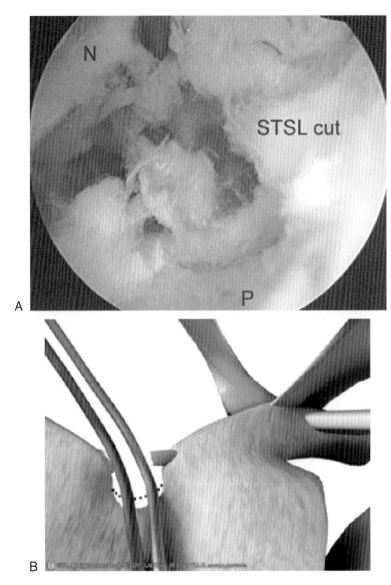

FIGURE 23.8. (A) Additional liberation of the suprascapular nerve (N) by notch plasty (P) (right shoulder, lateral view). (B) Schema of the endoscopic view in Figure 23.7(C): notch plasty (right shoulder, lateral view). (Reprinted with permission from Lafosse L, Tomasi A. Technique for endoscopic release of suprascapular nerve entrapment at the suprascapular notch. Techniques in Shoulder and Elbow Surgery 2006 Mar; 7(1):1–6.)

with a rotator cuff rupture had a postoperative CT arthrogram to assess the quality of the repair.

Of the 18 patients, ten patients had an isolated SSN entrapment and eight patients were associated with a retracted supraspinatus and infraspinatus tear. At follow-up, the abduction and external rotation strength was improved in all patients on manual muscle testing. All cases had improvement of the strength, but may remain slightly weaker than the contralateral shoulder.

The clinical results assessed by constant score evaluation between surgery and last evaluation showed an average improvement of 23 points (60.3–83.4 points) in isolated release, and 31 points (45.9–77.3 points) when associated with RCR. All eight cases of RCR who underwent an arthro-CT scan six months after surgery were shown to have had an intact repair.

EMG study performed at an average of six months after surgery demonstrated resolution of nerve compression in 15 patients with a normalization of the latency in the motor fibers of the suprascapularis nerve and normal function of the voluntary innervation of both the supraspinatus and infraspinatus muscles. One patient, who described his result as good, was found to have partial improvement on EMG with residual axonal deficit. Upon further assessment, patient recovery is gradual and the final result is pending.

All patients were treated as ambulatory cases, and there was no problem with postoperative scars, hematoma, or nerve damage. There were no complications from surgery in either the early or medium postoperative periods, and all patients operated on for isolated nerve entrapment reported minimal pain during the first 24 hours after surgery. Patients indicated that they were very satisfied with the procedure and outcome, and all stated that they would have the procedure again.

With regard to the eight cases with associated rotator cuff tear, it is noted that the follow-up, at present, is too short to draw valid conclusions, but the outlook is impressive. For those five patients who had both an EMG and Arthro-CT scan postoperatively, the SSN release and cuff repair resulted in significant improvement at six months.

23.8. Conclusion

Further follow-up and experience is required to prove the reliability and durability of our short-term good results. However, the initial results look extremely promising.

This new endoscopic technique for the release of the SSN at the suprascapular notch enables the surgeon to have excellent visualization of the lesion and of the surrounding anatomy. It also enables comprehensive assessment of the nerve and its compression without detachment of the trapezius muscle, thus avoiding its associated complications. Open decompression via the standard superior approach demands dissection through the trapezius muscle, which can be difficult between the spine and the clavicle, and the dissection of the nerve under the ligament is deep.

The new SSN portal avoids any trapezius and supraspinatus damage and no associated complications have been reported. There is a learning curve with this procedure, as with all techniques, and while the mean time of surgery was around one hour, the nerve release at present does not take more than ten minutes, which is significantly shorter than with open surgery.

In conclusion, we have demonstrated a new method of endoscopic SSN decompression which is an effective alternative to the open approach with reduction of perioperative morbidity.

References

1. Thompson WAL, Koppel HP. Peripheral entrapment neuropathies of the upper extremity. *N Engl J Med* 1959;260:1261–1265.
2. Pecina M. Who really first described and explained the suprascapular nerve entrapment syndrome? *J Bone Joint Surg Am* 2001;83-A(8):1273–1274.
3. Alon M, Weiss S, Fishel B, et al. Bilateral suprascapular nerve entrapment syndrome due to an anomalous transverse scapular ligament. *Clin Orthop* 1988;234:31–33.
4. Ganzhorn RW, Hocker JT, Horowitz M, et al. Suprascapular nerve entrapment. A case report. *J Bone Joint Surg Am* 1981;63A:491–492.
5. Hirayama T, Takemitsu Y. Compression of the suprascapular nerve by a ganglion at the suprascapular notch. *Clin Orthop* 1981;155:95–96.
6. Nevaiser TJ, Ain B, Nevaiser RJ. Suprascapular nerve denervation secondary to attenuation by a ganglionic cyst. *J Bone Joint Surg Am* 1986;68A:627–628.
7. Ogina T, Minami A, Kato H, et al. Entrapment neuropathy of the suprascapular nerve by a ganglion. A report of 3 cases. *J Bone Joint Surg Am* 1991;73A:141–147.
8. Ticker JB, Djurasovic M, Strauch R, et al. The incidence of ganglion cysts and other variations in anatomy along the course of the suprascapular nerve. *J Shoulder Elbow Surg* 1998;7(5):472–478.
9. Rengachary SS, Burr D, Lucas S, et al. Suprascapular entrapment neuropathy: a clinical, anatomical and comparative study. Part 2: anatomical study. *Neurosurgery* 1979;5:447–451.
10. Yoon TN, Grabois M, Guillen M. Suprascapular nerve injury following trauma to the shoulder. *J Trauma* 1981;21:652–655.
11. McIlveen SJ, Duralde XZ, D'Alessandro DF, et al. Isolated nerve injuries about the shoulder. *Clin Orthop* 1994;306:54–63.
12. Sandow MJ, Ilic J. Suprascapular nerve rotator cuff compression in volleyball players. *J Shoulder Elbow Surg* 1998;7(5):516–521.

13. Cummins CA, Bowen M, Anderson K, et al. Suprascapular nerve entrapment at the spinoglenoid notch in a professional baseball pitcher. *Am J Sports Med* 1999;27(6):810–812.
14. Asami A, Sonohata M, Morisawa K. Bilateral suprascapular nerve entrapment syndrome associated with rotator cuff tear. *J Shoulder Elbow Surg* 2000;9(1): 70–72.
15. Warner JJP, Krushell RJ, Masquelet A, et al. Anatomy and relationships of the suprascapular nerve: anatomical constraints to mobilization of the supraspinatus and infraspinatus muscles in the management of massive rotator cuff tears. *J Bone Joint Surg Am* 1992;74A:36–45.
16. Albritton MJ, Graham RD, Richards RS II, Basamania CJ. An anatomic study of the effects on the suprascapular nerve due to retraction of the supraspinatus muscle after a rotator cuff tear. *J Shoulder Elbow Surg* 2003;12: 497–500.
17. Lafosse L, Tomasi A. Technique for endoscopic release of suprascapular nerve entrapment at the suprascapular notch. *Techniques in Shoulder and Elbow Surg* 2006;7(1):1–6.
18. Callahan JD, Scully TB, Scott a, et al. Suprascapular nerve entrapment: a series of 27 cases. *J Neurosurg* 1991;74:893–896.

24
Mechanics and Healing of Rotator Cuff Injury

Miltiadis H. Zgonis, Nelly A. Andarawis, and Louis J. Soslowsky

Rotator cuff injuries are among the most prevalent and poorly delineated musculoskeletal problems facing orthopedic surgeons. Cadaveric studies of asymptomatic individuals have shown the prevalence of rotator cuff tears to be between 30% and 50% and this prevalence increases with age.[1,2] Occupational injury of the shoulder, and of the rotator cuff in particular, is second only to neck and back pain with regard to frequency of presentation.[3] The critical functions of the rotator cuff underscore the need to understand the basic biological and mechanical features that shape the healthy rotator cuff and their roles in injured and healing tendon. This chapter provides an overview of these factors as they relate to healthy, injured, and healing rotator cuff.

24.1. Biology and Biochemistry of Healthy Tendon

The primary cell type recognized in all tendons is the tenocyte, also known as the fibroblast, which is responsible for the elaboration and maintenance of the extracellular matrix (ECM).[4] As the rotator cuff tendons do not have a true synovial sheath or paratenon, they receive their blood supply from their respective muscles. Although blood is present to some extent in tendons, tenocytes produce energy primarily through anaerobic pathways, an adaptive mechanism suited for long periods of compressive load they may experience within the tendon midsubstance.[5] In the supraspinatus tendon in particular, a critical zone of relative hypovascularity about 1 cm from its insertion at the greater tuberosity has been described.[6]

The normal ECM of tendon is comprised of a variety of structural proteins and proteoglycans. The most abundant of these by far is collagen type I, comprising 95% of all collagens and 65% to 80% of the dry mass of tendon.[5] Other forms of collagen are also present in normal tendon in small quantities but can play an important role in tendon homeostasis. An example is collagen V and other minor collagens, which have been implicated in regulating fibril diameter during aging and in fibrillogenesis of collagen I. The combination of proteoglycans and glycosaminoglycans

(GAGs) found in the supraspinatus tendon reflect its complex loading environment that consists not only of tension but of compression and shear as well.[7–9] For example, aggrecan, a large proteoglycan mostly associated with compressive strength in cartilage, is found in the supraspinatus. Normal rotator cuff tendons contain approximately 2.5 times the GAG content of the distal biceps tendon,[7] and, incidentally, GAG content has shown to be well correlated with collagen content, mean fibril diameter, and overall mechanical properties.[9]

The supraspinatus is well adapted to its mechanical environment not only through its elaborate composition but also through its role in the complicated architecture of the rotator cuff. Clark and colleagues revealed that the rotator cuff in this area is actually composed of five distinct layers, as depicted in Figure 24.1.[10] The superficial layers (layers 1–2) show cuff

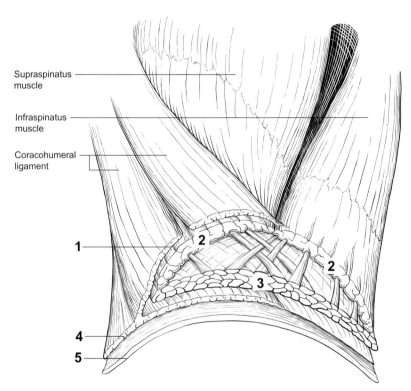

FIGURE 24.1. Five-layer structure of the cuff sectioned transversely at various sites in the supraspinatus, infraspinatus, and coracohumeral ligament. Fiber orientation in the layers is indicated by the lines on their surfaces. Layer 1 and 2 are superficial and contain superficial portions of the coracohumeral ligament and cuff tendons, respectively. Note that in layer 3, the supraspinatus tendon fibers intermingle with those of the infraspinatus and of the subscapularis (not shown). Layer 4 and 5 show the deep fibers of the coracohumeral ligament and the shoulder capsule, respectively.

tendons with discrete insertions, as taught to us by traditional anatomy. However, the deeper layers (layers 3–5) show that all the cuff tendons, ligaments, and joint capsule are fused together by intricate interdigitations that form a common humeral insertion. These help the cuff function in a unified manner to mechanically stabilize the dynamic motion of the glenohumeral joint.

24.2. Mechanical Properties of the Supraspinatus Tendon

The supraspinatus tendon plays a critical role in motion and stabilization of the shoulder joint.[11] The versatile motion of the rotator cuff joint regularly subjects the supraspinatus tendon to complex loads, causing it to have the highest incidence of tearing amongst the other portions of the rotator cuff.[12,13] Due to the importance of the supraspinatus and its frequent pathology in its high-demand mechanical environment, an understanding of tendon mechanics is essential.

The width of the supraspinatus tendon can be divided into anterior, middle, and posterior. The greater cross-sectional area of the anterior portion of the tendon supports its higher ultimate load to failure and modulus of elasticity in comparison to the middle and the posterior regions. The middle and posterior regions of the tendon are mechanically inferior to the anterior portion of the tendon.[14] It is believed that the anterior portion transmits most of the loads experienced by the tendon. Similarly, the articular side has a higher modulus of elasticity but a lower yield strain than the bursal side,[15] which is information that contributes to our understanding of regions of tear initiation and progression.

24.3. Types of Rotator Cuff Injury

Rotator cuff injury is a common disorder of the shoulder that is responsible for 8% to 13% of all athletic injuries.[16] Injury involves the supraspinatus tendon most frequently (96.6%) and the infraspinatus (60.4%), the subscapularis (28%), and the teres minor (16.1%) less often.[17] The high incidence of injury of the supraspinatus has triggered many studies on the loading environment and the mechanics of this tendon. An understanding of the pathological changes that may accompany rotator cuff diseases is essential to a full understanding of the disease.

The severity of rotator cuff diseases varies widely. Fukuda and coworkers used a three-group system of classification. Grade I rotator cuff disease consisted of a pre-tear stage characterized by initial tendon weakening. The disruptions of fascicles stimulate a healing response from the body in the form of cell infiltration or vascular proliferation causing tendon inflammation and edema. Although the overall degenerative changes of the tendon decrease the ultimate stress of the supraspinatus, this condition may not worsen and the vascularity on the bursal half of the tendon is sufficient to stimulate healing.[18] Continuous aggravation of the tendon can result in chronic partial- or full-thickness tears, classified as grade II and grade III, respectively. In contrast to chronic tears, acute tears result from an incidence of trauma or a specific tendon injury. Most diagnosed rotator cuff injury patients suffer from chronic rotator cuff tears. A study conducted in the Mayo Clinic over the course of 24 years showed that only 8% of rotator cuff injury patients recalled a specific incident that propagated their shoulder pain.[19]

Debates regarding the causes of rotator cuff tears are ongoing. Codman proposed an intrinsic mechanism, suggesting that hypovascularity of the tendon near its insertion site predisposes to degeneration in the tendon and is accelerated by its loading environment.[20] In contrast, Neer's popularized extrinsic mechanism suggests that tendon injury is not an innate degenerative process and that acromial impingement during shoulder motion can account for 95% of rotator cuff injury.[21] The success of anterior acromioplasty supports the conclusions supported by Neer. Bigliani and colleagues correlated a change in the acromial shape with rotator cuff tears. They found that hooked acromions and acromions with anterior spurs and a greater angle of anterior slope were more often associated with rotator cuff tears than flat and curved acromions.[22] However, if extrinsic factors were solely responsible for rotator cuff injury, then degenerative changes on the undersurface of the acromion would be found in the presence of any rotator cuff tear. As expected, acromial changes were found only in association with full-thickness and bursal-side tears not in patients with articular-side tears.[23] This supports the multifactorial model of rotator cuff tears wherein both intrinsic and extrinsic factors contribute to tear initiation and progression and the specific initiating factor is often difficult to ascertain.

Macroscopic tears are not the only types of injury that can occur in tendon. There is also the common diagnosis of tendinitis, a condition resulting from chronic microtrauma of tendon. This is thought to be a result of repetitive mechanical load, such as in overuse conditions, which may heal or may progress to chronic degeneration.[24,25] The suffix -itis denotes the presence of inflammation within the tendon as a result of this trauma. However, many human studies of chronic tendinitis have shown little or no evidence of histological inflammatory change.[26] This is also true in animal models where detailed characterization of the response over time to overuse can be evaluated.[27] Many authors and clinicians are now advocating the use of the term tendinosis, which denotes a chronic degenerative condition featuring a decrease in collagen and decreased fiber orientation, rather than an inflammatory condition of the tendon substance. Figure 24.2 shows the characteristic histological appearance of tendinosis, with a typical lack of inflammatory cells in the tissue. There are tissues associated with other tendons that can become truly inflamed in overuse, including the synovial sheath and the

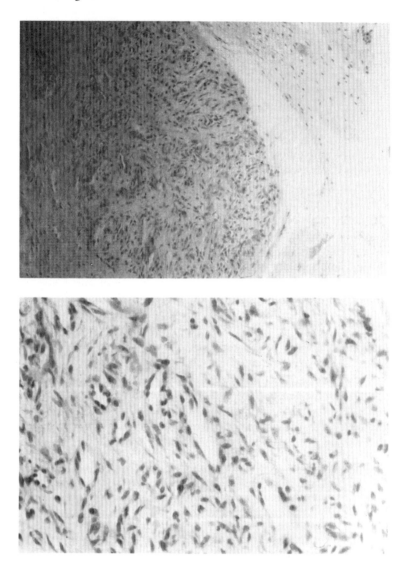

FIGURE 24.2. Angiofibroblastic tendinosis. Characteristic microscopic appearance of chronic tendinosis. Note the absence of inflammatory cells. (Reprinted with permission from Leadbetter et al., eds. Sports-induced inflammation. Park Ridge, IL: Clinical and basic science concepts. American Academy of Orthopaedic Surgeons; 1990.)

paratenon. A study by Backman and colleagues in 1990 showed tendinosis and paratenonitis coexisting in a rabbit overuse model.[28]

Etiological studies have shown that intrinsic, extrinsic, and overuse injury can individually cause tendinosis to occur in an animal model of rotator cuff injury.[22,27,29] Furthermore, the effects of these pathogenetic factors on tendinosis appear to be additive. In a recent study, this effect was measured in a rat rotator cuff model by combining the effect of overuse with extrinsic injury.[30] The result was a significant increase in cross-sectional area and a significant decrease in maximum stress and tissue modulus in the combined overuse/extrinsic injury group over control and over either overuse or extrinsic injury alone, as shown in Table 24.1. This and other findings support the multifactorial nature of the disease process.

In contrast to tendon degeneration, a tear is marked by fraying of the fibers and loss of tendon substance and must involve at least one quarter of the thickness or the width of the tendon.[12] Because early diagnosis of a rotator cuff tear is difficult and infrequent, many acute tears share the similar accompanying pathological cuff changes as chronic tears at the time of diagnosis.[19] Additionally, repetitive microtrauma is also a cause of chronic tendon tears. Irreversible degenerative cuff changes, such as muscle atrophy and fatty infiltration, impose added complexity in the treatment of chronic tears.[31] The presence of a chronic tendon tear diminishes the overall mechanical integrity of the tendon.[18] In contrast to chronic tears, acute tears result from a nonpenetrating blunt injury or laceration by a sharp object. Some believe that severe acute tears are more likely to enlarge and extend over time than chronic tears, while others maintain that acute tears occur in an already diseased tendon and thus early repair may unnecessarily subject the patient to an invasive procedure.[19]

Acute and chronic rotator cuff injury can cause partial- and full-thickness tears. Partial-thickness tears have a higher incidence of occurrence than full-thickness tears and are thought to affect 13% to 37% of the population. Figure 24.3 shows variations of partial tears of the rotator cuff. The longitudinal tendon bundles composing the bursal side of the tendon are more capable of dispersing tensile loads than the interlaced, thinner fibers found in the articular side of the tendon.[15] Therefore, the fibers on the articular side of the tendon are more likely to experience a greater tensile load than that experienced by the fibers on the bursal side.[32] This effect is further magnified under abduction as the articular side of the rotator cuff is believed to be closer to its yield strain than the bursal side.[32,33] Mathematical models further support the experimental findings and imply that the stress concentration moves from the articular surface closer to the insertion site with increasing abduction angle.[32] However, the

TABLE 24.1. Summary of Histological, Geometric, and Biomechanical Changes between Exercise (E), Overuse (OV), and both Together (OV/E) Relative to Appropriate Control Groups.

	Histology	Cross-sectional area	Maximum stress	Tissue modulus
E	Slight changes	↔	↔	↔
OV	Slight changes	↑	↓	↓
OV/E	Slight changes	↑↑	↓↓	↓↓

Source: Soslowsky LJ, et al. Rotator cuff tendinosis in an animal model: role of extrinsic and overuse factors. Ann Biomed Eng 2002;30:1060. Reprinted with kind permission of Springer Science and Business Media.

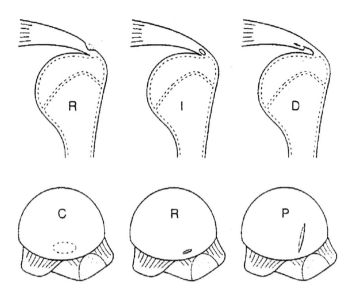

FIGURE 24.3. Partial tear of the rotator cuff (schema). Abbreviations: R, rim tear; I, intratendinous tear; D, deep surface tear; C, concealed tear; P, Posterior tear. (From Nobuhara, ed. The shoulder: its function and clinical aspects. Singapore: World Scientific; 2003, with permission from World Scientific.)

presence of an articular-side tear is thought to weaken the remaining intact portion of the insertion site and thus increase the risk of tear progression.[34] Intratendinous tears are completely contained within the tendon. The pathology of intratendinous tears is thought to differ from that of bursal- or articular-side tears, because degeneration due to shearing forces is thought to be the culprit for this type of tear.[18] Bursal-side tears are significantly more painful than articular or intratendinous tears.[12] This may relate to the presence of fluid in the joint that is more commonly associated with this type of partial-thickness tear.

Simply defined, a full-thickness tear is a gap in the tendon that encompasses the full thickness of the tendon. The incidence of full-thickness tears has been reported as 8% to 26%. Full-thickness tears can assume various morphologies and can initiate on the anterior, posterior, or middle portion along the width of the tendon. A transverse full-thickness tear exposes the insertion site of the tendon, in contrast to a longitudinal rent that occurs along the torn tendon fiber.[17] Despite the mechanical superiority of the anterior portion of the tendon, it is the location of almost 90% of rotator cuff tears in patients over the age of 35.[35]

Typically, radiography is used as a first-attempt approach to diagnose a shoulder injury patient.[36] While X-ray images can effectively show dystrophic calcification or spurs that may result in impingement, their success at showing tendon tears is limited and heavily depends on the expertise of the operator.[37] In contrast to the less subjective X ray, arthrography is a well-established objective technique that can be used to diagnose full-thickness tears and articular-side partial tears in the supraspinatus tendon with great accuracy.[38] Standard arthrography has been further enhanced by the addition of air for double contrast technique. In this technique, fluoroscopically guided intra-articular injection of room air supplements the standard intra-articular injections of a water soluble contrast material. Fluoroscopy successfully detects the location and extension of the cuff defect. Despite the accuracy of diagnosis of arthrography, its invasive nature motivates the quest for other less invasive methods of diagnosis and methods that can more accurately diagnose bursal-side tears and intratendinous tears.

Ultrasound provides a less costly, noninvasive method for the diagnosis of rotator cuff tears. Studies have shown that office-based ultrasound can correctly identify approximately 70% of full-thickness cuff tears [95% confidence interval (95% CI), 55%–84%].[39] Our limited knowledge of the optimal use of ultrasound has hindered its use as an independent diagnostic modality and mandated its coupling with findings from arthroscopic diagnosis.

Magnetic resonance imaging (MRI) is a more costly but promising diagnostic modality. MRI has successfully been used to diagnose complete tears, with an 80% to 97% sensitivity and a 94% specificity.[37] MRI is less successful in diagnosing partial tears, which are often misdiagnosed as impingement tendinopathy or full-thickness tears. MR arthrography is an advance over unenhanced MRI in diagnosis of shoulder injury. MR arthrography allows finer anatomical differentiation, thus improving diagnostics of partial thickness rotator cuff tears.

Appropriate methods of treatment of rotator cuff tears have not been finalized. Generally, the goal of treatment of tears is to minimize discomfort and avoid further loss of range of motion. The current clinical approach does not mandate surgical intervention for rotator cuff tears that encompass less then 50% of the tendon but instead prescribes more conservative treatment approaches. Tears that involve more than 50% of the tendon are surgically extended through the remaining normal tissue; then the tendon stump is sutured to the greater tuberosity.[40] The exclusion of tears that encompass less than 50% of the tendon from surgical treatment is solely based on clinical experience and not on any fundamental knowledge of which tears would progress without surgical intervention and which tears do not pose a risk of progression. Therefore, studies by Bey and colleagues have investigated the use of MRI with image processing techniques to obtain intratendinous strain information noninvasively. Assuming that an increase in tendon strain indicates an increase in the risk of tear progression, the studies investigated the intratendinous strains in relation to different types of tears in different locations of the tendon. Specifically, Bey and colleagues conducted studies examining the effect of joint position on strains in the tendon, both in the presence and absence of an articular-side partial thickness tear.[41] They concluded from these studies that the presence of a tear caused an increase in strain at 30°, 45°, and 60° of abduction but had no effect at 15°. They also found that the strains of the superior, middle, and inferior portions of the tendon were affected differently by the presence of a tear or the increase in the abduction angle, further supporting the notion that the location of the tear should be considered when prescribing treatment.[33] Figure 24.4 shows strain variations in an intact and torn tendon at four different abduction angles. The success of these studies and similar ongoing studies using this technology will provide clinicians with the means to treat tears surgically or conservatively on the basis of risk of tear progression specific to the individual patient.

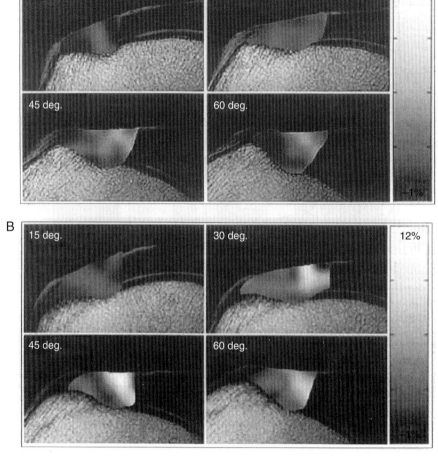

FIGURE 24.4. Representative specimen demonstrating a map of maximum principal strain throughout the intact (A) and torn (B) supraspinatus tendon at four glenohumeral abduction angles. (Reprinted from Bey et al., (41) with permission from the Journal of Shoulder and Elbow Surgery Board of Trustees.)

24.4. Mechanisms of Healing

Tendon healing generally occurs by two separate mechanisms depending on the source of the regenerative cells, namely intrinsic (cells from within the existing tendon) and extrinsic (cells from paratenon, periosteum, etc.). Both are usually occurring concurrently, although some studies have shown that the extrinsic mechanism has a more robust inflammatory response, acts earlier than the intrinsic mechanism, and reacts more vigorously to inflammatory cytokines produced in the initial phase of healing.[42–44] This vigorous response by the extrinsic mechanism is thought to contribute significantly to adhesion formation and subsequent decreased tendon excursion.

Healing occurs in three overlapping phases: the inflammatory phase, the fibroblastic phase, and the remodeling phase,[45] as depicted in Figure 24.5. The acute inflammatory phase occurs in the first week after injury and is characterized by the deposition of fibrin and fibronectin by platelets, which also secrete potent growth factors and chemotactic agents such as insulinlike growth factor (IGF-1), platelet-derived growth factor (PDGF), and transforming growth factor beta (TGF-β). These act to recruit fibroblasts and inflammatory cells like macrophages and neutrophils into the wound area to phagocytize necrotic debris and to induce further inflammation. This phase establishes the initial strength necessary to sustain the growing and remodeling matrix that will soon be deposited.

The second, or fibroblastic, phase begins at 48 h and can last up to 8 weeks. The primary feature of this phase is the deposition of collagen by migrated fibroblasts and intrinsic tenocytes, starting with type III, and eventually shifting to type I collagen. Collagen III is deposited as a temporary structure in random meshwork of uncrosslinked, small-diameter fibrils. Collagen III is also a known constituent of the rotator cuff, and plays a role in healing of the supraspinatus.[46] This has also been shown to occur in supraspinatus tendon after acute injury in a rat animal model.[47]

The third, or remodeling, phase is characterized by decreased synthetic activity by fibroblasts with a concomitant increase in collagen orientation and matrix organization. Although the result of the repair process is an intact tendon, the biomechanical properties of the repaired tissue will always be inferior to that of the uninjured tendon. This phenomenon has also been shown to be true in the same rat supraspinatus tendon model as above.[48,49] The above details the healing of generic tendon when the torn ends are approximated as in a partial tendon tear or after an acute repair. However, chronic, full-thickness tears of supraspinatus tendons are known to retract away from their insertion site at the greater tuberosity, the most common area to experience tearing.[6] This is associated with an increase in repair tension required to re-approximate the tendon edge to its bony insertion.[50] Figure 24.6 shows how repair tension increases with time after injury.

Even if a surgeon succeeds in re-approximating the tendon to the insertion site, recent evidence shows that delayed repair of tendon-to-bone

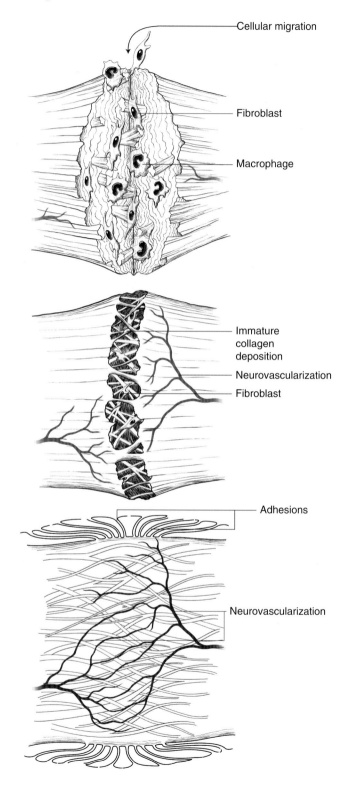

Cellular migration

Fibroblast

Macrophage

Immature collagen deposition

Neurovascularization

Fibroblast

Adhesions

Neurovascularization

FIGURE 24.5. Cellular phases of tendon healing. (A) Inflammatory phase (1 week postinjury): Extrinsic and intrinsic fibroblasts and macrophages travel to the injury site. Elimination of any clot or necrotic tissue through phagocytosis and initial deposition of extracellular matrix occurs during this phase. (B) Fibroblastic phase (3 weeks postinjury): This phase is marked by proliferation of fibroblasts at the injury site. This is followed by pronounced collagen deposition and revascularization at the site of injury. (C) Remodeling phase (8 weeks postinjury): Deposited collagen fibers become organized along the axis of the tendon, while adhesions between injured tendon and surrounding sheath become more prominent.

---

injuries exhibits decreased biomechanical properties of the tendon and loss of bone quality at the humeral head,[51] potentially contributing to a poor union and subsequent failure. In studies of massive tears, the rate of failure has been reported as between 50% to 70% by MRI.[52]

In addition to pretension experienced by the tendon due to existing muscular elasticity and tone, fibroblasts involved in wound repair exhibit contractile properties as they do in other types of wounds.[53] This may deter more than help a tear in the supraspinatus from coming together, as the tendon is already experiencing tensile forces at complete adduction, and the contracting fibroblasts might be pulling the edges of the wound further away from each other in this situation.

Conventional thinking with regard to postoperative rehabilitation has been to remobilize using passive motion soon after surgical reattachment of the supraspinatus tendon to bone.[19] While this may appear to decrease

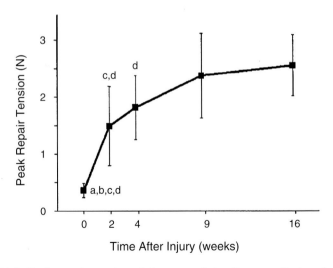

FIGURE 24.6. Peak repair tension of the musculotendinous unit at various times after injury. (From Gimbel JA, et al. The tension required at repair to reappose the supraspinatus tendon to bone rapidly increases after injury. Clin Orthop 2004;426:258–265, with permission from Lippincott Williams and Wilkins.)

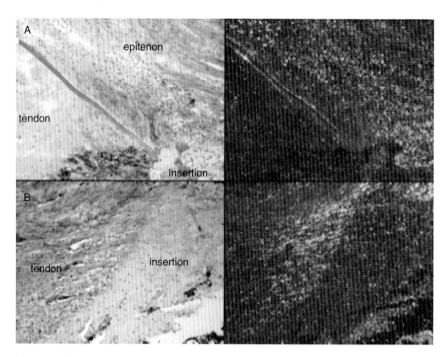

FIGURE 24.7. Type III collagen expression in the IM (A) and EX (B) groups at 16 weeks. Light-field images are presented on the left, dark-field images are presented on the right (10× objective). Note the increased levels of type III collagen in the EX (B) specimen compared to the IM specimen (A). (Reprinted from Thomopoulos et al., (54) with permission from ASME International.)

early postoperative stiffness and pain clinically, recent research in an animal shoulder model studying activity levels after acute injury has shown that postinjury insertion site biochemistry and biomechanical properties more closely mimic uninjured insertion sites after a period of immobilization.[54] Figure 24.7 demonstrates this phenomenon by showing less collagen III, an injury associated collagen, in the immobilized group than in the exercised group. This finding suggests that, clinically, a period of immobilization prior to remobilization may produce a superior quality tendon-to-bone union and reduce the number of failures seen by surgeons due to poor healing.

24.5. Future Directions

There is much left to learn in the healing of rotator cuff pathology. Studies will focus on many areas; of particular interest will be direct comparisons of postrepair tendon-to-bone healing between passive motion and immobilization. Furthermore, we must strive to understand and optimize the temporal relationship between insertion site healing and remobilization to provide surgeons with the best postoperative rehabilitation data available for the creation of novel and better clinical outcomes.

New avenues to explore also include muscle adaptation after rotator cuff tear. Retraction of the supraspinatus musculotendinous unit in the chronic tear condition is a common problem leading to increased repair tension and possible failure.[50,55] Understanding this process in the context of the complete musculotendinous complex will be important in possible future interventions directed at decreasing tension and subsequent failure of repairs.

References

1. Sher JS, Uribe JW, Posada A, Murphy BJ, Zlatkin MB. Abnormal findings on magnetic resonance images of asymptomatic shoulders. J Bone Joint Surg Am 1995;77(1):10–15.
2. Tempelhof S, Rupp S, Seil R. Age-related prevalence of rotator cuff tears in asymptomatic shoulders. J Shoulder Elbow Surg 1999;8(4):296–299.
3. Bureau of Labor Statistics, Occupational injuries and illnesses in the United States by industry. Bulletin 2468. August 1990.
4. O'Brien M. Structure and metabolism of tendons. Scand J Med Sci Sports 1997;7(2):55–61.
5. Amiel D, Frank C, Harwood F, Fronek J, Akeson W. Tendons and ligaments: a morphological and biochemical comparison. J Orthop Res 1984;1(3):257–265.
6. Codman E. The Shoulder. Boston: Thomas Todd Co. 1934.
7. Berenson MC, Blevins FT, Plaas AH, Vogel KG. Proteoglycans of human rotator cuff tendons. J Orthop Res 1996;14(4):518–525.
8. Derwin KA, Soslowsky LJ, Kimura JH, Plaas AH. Proteoglycans and glycosaminoglycan fine structure in the mouse tail tendon fascicle. J Orthop Res 2001;19(2):269–277.
9. Robinson PS, Lin TW, Jawad AF, Iozzo RV, Soslowsky LJ. Investigating tendon fascicle structure-function relationships in a transgenic-age mouse model using multiple regression models. Ann Biomed Eng 2004;32(7):924–931.
10. Clark JM, Harryman DT. 2nd. Tendons, ligaments, and capsule of the rotator cuff. Gross and microscopic anatomy. J Bone Joint Surg Am 1992;74(5):713–725.
11. Itoi E, Hsu HC, An KN. Biomechanical investigation of the glenohumeral joint. J Shoulder Elbow Surg 1996;5(5):407–424.
12. Fukuda H. Partial-Thickness Rotator Cuff Tears: A Modern View on Codman's Classic. J Shoulder Elbow Sur 2000;9:163–168.
13. Lee SB, Nakajima T, Luo ZP, Zobitz ME, Chang YW. An KN, The bursal and articular sides of the supraspinatus tendon have a different compressive stiffness. Clin Biomech (Bristol, Avon) 2000;15(4):241–247.
14. Itoi E, Berglund LJ, Grabowski JJ, et al. Tensile properties of the supraspinatus tendon. J Orthop Res 1995;13(4):578–584.
15. Nakajima T, Rokuuma N, Kazutoshi H, Tomastu T, Fukuda H. Histologic and Biomechanical Characteristics of the Supraspinatus Tendon: Reference to Rotator Cuff Tearing. J Shoulder Elbow Surg 1994;3:79–87.
16. Maday M, Harner C, Warner J. Shoulder Injuries In Fu SDA, Freddie H, eds. Sports Injuries. Baltimore: Williams & Wilkins; 1994:895–921.
17. Nobuhara K. Diseases of the shoulder, In The Shoulder, its Function and Clinical Aspects. World Scientific: Singapore. 2003:208–237.

18. Uhthoff HK, Sano H. Pathology of failure of the rotator cuff tendon. Orthop Clin North Am 1997;28(1):31–41.
19. Cofield RH. Rotator cuff disease of the shoulder. J Bone Joint Surg Am 1985;67(6):974–979.
20. Codman E, Akerson I. The pathology associated with rupture of the supraspinatus tendon. Ann. Surg 1931;93:348–359.
21. Neer CS. 2nd. Impingement lesions. Clin Orthop Relat Res 1983(173):70–77.
22. Bigliani LU, Ticker JB, Flatow EL, Soslowsky LJ, Mow VC. The relationship of acromial architecture to rotator cuff disease. Clin Sports Med 1991;10(4): 823–838.
23. Ozaki J, Fujimoto S, Nakagawa Y, Masuhara K, Tamai S. Tears of the rotator cuff of the shoulder associated with pathological changes in the acromion. A study in cadavera. J Bone Joint Surg Am 1988;70(8):1224–1230.
24. Clancy W. Tendon trauma and overuse injuries. In W, ed. Sports-induced Inflammation. Leadbetter Park Ridge, IL: American Academy of Orthopaedic Surgeons 1990:609–618.
25. Clement DB, Taunton JE, Smart GW. Achilles tendinitis and peritendinitis: etiology and treatment. Am J Sports Med 1984;12(3):179–184.
26. Almekinders LC, Temple JD. Etiology, diagnosis, and treatment of tendonitis: an analysis of the literature. Med Sci Sports Exerc 1998;30(8):1183–1190.
27. Soslowsky LJ, Thomopoulos S, Tun S, et al. Neer Award 1999. Overuse activity injures the supraspinatus tendon in an animal model: a histologic and biomechanical study. J Shoulder Elbow Surg 2000;9(2):79–84.
28. Backman C, Boquist L, Friden J, Lorentzon R, Toolanen G. Chronic achilles paratenonitis with tendinosis: an experimental model in the rabbit. J Orthop Res 1990;8(4):541–547.
29. Carpenter JE, Flanagan CL, Thomopoulos S, Yian EH, Soslowsky LJ. The effects of overuse combined with intrinsic or extrinsic alterations in an animal model of rotator cuff tendinosis. Am J Sports Med 1998;26(6):801–807.
30. Soslowsky LJ, Thomopoulos S, Esmail A, et al. Rotator cuff tendinosis in an animal model: role of extrinsic and overuse factors. Ann Biomed Eng 2002;30(8):1057–1063.
31. Goutallier D, Postel JM, Laveau L, Voison MC. Fatty muscle degeneration in cuff ruptures. Pre- and postoperative evaluation by CT scan. Clin Orthop 1994;304:78–83.
32. Wakabayashi I, Itoi E, Sano H, et al. Mechanical environment of the supraspinatus tendon: a two-dimensional finite element model analysis. J Shoulder Elbow Surg 2003;12(6):612–617.
33. Bey MJ, Song HK, Wehrli FW, Soslowsky LJ. Intratendinous strain fields of the intact supraspinatus tendon: the effect of glenohumeral joint position and tendon region. J Orthop Res 2002;20(4):869–874.
34. Reilly P, Amis AA, Wallace AL, Emery RJ. Mechanical factors in the initiation and propagation of tears of the rotator cuff. Quantification of strains of the supraspinatus tendon in vitro. J Bone Joint Surg Br 2003;85(4):594–599.
35. Tuite MJ, Turnbull JR, Orwin JF. Anterior versus posterior, and rim-rent rotator cuff tears: prevalence and MR sensitivity. Skeletal Radiol 1998;27(5): 237–243.
36. Miniaci A, Salonen D. Rotator cuff evaluation: imaging and diagnosis. Orthop Clin North Am 1997;28(1):43–58.

37. Guckel C, Nidecker A. Diagnosis of tears in rotator-cuff-injuries. Eur J Radiol 1997;25(3):168–176.
38. Mink JH, Harris E, Rappaport M. Rotator cuff tears: evaluation using double-contrast shoulder arthrography. Radiology 1985;157(3):621–623.
39. Iannotti JP, Ciccone J, Buss DD, et al. Accuracy of office-based ultrasonography of the shoulder for the diagnosis of rotator cuff tears. J Bone Joint Surg Am 2005;87(6):1305–1311.
40. Flatow EL, Altchek DW, Gartsman GM, et al. The rotator cuff. Commentary. Orthop Clin North Am 1997;28(2):277–294.
41. Bey MJ, Ramsey ML, Soslowsky LJ. Intratendinous strain fields of the supraspinatus tendon: effect of a surgically created articular-surface rotator cuff tear. J Shoulder Elbow Surg 2002;11(6):562–569.
42. Khan U, Edwards JC, McGrouther DA. Patterns of cellular activation after tendon injury. J Hand Surg [Br] 1996;21(6):813–820.
43. Khan U, Kakar S, Akali A, Bentley G, McGrouther DA. Modulation of the formation of adhesions during the healing of injured tendons. J Bone Joint Surg Br 2000;82(7):1054–1058.
44. Khan U, Occleston NL, Khaw PT, McGrouther DA. Differences in proliferative rate and collagen lattice contraction between endotenon and synovial fibroblasts. J Hand Surg Am 1998;23(2):266–273.
45. Beredjiklian PK. Biologic aspects of flexor tendon laceration and repair. J Bone Joint Surg Am 2003;85-A(3):539–550.
46. Blevins FT, Djurasovic M, Flatow EL, Vogel KG. Biology of the rotator cuff tendon. Orthop Clin North Am 1997;28(1):1–16.
47. Yokota A, Gimbel JA, Williams GR, Soslowsky LJ. Supraspinatus tendon composition remains altered long after tendon detachment. J Shoulder Elbow Surg 2005;14(1 Suppl S):72S-78S.
48. Carpenter JE, Thomopoulos S, Flanagan CL, DeBano CM, Soslowsky LJ. Rotator cuff defect healing: a biomechanical and histologic analysis in an animal model. J Shoulder Elbow Surg 1998;7(6):599–605.
49. Gimbel JA, Van Kleunen JP, Mehta S, Perry SM, Williams GR, Soslowsky LJ. Supraspinatus tendon organizational and mechanical properties in a chronic rotator cuff tear animal model. J Biomech 2004;37(5):739–749.
50. Gimbel JA, Mehta S, Van Kleunen JP, Williams GR, Soslowsky LJ. The tension required at repair to reappose the supraspinatus tendon to bone rapidly increases after injury. Clin Orthop Relat Res, 2004(426):258–265.
51. Galatz LM, Rothermich SY, Zaegel M, Silva MJ, Havlioglu N, Thomopoulos S. Delayed repair of tendon to bone injuries leads to decreased biomechanical properties and bone loss. J Orthop Res 2005;28:28.
52. Gerber C, Fuchs B, Hodler J. The results of repair of massive tears of the rotator cuff. J Bone Joint Surg Am 2000;82(4):505–515.
53. Premdas J, Tang JB, Warner JP, Murray MM, Spector M. The presence of smooth muscle actin in fibroblasts in the torn human rotator cuff. J Orthop Res 2001;19(2):221–228.
54. Thomopoulos S, Williams GR, Soslowsky LJ. Tendon to bone healing: differences in biomechanical, structural, and compositional properties due to a range of activity levels. J Biomech Eng 2003;125(1):106–113.
55. Reilly P, Bull AM, Amis AA, et al. Passive tension and gap formation of rotator cuff repairs. J Shoulder Elbow Surg 2004;13(6):664–667.

25
Postoperative Rehabilitation Following Arthroscopic Rotator Cuff Repair

Jonathan B. Ticker and James J. Egan

25.1. Principles of Rehabililtation

Although the arthroscopic techniques described in the previous chapters have altered our approach to rotator cuff repairs and have improved upon the open procedures previously considered the gold standard, the principles of rehabilitation have not changed as dramatically. As Neer stated, "It is not enough to perform a technically perfect, clean shoulder reconstruction. The shoulder surgeon must have an equal fervor for preventing adhesions and strengthening muscles while preserving the integrity of his or her repair."[1] In addition, "because a good rehabilitation program is critical ... in restoring optimum function in this complex joint, the shoulder surgeon must not only understand this type of rehabilitation but also remain actively involved with the patient and therapist to make it work." There is now more science available to guide the shoulder surgeon and physical therapist, but there remains an art to the process.

The postoperative rehabilitation following arthroscopic rotator cuff repair begins preoperatively when the shoulder surgeon explains to the patient the planned operative procedure, the peri-operative course, and the demands of postoperative rehabilitation. Questions about the planned procedure and any intraoperative decisions to be made are answered. In this manner, the patient's and the shoulder surgeon's expectations are understood by both parties. This includes a frank discussion of the benefits and risk, including the risk for re-tear. The initial postoperative home exercise regimen can be reviewed at this time. In addition, the outpatient pain management program is discussed, including the senior author's preference for anesthetic infusion with lidocaine into the subacromial space for approximately 48h following surgery.[2] If there are any concerns that the patient cannot, or will not, comply with the postoperative course outlined for the planned procedure, addressing this preoperatively is clearly more desirable.

The primary goal of a postoperative rehabilitation program is to control pain, protect repaired tissue during the healing process, restore function, and avoid recurrence of symptoms.

The size of the tear, the quality of the tissue and bone, and the quality of the repair, as well as the patient's abilities and motivation, are taken into account by the shoulder surgeon as the rehabilitation program is initiated and progressed. The approach to rehabilitation following a secure repair in a young patient with strong bone and healthy tendon should differ from the approach in an older patient having a repair of the same size tear with tendon and bone that is of poorer quality. Thus, general principles are applied to each patient and the repair in an individualized fashion.

Typically, the sling is worn for 4 to 6 weeks, with the longer time period required for large and massive tears. (Abduction pillows for large and massive tears may decrease tendon contact to the prepared sulcus and are not used for arthroscopic repairs at this time by the senior author, including the setting of a double row repair.) Passive range-of-motion (ROM) exercise usually begins within the first 24 to 48h in small- and medium-sized tears, based on patient ability and comfort. The shoulder surgeon and physical therapist perform ROM on the patient in the supine position, within the limits determined at the time of surgery. With repair of a small tear, the limits on elevation and external rotation may be present for only the first few weeks following surgery. However, in medium and larger tears, the limits determined at the time of surgery must be respected for a longer period of time. Limited active-assisted ROM exercises begin as pendulum exercises and initial supine self-assisted exercises. This is delayed in large tears, and massive tears are delayed even longer, again depending upon factors noted above.

Pain will interfere with the recovery, and steps to diminish pain are essential. Analgesics are utilized to allow for earlier progression of motion. Initially, avoiding internal rotation (IR), arm extension, and reaching behind the back following a rotator cuff repair is helpful to limit tension on the repair and to decrease pain. Cryotherapy is essential initially to control pain and swelling, and following exercises and activities during the healing process to diminish muscle soreness. Cautioning patients on specific activities to avoid is advantageous.

A physician-supervised physical therapy rehabilitation program is an important component of the recovery process. The shoulder surgeon must communicate with the physical therapist to set the initial limits, based on the intraoperative impression of the repair, and to advance the rehabilitation. This interaction between the shoulder surgeon and treating physical therapist will allow the therapist to fully understand the type of procedure, size of the tear, quality of repair, any concomitant procedures performed, and the shoulder surgeon's rehabilitation guidelines for each rotator cuff repair. The physical therapist is the eyes and ears for the shoulder surgeon during the rehabilitation process and must communicate back to the shoulder surgeon any necessary information regarding the patient's progress, or lack thereof.[3] It is imperative for the treating physical therapist to understand the biomechanics of the shoulder and the forces that are placed on the rotator cuff during specific exercises. These principles will allow the physical therapist to use the general postoperative guidelines to develop an appropriate and individualized program for the patient that will allow the repair to heal properly and restore ROM and strength, as well as maintain glenohumeral stability and proprioception, which is essential for normal shoulder function. Programs must also be tailored to the individual patient for return to previous activity. The shoulder surgeon and physical therapist must also serve to advise, encourage, and even caution the patient throughout the recovery.

During the initial stages of healing following a repair, gaining motion is the focus of rehabilitation. Phase I, or the acute or protective stage, is generally designed to manage postoperative pain and inflammation, as well as protect the repair, initiate passive ROM then active-assisted ROM exercises for the involved joint, initiate isometrics for the unaffected muscles, and resume motion to the uninvolved joints, especially the elbow, wrist, and hand. Initial motion limits are based on the shoulder surgeon's intraoperative assessment of the safe zone for motion following the repair. For example, the secure repair of a medium-sized tear in a young patient with good quality bone and tendon may be allowed a greater passive ROM than the repair of a medium-sized tear in an elderly patient with poorer quality bone and tendon. Advancing these limits as tissue healing progresses is based on the shoulder surgeon's assessment of the patient's overall progress. The duration of this phase varies by the size of the repair. Pulley exercises are only initiated toward the end of this phase to avoid active muscle recruitment that can occur when started too early.[4]

Phase II, the subacute or recovery stage, begins when sufficient tissue healing is achieved, again depending upon the size of the tear and the quality of the tissue and its repair. The timing is clearly much sooner following a repair of a small 1-cm rotator cuff tear than following repair of a large, 4-cm rotator cuff tear. One might also be more confident with advancing the rehabilitation in the setting of a secure double row repair compared with a single row repair in a similar-sized tear. This phase includes active ROM exercises, advanced stretching to restore full motion, and light, then more advanced, strengthening of the affected muscles and the entire shoulder girdle. Judicious application of heat promotes soft tissue flexibility and facilitates stretching. Application of cold following exercises and activities is encouraged to diminish pain and swelling. Posterior capsular tightness should not be overlooked and should be addressed with specific stretching exercises of the posterior capsule. In addition, joint mobilization techniques for the posterior capsule can be used. Slow, gradual stretching exercises are preferred over rapid, ballistic-type movements. Pain control should be re-assessed at many intervals during the recovery to ensure the patient's needs are met. Slow down if the patient's pain does not allow steady progress. Steady encouragement and positive reinforcement is essential, especially if the patient expresses frustration with the perceived slow recovery.

Phase III, or the functional stage, maximizes stretching and strengthening and adds sports- or activity-related exercises, as well as a maintenance program. Activities are resumed in stages, based upon the demands such activities will place on the repair. Ensure the patient understands that postoperative gains do not always follow a smooth and steady progression, and that the course can fluctuate with the addition of new exercises and advancing to a new stage, as well as with added activities of daily living. If the patient can look back week by week and appreciate his or her progress, this can be an encouraging perspective.

A diligent home exercise program is of equal importance to the physical therapy visits. There are specific exercises at each stage that complement the supervised program to maintain and build upon the gains achieved thus far. The physical therapist, as well as the shoulder surgeon, guides the patient with the individualized home exercise program. As a general guideline, ROM exercises should be performed more frequently on a daily basis than strengthening exercises. Rehabilitation tools, such as a stick, a pulley, and, eventually, weights and elastic bands facilitate the home exercise program.

Specific accommodations are made when a biceps tenotomy or tenodesis is performed and when a subscapularis repair is performed. When the biceps is treated as part of an arthroscopic rotator cuff repair, either at its superior glenoid anchor or along the course of the tendon with a tenodesis or tenotomy, biceps-active components of the program are not started until healing progresses. The subscapularis is more often fixed as part of an arthroscopic repair of the posterosuperior rotator cuff than as an isolated repair. Under these circumstances, passive external rotation (ER) is progressed more slowly and active IR is delayed.[5] More emphasis is placed on the specific arthroscopic subscapularis repair protocol if it is repaired in the setting of a small supraspinatus repair than if the subscapularis is repaired in the setting of a massive supraspinatus and infraspinatus repair. In addition, the repair of a full-thickness subscapularis tear that involves 100% of the tendon is progressed more slowly than a full-thickness subscapularis tear that involves only the upper 50% of the tendon. This is similar in concept to the rehabilitation approach following the repair of a large or massive tear involving the supraspinatus and infraspinatus compared with the approach for a small or medium tear of the supraspinatus.

An understanding of a tissue's response to injury and its mechanisms of repair is quite helpful when designing a rehabilitation program. The healing process is much the same for all soft tissues, with a surgical repair creating a more controlled healing environment.[6] The initial inflammatory phase is followed by a reparative phase. This healing tissue is weaker and at risk of re-tear early on, so a careful regimen to avoid overstressing the repaired tissue is essential. A 6-week time frame for this initial period has been described. The remodeling phase then progresses for many months and will influence decisions regarding progression of the rehabilitation program and return to activities.

25.2. Suggested Postoperative Protocols

The protocols are divided into sections as follows: repair of small tears (<1 cm), medium tears (1–3 cm), large (3–5 cm), and massive tears (>5 cm), subscapularis tears, and biceps tears. (The indications of tear size for separate categories are general approximations.) Postoperative rehabilitation for repair of a small rotator cuff tear repaired arthroscopically is described in full detail. Postoperative rehabilitation of medium, large, and massive rotator cuff tears repaired arthroscopically is described by how it differs from the protocol for repair of a small tear. Postoperative protocols in outline form can be viewed at www.LIshoulder.com/ARCRrehab.htm. The suggested protocols are not intended to include each and every detail for each time period described but are intended to include the most relevant steps. The time period refers to the 7 days of the particular week noted. As examples, Post-op Week 1 includes days 1 to 7 and Post-op Week 7 includes days 43 to 49.

25.2.1. Arthroscopic Repair of Isolated Small Tear Protocol

During Post-op Week 1, there is a necessary focus on pain control for patient comfort. Application of cryocompression to decrease pain and swelling, including the extravasated arthroscopic fluid, is routine. Pendulum exercises begin as simply dangling of the arm, and then progress. Gentle pain-free passive ROM by the shoulder surgeon and physical therapist begins in the supine position within the defined limits. During Post-op Week 2, supine active-assisted ROM in ER with a stick and in self-assisted elevation is started (Figure 25.1). External rotation should be initiated with the arm abducted 30° to 45° from the body to diminish tension on the repair.[7] Active ROM of the wrist and hand, as well as active ROM of the elbow, assuming the biceps tendon or the superior labrum is not involved in the repair, is instructed. Modalities, such as electrical stimulation, can be utilized for pain modulation. Clear instructions about restrictions include avoiding any lifting, pushing, pulling, carrying, or any active ROM. To prevent extension of the arm, particularly in the supine position, a pillow is placed behind the elbow to keep the arm more level with the abdomen. Internal rotation beyond the stomach and sleeping on the operated shoulder are also avoided.

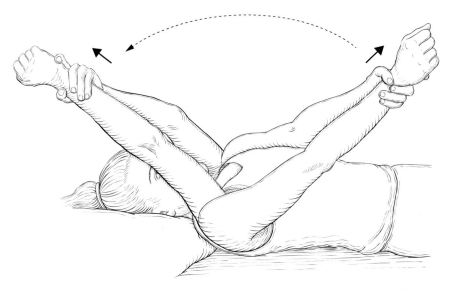

FIGURE 25.1. Supine self-assisted elevation is demonstrated, with the well arm elevating the operated arm. The operated arm starts away from the body toward the scapula plane.

During Post-op Weeks 3 and 4, pain control and the various alternatives available to the patient, are more established and better understood by the patient. Pendulum exercises continue, and supine active-assisted ROM in ER with a stick and in self-assisted elevation are progressed within the determined ranges. The use of the pulley in the scapular plane can be considered if there is quality ROM (with minimal scapula hike indicating limited scapula substitution pattern) and if its use does not cause substantial pain. Pain-free submaximal isometrics of the uninvolved tendons can also be added. Scapula control exercises in the side-lying position with the physical therapist are added to restore the scapula musculature necessary to re-establish scapula stability and the force couples needed for arm elevation.[8,9] Active ROM of the elbow, wrist, and hand continues. Restrictions from Post-op Week 1 are maintained.

During Post-op Weeks 5 and 6, the patient should work toward achieving near-full ROM. Moist heat may be utilized prior to ROM exercises. If the patient is having difficulty restoring ROM, pain can often be a limiting factor that must be addressed or the rehabilitation slowed down. Premedication with analgesics prior to exercises should be utilized. Supine stick active-assisted elevation is added and previous active-assisted ROM exercises are continued. Glenohumeral and rhythmic stabilization exercises are initiated to restore proprioception and neuromuscular control of the shoulder.[10] Prone row and prone extension active ROM to neutral without weight may begin, and active ROM in the side-lying position for internal and external rotation may be considered in this stage. Lifting restrictions continue, as well as continued avoidance of both extension beyond neutral and IR. Patients who feel they should be progressing faster are informed of the healing process, reminded of the gains they have made, and cautioned against advancing beyond the instructed limits.

During Post-op Week 7, the next phase begins and the emphasis of the rehabilitation program transitions to restoring active ROM. Active ROM with elevation in the scapula plane is initiated, beginning with gravity-eliminated (supine and possibly side-lying) positions and progressed (to semi-recumbent, sitting, and/or standing).[3] Elevation, with the elbow flexed initially to shorten the lever arm, will minimize the demand on the glenohumeral musculature.[11,12] Supported active ROM exercises have been demonstrated to have less electromyographic activity on the supraspinatus than unsupported exercises and, therefore, should be used initially to restore active ROM.[12] These principles are even more important with larger tears. Rarely, active ROM is added earlier than Week 7, based on the milestones achieved and the shoulder surgeon's comfort. No weights or resistive bands are used at this point. The weight of the arm, especially in a large individual, is sufficient. Passive ROM and active-assisted ROM are added for internal rotation and extension. Passive ROM and active-assisted ROM for all planes of motion are continued and advanced to maximize and maintain ROM. Light biceps (if not contraindicated) and triceps strengthening is added.

During Post-op Weeks 8 and 9, light resistive shoulder strengthening exercises are initiated if the patient demonstrates normal active ROM in these planes without abnormal or substituted movement patterns.[8] Starting with a 1-lb dumbbell, side-lying IR and ER exercises, prone extension and row exercises, and supine scapula protraction (punches) exercises are added. Elastic bands, beginning with the least resistance, are used for ER, IR, shoulder extension to neutral, scapula retraction, and advanced scapula protraction exercises (standing scapula punches and dynamic hug).[13] Elevation in the scapula plane in the "open can," thumb-up, position (Figure 25.2) is performed initially without weight.[14,15] Only when normal active ROM without substitution patterns (scapula hike) is present is resistance added in the form of light weights or low resistance bands. Repetitions and sets of exercises are increased before weight or resistance is increased. Scapula stabilization exercises are continued and progressed. An upper body ergometer (UBE) is added later, which helps with motion but also contributes to muscular endurance. Closed chain exercises are also performed. Advanced stretching in all planes is encouraged, especially for the posterior shoulder and capsule, such as with the sleeper stretch (Figure 25.3).

During Post-op Weeks 10 and 11, the strengthening program is progressed based on the patient's achievements. Stretching and closed chain exercises continue, and proprioceptive neuromuscular facilitation (PNF)

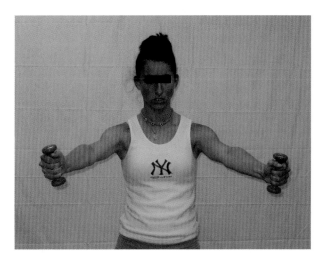

FIGURE 25.2. Elevation in the scapula plane in the "open can," thumb-up position.

patterns are started carefully. By Post-op Weeks 12 and 13, strengthening exercises are advanced, as are the open and closed chain exercises. Range of motion in all planes is monitored to ensure motion is maintained. Any deficiencies are addressed. Exercises directed at specific functional

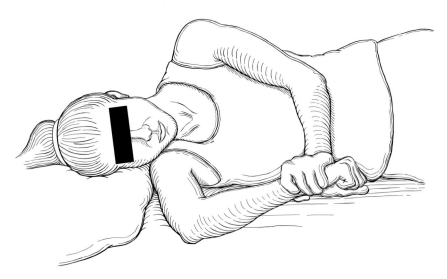

FIGURE 25.3. The sleeper stretch is used to stretch the posterior shoulder and capsule. The patient is lying on the operated side, which stabilizes the scapula, and the shoulder and elbow are at 90° angles. The well arm is used to internally rotate the operated arm toward the table until the stretch is felt in the posterior shoulder; then the position is held for 15 to 30s.

activities are added as appropriate, with considerations given for return to work. Sports-specific activities and plyometrics are added. For the recreational athlete, return to lower-extremity sports can be considered by 4 to 5 months, with upper extremity sports involving the operated extremity delayed to 7 to 9 months, if strength, endurance, and motion allow. Elite athletes will require additional training and preparation for return to sports participation, and these programs are not addressed here.

As far as work is concerned, return to work in a sling can begin when desired. An executive who can be driven to work and perform the required duties while maintaining the sling can start within the first weeks. However, the sooner a patient returns to work, the less time he or she has available to focus on the important recovery process. Return to work for a manual laborer who does not have a light duty job option that precludes lifting with the operated arm should be delayed until the milestones are achieved that will allow him or her to perform the particular work duties required. These include, primarily, the weight requirements, activity in the overhead position, or frequency of repetitions that certain jobs entail. The earliest this should be achieved is 4 months, but it often takes 5 to 6 months to achieve the necessary fitness for return to work with limited risk for the heavy duty manual laborer.

25.2.2. Arthroscopic Repair of Isolated Medium Tear Protocol

The general guidelines for rehabilitation following repair of a medium tear include the same steps as the repair protocol following a small tear, but introduce many steps at later stages. Post-op Weeks 1 and 2, the guidelines are the same, except self-assisted supine elevation is delayed until Post-op Weeks 3 and 4. Range of motion is often limited more with repair of medium tears, based on the intraoperative assessment, than with repair of small tears. The shoulder surgeon needs to guide the physical therapist and instruct the patient more carefully about advancing ROM limits in the earlier stages, and all should expect the return of motion to take longer with tears of greater size. Isometrics and pulley exercises are delayed from Post-op Weeks 3 and 4 to the next time period. Glenohumeral and rhythmic stabilization exercises, as well as prone row and prone extension to neutral, can begin in Post-op Week 7, but side-lying IR and ER active ROM exercises are delayed until the next time period. The sling is now used only for activity in public, but restrictions on lifting continue. Initiating active ROM in the supine position may begin Post-op Weeks 8 and 9 in some repairs of medium tears, but this might be delayed in others, and ROM is always progressed at a slower pace. This trend continues into Post-op Weeks 10 and 11. Stretching continues with particular attention paid to the posterior capsule. Strengthening of tendons not involved in the repair is started by now, but strengthening for elevation is usually delayed into

Post-op Weeks 12 and 13, and only if nearly normal active ROM, without substitution patterns, has been achieved. Introduction of PNF patterns, closed chain exercises, and the UBE may also begin in this time period, again if nearly normal active ROM, without substitution patterns, has been achieved. Guidelines for Post-op Weeks 14 and 15 include light functional activity as appropriate. Considerations for return to work in light duty manual labor settings are made, but heavy duty manual labor is usually delayed, until at least 5 to 6 months following repair, with erring on the side of caution.

25.2.3. Arthroscopic Repair of Isolated Large and Massive Tear Protocol

The general guidelines for rehabilitation following repair of large and massive tears include the same steps as the protocol following repair of small tears but introduce most steps at later stages. Post-op Weeks 1 and 2 include only wrist and hand exercises and elbow exercises if not contra-indicated. The postoperative course is much slower, with dangling the arm at the side only allowed for showering. In many cases, a supervised therapy program is not initiated until 5 to 8 weeks postoperatively. In these types of repairs, intraoperative assessment and patient issues are more important factors to consider concerning the start of the supervised rehabilitation program. Therefore, large repairs might begin pendulums and passive ROM exercises by Post-op Weeks 5 and 6 within determined limits, such as 120° of elevation and 30° of ER. For massive tears, this could be Post-op Week 7 or later. However, if the patient has stiffness that concerns the shoulder surgeon on follow-up at about Post-op Week 4, that is, substantial limitations of supine elevation and external rotation, gentle passive ROM may be initiated sooner. By Post-op Weeks 8 and 9, supine active-assisted ER exercises are often started prior to elevation exercises to protect the repair. Slow, incremental increases in the ROM limits are observed. This is when communication between the shoulder surgeon and physical thera-pist is even more important. If ROM exceeds the set limits by a substantial amount, the integrity of the repair may be compromised. Pulleys can be considered if there is minimal pain and sufficient ROM to perform this exercise. Scapula controlled exercises with the physical therapist can begin, as well as submaximal isometrics of uninvolved tendons. Restrictions often continue until post-op Weeks 10 and 11, including avoiding extension, IR, active ROM, lifting, pushing, pulling, and carrying.

Glenohumeral and rhythmic stabilization exercises, as well as prone row and prone extension to neutral can begin in Post-op Weeks 10 and 11. Gravity-eliminated active ROM exercises for elevation, ER and IR, are considered if patient progress allows. Light biceps and triceps strengthen-ing exercises are also started now, and delayed until this point simply to keep weights and bands away from the patient. By Post-op Weeks 12 and

13, restoring full passive ROM is a goal. Active ROM is progressed to include gravity-resisted positions. Weights and bands are not added until nearly normal active ROM is achieved. However, side-lying IR and ER exercises, as well as scapula strengthening exercises, may begin without nearly normal active ROM, as these exercises will assist with gaining strength in elevation. Stretching continues, with particular attention paid to the posterior capsule. By Post-op Weeks 14 and 15, active ROM in elevation is progressed with light resistance as able, and PNF patterns, closed chain exercises, and UBE are considered. The extended rehabilitation into later weeks includes adding, when able, light functional activities. As opposed to repairs of small and medium tears, the patient must continue both stretching exercises, to maintain ROM and flexibility, and strengthening exercises for a longer period of time. Patients should not expect full return of strength and endurance, particularly if the tear is longstanding. However, substantial improvement over the preoperative function is usual with successful repairs, even including light activities in the overhead position. Light duty manual labor may resume by 5 to 6 months. Patients with heavy duty manual labor jobs may never return to their previous level of function.

The above protocol is not altered when the subscapularis is involved in the repair. The restrictions on passive ER into Post-op Weeks 8 and 9, and active IR into Post-op Weeks 10 and 11, afford the necessary protection of the subscapularis repair. It is important that the physical therapist is aware of this component of the repair. There are occasions when 3.5-cm tear, technically defined as large, that can be easily mobilized and securely repaired, will be advanced during the mid to late stages of rehabilitation at a slightly faster pace when compared to the rehabilitation of a chronic tear greater than 5-cm, technically defined as massive, following its repair. This highlights the importance of good clinical judgment and continued communication between the shoulder surgeon and physical therapist.

25.2.4. Arthroscopic Repair of Isolated Subscapularis Tear Protocol

The general guidelines for rehabilitation following repair of an isolated subscapularis tear vary based on both the amount of tendon involved in the tear pattern and the repair. The repair of an isolated subscapularis tear that involves 50% of the tendon should be more secure than repair of an isolated subscapularis tear that involves 100% of the tendon. Therefore, the protocols are divided into these two categories.

During Post-op Weeks 1 and 2 following the repair of an isolated subscapularis tear that involves 50% of the tendon, passive ROM is begun within limits, especially ER, as determined by the shoulder surgeon's intraoperative assessment, which must be communicated to the physical therapist. Supine active-assisted ER is maintained within the established limits. Supine active-assisted elevation is started and advanced as tolerated, unless limits are established by the shoulder surgeon. Wrist and hand active ROM begins, and the elbow is included if the biceps is not involved in the repair. Restrictions include any active ROM, especially IR; extension and IR beyond the stomach; sleeping on the involved side; and any lifting, pushing, pulling, and carrying. In Post-op Weeks 3 and 4, passive and active-assisted ROM in elevation is usually advanced. Limits are maintained for ER as previously established. Pulley exercise in the scapula plane is added if there is quality ROM (limited scapula hike) and minimal pain. Scapula-control exercises in the side-lying position can begin. Submaximal isometrics, excluding IR, are initiated. Otherwise, the same restrictions from Post-op Weeks 1 and 2 continue.

In Post-op Weeks 5 and 6, active ROM is started in all planes, except IR, beginning with gravity-eliminated positions. For example, this includes ER, as the posterosuperior cuff was not involved in the repair. Limits in ER, and possibly elevation, can be increased by the shoulder surgeon but still need to be monitored. Rhythmic stabilization exercises are started, with the exception of those involving IR. Lifting, pushing, pulling, and carrying continue to be restricted, as is active IR. At Post-op Week 7, the limits of passive and supine active-assisted ER can be advanced as tolerated. Active and passive extension past neutral and passive IR beyond the stomach are added. Strengthening of the posterior shoulder muscles (external rotators, posterior deltoid, and scapula muscles) maybe added when nearly full active ROM, excluding IR, is achieved, beginning with light resistance and progressed over time. Light biceps (if not contraindicated) and triceps strengthening are added. Active IR is carefully added in a gravity-eliminated position, such as sitting. At this point, the sling is usually discontinued.

During Post-op Weeks 8 and 9, a goal is to progress toward full passive, and active ROM in all planes. Stretching of the posterior capsule should be considered, though the patient may not tolerate these positions for stretching in this time period. Active IR is progressed from sitting to lying on the affected side to add the element of gravity. Strengthening of the uninvolved tendons is progressed, including the supraspinatus and deltoid, and UBE is added. Post-op Weeks 10 and 11 add resistive IR exercises and continues to maximize ROM and strength in all planes.[16] Closed chain exercises and PNF patterns can be added as tolerated. During Post-op Weeks 12 and 13, ROM is maintained and strengthening continues. Light functional activities are considered. For Post-op Weeks 14 and 15 and beyond, exercises directed at specific functional activities are added as appropriate, with considerations given for return to manual labor. Sports-specific activities and plyometrics are added. For the recreational athlete, return to lower-extremity sports can be considered by 4 to 5 months, with upper extremity sports involving the operated extremity delayed to 7 to 9 months, if strength, endurance, and motion allow.

Following the repair of an isolated subscapularis tear that involves 100% of the tendon, a slower course is followed. Passive and active-assisted ER might begin in Post-op Weeks 3 and 4 if the quality of the tissue and repair allow, but are often delayed until Post-op Weeks 5 and 6 within limits defined by the shoulder surgeon. These limits continue into Post-op Weeks

8 and 9, and possibly longer, again, if the quality of the tissue and repair dictates. However, active ER within these limits can start by Post-op Weeks 5 and 6. Passive and active-assisted elevation might also begin Post-op Weeks 3 and 4, but at times are delayed until Post-op Weeks 5 and 6 within limits defined by the shoulder surgeon. These limits continue into Post-op Week 7 and are progressed more slowly. Active elevation may be delayed until Post-op Weeks 8 and 9 and progressed only if quality ROM exists without substitution patterns. Passive and active-assisted IR, as well as extension beyond neutral, is delayed until Post-op Weeks 8 and 9. Furthermore, active IR is often delayed until Post-op Weeks 10 and 11.

Strengthening of the posterior shoulder muscles (external rotators, posterior deltoid, and scapula muscles) may be added when nearly full active ROM, excluding IR, is achieved, beginning with light resistance and progressed over time. This is often Post-op Weeks 10 and 11, but may be Post-op Weeks 8 and 9. Light biceps (if not contraindicated) and triceps strengthening are added at the same time. Post-op Weeks 12 and 13 add resistive IR exercises and continues to maximize ROM and strength in all planes. Closed chain exercises and PNF patterns can be added as tolerated. During Post-op Weeks 14 and 15, ROM is maintained and strengthening continues. Light functional activities are considered. For Post-op Week 16 and beyond, exercises directed at specific functional activities are added as appropriate, with considerations given for return to work by 4 to 5 months for light duty manual labor and later for heavy duty manual labor. Patients should not expect full return of strength and endurance, particularly if the tear is longstanding, though substantial improvement over the preoperative function is usual with successful repairs.

25.2.5. Arthroscopic Treatment of Isolated Long Head of Biceps Tear Protocol

Rehabilitation following an isolated biceps tenodesis would progress in a fashion somewhat faster than that of a repair of a small supraspinatus tear. Passive and active-assisted ROM are progressed as tolerated in all planes, except for extension in the first few weeks. Limitations for active motion include active and resistive elbow flexion and supination for 6 weeks, as well as resisted shoulder elevation.[17] At Post-op Week 7, active elbow flexion is initiated. During Post-op Weeks 8 and 9, light resistance can be added judiciously if there are no symptoms with active elbow flexion. Following an isolated biceps tenotomy, the limiting factor is pain in the biceps. As pain resolves, active elbow flexion is initiated, often by Post-op Weeks 5 and 6, followed by the addition of light resistance. When biceps tenodesis is performed in addition to a rotator cuff repair, the repair protocol is followed, except that active elbow flexion is delayed for 6 weeks. In the presence of biceps tenotomy and rotator cuff repair, active elbow flexion is delayed until biceps pain resolves.

25.3. Conclusions

Postoperative guidelines following arthroscopic repair of small, medium, large, and massive tears, as well as subscapularis repairs and biceps tenodesis or tenotomy, follow the same general principles that are introduced at different timeframes. However, the guidelines must be adapted to each individual patient and each specific tear to ensure the best possible outcome. While it clearly demands much of the patient during the postoperative recovery, postoperative rehabilitation also requires an investment of time by the shoulder surgeon and the physical therapist, along with a high level of trust and an open line of communication. The goals should be to promote healing of the repair first, then to restore mobility before strengthening is emphasized. Balancing these three important goals in each individual patient reflects the art of the process.

References

1. Neer CS II. Shoulder rehabilitation. In: The shoulder. Philadelphia: Saunders; 1990:487.
2. Savoie FH, Fields LD, Jenkins N, et al. The pain control infusion pump for postoperative pain control in shoulder surgery. Arthroscopy 2000;16: 339–342.
3. Leggin BG, Kelley MJ. Rehabilitation of the shoulder following rotator cuff surgery. The University of Pennsylvania Orthop J 2000;13:10–17.
4. McCann PD, Wooten ME, Kadaba MP, Bigliani LU. A kinematic and electromyographic study of shoulder rehabilitation exercises. Clin Orthop 1993;288:177–188.
5. Ticker JB, Warner JJP. Single-tendon tears of the rotator cuff: Evaluation and treatment of subscapularis tears and principles of treatment for supraspinatus tears. Orthop Clin North Am 1997;28:99–116.
6. Johnson DL, Ticker JB. Soft-tissue physiology and repair. In: Beaty JR, ed. Orthopaedic Knowledge Update 6. Rosemont, IL: AAOS Press; 1999: 1–18.
7. Hatakeyama Y, Itoi E, Pradhan RL, Urayama M, Sato K. Effect of arm elevation and rotation of the strain in the repaired rotator cuff tendon: a cadaveric study. Am J Sports Med 2001;29:788–794.
8. Magarey ME, Jones MA. Dynamic evaluation and early management of altered motor control around the shoulder complex. Man Ther 2003;8: 195–206.
9. Kibler WB. The role of the scapula in athletic shoulder function. Am J Sports Med 1998;26:325–339.
10. Wilk KE, Harrelson GL, Arrigo C. Shoulder rehabilitation. In: Andrews JR, Wilk KE, Harrelson GL, eds. Physical rehabilitation of the injured athlete, 3rd ed. Philadelphia: Elsevier; 2004:513–589.
11. Otis JC, Jiang CC, Wickiewicz TL, et al. Changes in the moment arms of the rotator cuff and deltoid muscles with abduction and rotation. J Bone Joint Surg Am 1994;76:667–676.

12. Wise MB, Uhl TL, Mattacola CG, et al. The effect of limb support on muscle activation during shoulder exercises. J Shoulder Elbow Surg 2004; 13:614–620.
13. Decker MJ, Hintermeister RA, Faber KJ, et al. Serratus anterior muscle activity during selected rehabilitation exercises. Am J Sports Med 1999;27: 784–791.
14. Poppen NK, Walker PS. Forces at the glenohumeral joint. Clin Orthop 1978;135:165–170.
15. Reinold MM. Biomechanical implications in shoulder and knee rehabilitation. In: Andrews JR, Wilk KE, Harrelson GL, eds. Physical rehabilitation of the injured athlete, 3rd ed. Philadelphia: Elsevier; 2004:34–50.
16. Decker MJ, Tokish JM, Ellis HB, et al. Subscapularis muscle activity during selected rehabilitation exercises. Am J Sports Med 2003;31:126–134.
17. Romeo AA, Mazzocca AD, Tauro JC. Arthroscopic biceps tenodesis. Arthroscopy 2004;20:206–213.

26
How to Avoid and Manage Complications in Arthroscopic Rotator Cuff Repair

Wesley M. Nottage

Complications associated with arthroscopic shoulder surgery have been reviewed by numerous authors. Where most review studies suggest the rate varies between 5.8% and 9.5%, all recent review studies published make note of underreporting of complications and lack of consensus over what is considered a complication, which makes accurate assessment of the true rate of complications difficult.

Shoulder arthroscopy presents an increased risk of complications over that of knee arthroscopy, specifically in terms of neurological and vascular injury; fluid extravasation; compromised airways; acquired postoperative stiffness; iatrogenic tendon, joint, or cartilage injury; and equipment failure. Newer techniques involving specific anchors and fixation devices tend to make the procedures more complex and lead to problems related to unique implant complications.

Shoulder arthroscopic complication rates have been described in the literature; the first report of complications for all arthroscopic surgery was made by Small in 1986.[1] He noted a complication rate of 5.3% in the shoulder, which he attributed to the use of shoulder stabilization staples, which decreased to a 0.7% incidence of complications with subacromial surgery. A subsequent study by Small in 1988[2] reviewed complications in arthroscopic surgery limited to experienced arthroscopists and noted a 5.2% incidence of complications. These initial studies established the relative safety of the procedures as well as a benchmark for shoulder arthroscopy. Complications following shoulder arthroscopy have ranged from 5.3% to 9.5%, but this accounts for all types of arthroscopic shoulder surgery.

Several review articles have addressed shoulder surgical complications. Curtis and colleagues reviewed 660 cases presented in abstract form, noting an overall complication rate of 6.5%.[3] McFarland and colleagues reviewed the literature in 1997 and noted complication rates for neurological injury from 0% to 30% and infection rates from 0.04% to 0.23%.[4] Rupp and colleagues reviewed specifically subacromial complications, noting in 108 procedures two infections (2%), adhesive capsulitis (3%), neurological injury (1%), and acromial fracture (1%).[5]

Berjan and colleagues reviewed 179 shoulder arthroscopies, noting a complication rate of 9.49% and a higher rate for arthroscopic procedures of 10.6% than for combined arthroscopic and open procedures (5.26%).[6]

Mohammed and colleagues reviewed 9 "unusual" complications in 4000 shoulder arthroscopies.[7] Nerve injuries were noted in three (two with ultimate improvement), three skin burns secondary to electrocautery, and two complications related to intraoperative swelling. One patient had late severe heterotopic ossification.

Muller and Landsiedl reported 846 shoulder arthroscopies, noting 48 complications in 44 patients for an incidence of 5.8%.[8] Complications included neurological injuries, stiffness, instrument breakage, and non-technical complications such as drug allergy, nerve injury secondary to scalene block, and infection; 43% of the total complications were related to infection (2.4% overall).

Comparison of these and other shoulder arthroscopy reviews is difficult because of underreporting. Definition of what exactly constitutes a complication differs as well; several authors do not consider stiffness a complication, where as other reviewers include it.

Shoulder arthroscopy complications can be divided into three groups: complications typical of all surgery, complications related specifically to arthroscopic shoulder surgery, and complications related specifically to arthroscopic rotator cuff repair.

26.1. Nonspecific Surgical Complications

26.1.1. Infection

The infection rate with shoulder arthroscopy is low; the benchmark was set by Johnson with an infection rate of 0.04% with all types of arthroscopies using glutaraldehyde sterilization.[9] Other authors have confirmed this: DiAngelo and Olgivie-Harris noted an infection rate of 0.23%; this was sufficient enough for them to suggest use of perioperative antibiotics.[10] Review articles have noted infection rates ranging from 0% to 3.4%. It seems wise to include prophylactic antibiotics for any shoulder arthroscopic procedure simply to lower the risk, as noted in this study.

26.1.2. Anesthetic-Related Complications

Anesthetic-related complications have received numerous anecdotal reports. Reported complications include fatal air embolism, tracheal compression (due to fluid extravasation), pneumothorax, quadriparesis with the beach chair position, complete airway obstruction secondary to extravasation of fluid in the mediastinum, potentially fatal epinephrine-induced arrhythmias, negative pressure pulmonary edema, and pneumomediastinum.[11-18] It is considered advisable not to perform gas arthroscopy in the shoulder. In a pump or gravity system, maintaining the inflow pressure at 60 mm Hg while the anesthesiologist maintains the systolic pressure around 90 mm Hg seems to provide a optimal compromise to maintain a visual field and control bleeding, while not pumping excessive fluid into the soft tissues.

Complications related to regional anesthesia are rare, but temporary and permanent neurological injuries have been reported due to direct nerve injury.[19] The ultimate choice of anesthesia and risk must be assessed by the patient, surgeon, and anesthesiologist.

26.2. Specific Shoulder Arthroscopy Complications

26.2.1. Neurological Injury

Neurological injury remains the primary area of concern with shoulder arthroscopy. The injury rate is reported as high as 30%, noting that most of these are believed to be neuropraxias. The reported mechanisms for injury include excessive traction in the lateral position, direct nerve injury, compression secondary to fluid extravasation, tourniquetlike problems associated with wrapping the operated extremity for arm traction, and regional sympathic dystrophy. Klein and colleagues reviewed the use of arm traction and noted that positions of increased extension and decreased abduction produced increased load on the brachial plexus.[20] The amount of axial arm traction in the lateral decubitus position also can affect plexus and forearm skin cutaneous nerve strain. Techniques have been reported using typically 10 to 12 lbs of axial arm traction in the decubitus position.

Decreasing plexus strain can be accomplished by proper head and neck support (restrained in slight lateral flexion towards the operative side) and by keeping the arm in a more forward flexed and abducted position (45–45) as a compromise to avoid excessive neurological traction and yet allow adequate visualization in lateral decubitus. A guideline is the appearance of relaxed skin folds on the operative side.

Lateral decubitus arm traction should really be "balanced suspension" commonly using 5 to 7 lbs of axial traction to counterbalance the arm weight and minimize the shear on the forearm skin nerves.

Lateral decubitus arthroscopy has had reported transient neurological injury in the dependent leg (peroneal nerve, lateral femoral cutaneous nerve), which can be minimized by appropriate attention to padding of the iliac wing and peroneal nerve.

Direct cutaneous shoulder nerve injury has been noted by Segmuller and colleagues, who described sensory deficits in 7% of their patients.[21] They also described cutaneous lesions of the shoulder and arm after arthroscopic shoulder surgery and specific involvement of branches of the axillary nerve as complications. Specifically, they noted that it may occur without motor branch involvement, describing a pattern of medial brachial cutaneous nerve, lateral brachial cutaneous nerve, and axillary posterior brachial cutaneous nerve from the radial and antebrachial cutaneous nerve from the radial nerve. This author hypothesized the most likely cause of injury was at the portal sites, noting that an overall complication rate was 7% in 304 patients.

Described mechanisms for nerve injury with shoulder arthroscopy include traumatic injury at the portal site, excessive traction, manipulation of the shoulder under general anesthesia, and extravasation of fluid with joint distension.

Permanent direct neurological injury from portals is unusual, but this possibility underscores the importance of careful portal placement. Although specific arthroscopic portals have been described in the literature in an attempt to minimize damage to nerves,[22] positioning of the patient's arm in surgery may change the position of the nerve relative to the portals, especially with arm abduction and the axillary nerve.

Reflex sympathetic dystrophy continues to be a poorly defined and problematic neurological syndrome that is rarely associated with shoulder arthroscopy.

Attention to proper head and neck positioning, avoidance of heavy and long amounts of arm traction, maintaining a lower plexus strain position for the arm in lateral decubitus, and limiting fluid extravasation by running lower inflow pressures (such as 60 mm Hg) all minimize complications. Appropriate padding in the traction device of the wrist and the dependent extremity is required to minimize other nerve injuries. Furthermore, care must be taken in portal placement and arm positioning with awareness at all times of adjacent neurological structures.

26.2.2. Portals

Abnormal portal placement or positioning has led to iatrogenic rotator cuff tears as well. Norwood and Fowler have described a case of iatrogenic rotator cuff tear due hypothesized to be due to portal placement in the infraspinatus tendon.[23]

26.2.3. Vascular Complications

Few vascular complications have been reported. Deep venous thrombosis in a patient with a hypercoaguable state was described by Burkhart.[24] Cameron reported a single venous pseudoaneurysm.[25] Curtis described cephalic vein laceration without residual morbidity.[3]

26.2.4. Fluid Dynamics

Fluid extravasation complications have been reported, producing problem-atic airways.[12,15] Although local increased pressures occur in the deltoid area with extravasation, little sequelae appear to occur from this. It is important, however, to avoid excessive extravasation that could, in rare instances, result in neurological or respiratory problems. Skin necrosis secondary to excessive swelling has been reported by Mohammed and colleagues.[7]

Maintaining a clear visual field can be challenging for the inexperienced arthroscopist, but this can be aided by minimizing openings into the opera-tive cavity, using gasketed portals, limiting suction on surgical devices, and maintaining a systolic blood pressure of 90 mm Hg with a matched inflow of 60 mm Hg.

Inflow pressures in the 60 mm Hg range seem to be a reasonable com-promise in controlling extravasation and allowing visualization. Avoid multiple portals to minimize leakage and use gasketed portals. Minimize suction whenever in a cavity to keep the distention in the cavity to aid in visualization and tamponade vessels.

26.2.5. Stiffness

Shoulder stiffness is one of the most common problems of shoulder surgery in general, as well in as shoulder arthroscopy, usually presenting as a post-operative morbidity that may have significant residuals. Although several authors do not consider this a complication, reviews suggest rates range from 2.7% to 15.0%. Stiffness can occur for numerous reasons, including the tightening of closing a cuff defect, the associated capsulitis with rotator cuff disease, and significant postoperative immobilization.

Analogous to knee surgery, early motion in protected directions seems to control this complication best, exhort the patient to establish early passive motion in safe directions as soon as possible. Subacromial surgery without cuff repair should allow immediate, complete, full active, and passive motion. A rotator cuff repair will limit the active range but should allow significant passive motion in multiple planes.

26.3. Complications

Arthroscopic rotator cuff repair is a technique still in evolution. Few pub-lications exist regarding the outcomes of this challenging technique as well as its specific complications. Complications reported include those of loose hardware in 0.75% and failure of the repair in 3%.

Savoie, Brisland, and Field have reported their complications in arthroscopic rotator cuff repairs.[26] They reviewed 263 patients undergoing shoulder arthroscopic rotator cuff repair and defined 12 complications for an incidence of 4.5%. Three were believed to be major complications, including one deltoid detachment and two anchor displacements. Minor complications, numbering nine, included three patients with stiffness, three patients with synovitis due to bioabsorbable cuff tacks, and three infections requiring oral antibiotics.

26.3.1. Subacromial Decompression

Arthroscopic rotator cuff repair commonly includes an arthroscopic subacromial decompression. Bonsell reported a complication for arthroscopic subacromial decompression of a case of deltoid detachment recognized intraoperatively and repaired open.[27] This can be minimized by releasing the coracoacromial ligament under direct vision before removing bone, using a small tip device for the release.

Reported complications of arthroscopic subacromial decompression include inadequate acromial resection, acromial fracture (Figure 26.1), acromioclavicular symptoms post–subacromial decompression, and heterotopic ossification.[26,28–30]

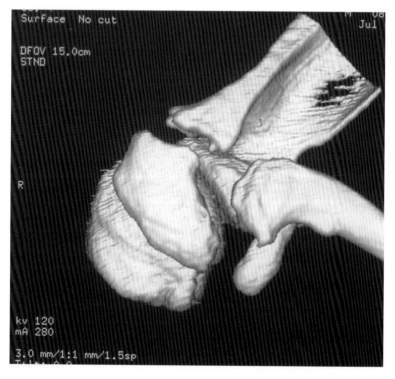

FIGURE 26.1. Acromial fracture post–subacromial decompression. (Reprinted from Arthroscopy, V18(2); Weber, Abrams, Nottage, Complications associated with arthroscopic surgery, pp 88–95, Copyright 2002, with permission from the Arthroscopic Association of North America.)

Fracture of the acromion has been associated with arthroscopic and open acromioplasty as part of an arthroscopic rotator cuff repair. This is usually due to technical error due to overzealous resection, especially in a patient with a thin acromion not recognized preoperatively. This can be minimized by careful attention to detail with assessment of acromial thickness on preoperative films and adherence to the "posterior cutting block" technique of acromial resection described by Sampson.[31]

Residual acromioclavicular joint symptoms secondary to violation of the acromioclavicular joint during acromioplasty have been described by Fischer and colleagues;[29] this complication remains relatively infrequent. The best way to address inferior acromioclavicular joint osteophytes remains unanswered. Several authors recommended complete acromioclavicular resection whenever the joint is exposed; others, however base the need for such resection on preoperative clinical symptoms.

26.3.2. Anchor-Related Complications

Bioabsorbable implants have become commonplace for the management of shoulder rotator cuff injuries. They are specifically designed to allow adequate time for healing as well as gradual resorption. Changes in the chemical make-up of these devices have favored fewer problems with resorption and synovitis. A case report provided by Glueck and colleagues described extensive osteolysis after rotator cuff repair of the bioabsorbable suture anchor [poly(L-lactide-co-D, L-lactide) (PLDLA) material].[32] Cummins and colleagues compared bioabsorbable screws with metal suture anchors in an in vivo and ex vivo study, noting poor outcomes and higher rate of secondary surgery with the bioabsorbable screws; however, they did not specifically address osteolytic changes.[33] The bioabsorbable screw chosen in this study was one in which the head of the screw is used to fix the tissue as opposed to a true suture anchor. Although unproven, authors have suggested that resorbable anchors may produce osteolysis not solely on the basis of resorption but in part due to the anchor's mechanical behavior, as opposed to a pure biological response. The complications related to resorption can be entirely avoided by the use of metal suture anchors.

Anchor displacement remains a frustrating problem that is generally tied to placement of anchors in the greater tuberosity area in osteoporotic bone. This is a technical problem that can be seen by the surgeon at the time of implantation. Improved fixation can be obtained by redirecting the anchors into the subchondral bone beneath the humeral head, which will generally provide good fixation (Figure 26.2). Following placement, anchor stability is tested with a firm pull on the sutures. Any evidence of poor fixation should be addressed immediately by redirecting the device.

The reverse problem, failure of the anchor to fully seat in the tuberosity bone and remain proud in the subacromial space, is uncommon and generally occurs in younger patients. An anchor that is directly screwed into bone without predrilling or tapping is at risk to have this happen. We recommend that in bone that will not accept an 18-gauge needle, the bone be predrilled or tapped before using this class of anchor to avoid this problem.

Anchor migration has been described by Mallik and colleagues, who noted the intra-articular migration of a sutureless arthroscopic rotator cuff fixation device in one case, suggesting that there was a learning curve associated with use of this device (Figure 26.3).[34]

The typical technical problem of "off loading an anchor" occurs when transferring a suture for a repair and pulling it through the eyelet of the anchor. This can be prevented by always directly viewing the eyelet with the arthroscope when transferring a suture. There should be no motion at that interface when making the transfer. If any occurs, let go of the suture limb being transferred and use the other suture limb.

Suture fraying and failure can be minimized by use of second generation suture materials, with an inner core covered with an outer lining (Fiber-Wire® or Ultrabraid®). The advent of these suture materials has significantly decreased the risk of premature suture failure. We recommend use of second generation suture materials in arthroscopic rotator cuff repair and reloading of the anchor if needed.

Knot failure and knot tying problems can be minimized by attending to detail and learning the nuances of arthroscopic knot tying. Newer devices are on the market that allow knotless fixation; these include "welding" devices and "knotless" anchors as an alternative. We recommend taking

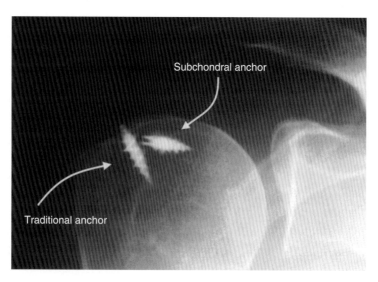

FIGURE 26.2. Correct positioning of anchor in subchondral bone when pullout occurs in cuff repair.

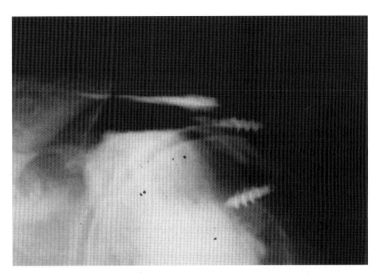

FIGURE 26.3. Loose subacromial anchor from rotator cuff repair. (Reprinted from Arthroscopy, Vol. 18(2); Weber, Abrams, Nottage, Complications associated with arthroscopic surgery, pages 88–95, Copyright 2002, with permission from the Arthroscopic Association of North America.)

the time to learn one sliding and one nonsliding arthroscopic knot and using these as your mainstay, rather than relying on a device to substitute for this surgical skill.

References

1. Small NC. Complications in arthroscopy: the knee and other joints. Arthroscopy 1986;2:253–258.
2. Small N.C. Complications in arthroscopy surgery performed by experienced arthroscopists. Arthroscopy 1988;4:215–221.
3. Curtis AS, Snyder SJ, DelPizzo W, Ferkel RD, Karzel RP. Complications of shoulder arthroscopy. Arthroscopy 1992;8:395.
4. McFarland EG, O'Neill OR, Hsu CY. Complications of shoulder arthroscopy. J South Orthop Assoc 1997;6:190–196.
5. Rupp S, Seil R, Muller B, et al. Complications after subacromial decompression. Arthroscopy 1998;14:445.
6. Berjano P, Gonzalez BG, Olmedo JF, et al. Complications in arthroscopic shoulder surgery. Arthroscopy 1998;14:785–788.
7. Mohammed KD, Hayes MG, Saies AD. Unusual complications of shoulder arthroscopy. J Shoulder Elbow Surg 2000;9:350–352.
8. Muller D, Landsiedl F. Arthroscopy of the shoulder joint, a minimally invasive and harmless procedure? Arthroscopy 2000;16:425.
9. Johnson LL, Schnieder DA, Austin MD, et al. Two percent glutaraldehyde: a disinfectant in arthroscopy in arthroscopic surgery. J Bone Joint Surg Am 1982;64:237–239.

10. DiAngelo CL, Olgivie-Harris DJ. Septic arthritis following arthroscopy with cost/benefit of antibiotic prophylaxis. Arthroscopy 1988;4:10–14.
11. Bauereis C, Schifferdecker A, Buttner J, et al. Fulminant air embolism in arthroscopy of the shoulder using CO2. Anathesiol Intensivmed Notfallmed Schmerzther 1996;31:654–657.
12. Borjat A, Bird P, Ekatodramis SG, et al. Tracheal compression caused by periarticular fluid accumulation: a rare complication of shoulder surgery. J Shoulder Elbow Surg 2000;9:443–445.
13. Burkhart SS, Barnett CR, Synder SS. Transient postoperative blindness as a possible affect of glycine toxicity. Arthroscopy 1990;6:112–114.
14. Ditzel DP, Ciullo JV. Spontaneous pneumothorax after shoulder arthroscopy: report of four cases. Arthroscopy 1996;12:199–202.
15. Hynson JM, Tung A, Guevara J. Complete airway obstruction during arthroscopic shoulder surgery. Anesthesia Anathes Analg 1993;76:875–878.
16. Karns JL. Epinephrine induced potentially lethal arrhythmia during arthroscopic shoulder surgery: a case report. AANA J 1999;67:419–421.
17. Langan NP, Michaels R. Negative pressure pulmonary edema, a complication of shoulder arthroscopy. Am J Orthop 1999;28:56–58.
18. Anderson AF, Alfrey D, Lipscomb AB. Acute pulmonary edema, an unusual complication following arthroscopy: a report of three cases. Arthroscopy 1990;6:235–237.
19. Rodeo SA, Forster RA, Weiland AJ. Neurological complications due to arthroscopy. J Bone Joint Surgery Am 1993;75:917–926.
20. Klein AH, France JC, Mutschler TA, et al. Measurement of brachial plexus strain in arthroscopy of the shoulder. Arthroscopy 1987;3:45–52.
21. Segmuller HE, Alfred SP, Zilio G, et al. Cutaneous nerve lesions of the shoulder and arm after arthroscopic surgery. J Shoulder Elbow Surg 1995; 4:254–258.
22. Nottage WM. Arthroscopic portals anatomy at risk. Orthop Clin Am 1993;24:19–26.
23. Norwood LA, Fowler HL. Rotator cuff tears. A shoulder arthroscopy complication. Am J Sports Med 1989;17:837–841.
24. Burkhart SS. Deep venous thrombosis after shoulder arthroscopy. Arthroscopy 1990;6:61–63.
25. Cameron SE. Venous pseudoaneurysm as a complication of shoulder arthroscopy. J Shoulder Elbow Surg 1996;5:44–46.
26. Savoie FH, Brislin KJ, Field LD. Complications of arthroscopic rotator cuff repairs. Arthroscopy 2004;20(suppl):4–5.
27. Bonsel S. Detached deltoid during arthroscopic subacromial decompression. Arthroscopy 2000;16:745–747.
28. Weber SC, Abrams JA, Nottage WM. Complications associated with arthroscopic shoulder surgery. Arthroscopy 2002;18(2) Suppl 1:88–95.
29. Fischer B, Gross RM, McCarthy JA, Arroyo JS. Incidence of acromioclavicular joint complications after arthroscopic subacromial decompression. Arthroscopy 1999;15:241–248.
30. Boyton MD, Anders TJ. Severe heterotopic ossification after arthroscopic acromioplasty, a case report. J Shoulder Elbow Surg 1999;8:495–497.
31. Sampson TG, Nisbet JK, Glick JM. Precision acromioplasty in arthroscopic subacromial decompression of the shoulder. Arthroscopy 1991;7:301–307.

32. Glueck D, Wilson TC, Johnson DL. Extensive osteolysis after rotator cuff repair with a bioabsorbable suture anchor: a case report. Am J Sports Med 2005;33:742–744.
33. Cummins CA, Strickland S, Appleyard RC, et al. Rotator cuff repair with bioabsorbable screws: An in vivo and ex vivo investigation. Arthroscopy 2003;19:239–248.
34. Mallik K, Barr MS, Anderson MW, et al. Intra-articular migration of a sutureless arthroscopic rotator cuff fixation device. Arthroscopy 2003; 19:6, 50.

Index

A

A. *See* Anterior portal

AAC. *See* Anterior acromioclavicular portal

Abduction testing, anterosuperior cuff tear evaluation with, 230

Accordion biceps, 293

A-C joint. *See* Acromioclavicular joint

Acromioclavicular joint (A-C joint)
  ASAD with, 88–89
  suture anchor repair with, 163

Acromioplasty
  rotator cuff repair with, 214
  suture anchor repair with, 162
  tendon-to tuberosity repair with, 121

Adjunctive pain management, 26

AL. *See* Anterolateral portal

Anchor portal, suture anchor repair with, 161

Anchors. *See also* Suture anchor repair
  anchor material/removal in, 38–39
    PDLLA, 38–39
    PLLA, 38
  anterosuperior cuff tears surgery with, 234, 237
  arthroscopic repair complications with, 369–371
  arthroscopic repair with, 17–18
  characteristics of good, 35
  developments in, 41–52
    Arthrex, 41–43
    Arthrocure, 43–44
    Bio-Corkscrew™, 41–43
    BioRaptor™, 46, 48–49

BioZip™, 50–52
    Depuy Mitek, 44–46
    Duet™, 46, 47
    Fastin RC, 44–46
    Impact™, 46
    Linvatec, 46
    Magnum™, 43–44
    Smith & Nephew Endoscopy, 46–50
    SpiraLok™, 44–46
    Stryker Endoscopy, 50–52
    Super Revo™, 46, 47
    Twinfix™ AB, 47–49
    Twinfix™ Quick T, 49–50
    Twinfix™ Ti, 49
  disadvantages with, 36
  evaluation for, 35–36
  eyelet with, 37–38
    load-to-failure force in, 37
  failure in, 40
  glenohumeral stabilization v. rotator cuff in, 34
  history of, 34
  options for, 34–52
  placement in, 39–40
    MRI for, 39
  rehabilitation with, 40–41
  shape of, 36–37
  size of, 36
  suture anchor repair placement of, 162–163
  suture material with, 38
    Dynema, 38
    FiberWire®, 38
    UHMW polyethylene, 38

Anchors (*cont.*)
 tendon-to tuberosity repair
  placement of, 123, 133–134, 136,
   139–140
  selection for, 122–123
 ThRevo®, 110, 112
Anesthesia, 26–27
 adjunctive pain management with,
  26
 arthroscopic repair complications
  with, 364–365
 beach chair orientation with, 26
 bupivacaine with, 26
 endotracheal intubation, 26
 general, 26–27
 interscalene regional block, 26
 laryngeal mask airway, 26
 lateral decubitus orientation with,
  25
 nausea with, 26
 suprascapular nerve with, 26
 tendon-to tuberosity repair with,
  120
Antegrade suturing, 58–62
 advantages of, 58
 cost awareness with, 61–62
 disadvantages of, 58
 FiberWire® for, 58
 instruments for, 58–60
 long-needle technique for, 58–60
 Scorpion™ for, 58–60
 suture hook with, 61
Anterior acromial protuberance, 90
Anterior acromioclavicular portal
  (AAC), 32, 33
 entry site for, 33
 field of view with, 33
 path with, 33
 structures transgressed with, 33
 uses for, 33
Anterior portal (A), 29
 entry site for, 29
 field of view with, 29
 path with, 29
 structures transgressed with, 29
 uses for, 29
Anterior subacromial portal (ASA),
  29
Anterior subcoracoid impingement, 86

Anterolateral portal (AL), 32
 entry site for, 32
 field of view with, 32
 path with, 32
 structures transgressed with, 32
 uses for, 32
Anterosuperior bursectomy, long head
  of biceps tendon disorder
  with, 279
Anterosuperior cuff tears, 228–244
 arthroscopic evaluation of, 233–235
  biceps pulley in, 233–234
  biceps tendon in, 233
  bursoscopy in, 233, 234
  posterior viewing portal in, 233
  supraspinatus in, 233–234
 clinical evaluation of, 229–232
  abduction testing in, 230
  belly press signs in, 230
  biceps testing in, 230
  imaging studies in, 230
  lift off testing in, 230
  MRI in, 230
  passive external rotation testing
   in, 230
  range of motion testing in, 230
  strength testing in, 230
 hidden lesion as, 229
 incidence of, 228
 literature reports on, 228
 results with, 240–244
 surgical technique for, 234–241
  articular suture in subscapularis,
   234
  biceps problems in, 234, 237
  bursal repair in, 237
  PASTA repair, 234, 236
  percutaneous anchor in, 234, 237
Anterosuperior portal (AS), 32
 entry site for, 32
 field of view with, 32
 path with, 32
 structures transgressed with, 32
 uses for, 32
Ariadne guide suture (PDS), 301
Arthrex, 41–43
Arthro-CT. *See* Arthroscopic
  computerized tomography
Arthrocure, 43–44

Arthrography, repairability assessed with, 2, 4
Arthroscopic cannulae, arthroscopic repair with, 17
Arthroscopic computerized tomography (Arthro-CT), suprascapular nerve entrapment diagnosis with, 329
Arthroscopic repair
  complications with, 22–23, 363–371
    anchor-related, 369–371
    anesthetic-related, 364–365
    fluid dynamics, 367
    infection, 364
    neurological injury, 365–366
    nonspecific surgical, 364–365
    portals, 366
    rates of, 363
    specific shoulder arthroscopy, 365–367
    stiffness, 367
    subacromial decompression, 368–369
    vascular, 366
  contraindications for, 16
  indications for, 16
  instrumentation for, 17–18
    anchors as, 17–18
    arthroscopic cannulae as, 17
    inserters as, 17–18
    suture passing devices as, 18
    sutures as, 17–18
    tissue grasper as, 17
  interval release for contracted rotator cuff tears, 208–216
  knot tying for, 68–82
    cannula use with, 80
    definitions for, 68–69
      post limb, 68
      wrapping limb, 68
    dry land training with, 80
    Duncan loop, 69, 70
    knot types with, 69–70
    loop with, 68–69
    lost suture finding with, 81
    Nicky's knot, 69, 70, 78
    retrieving sutures with, 80–81
    Revo knot, 69–70
    Roeder knot, 69, 70, 76–80
    security with, 68
    sliding knot, 69–70, 76–80
    SMC knot, 69, 70
    static knot, 70–76
    surgeon's knot, 70–76
    suture sliding determination with, 81
    Tennessee slider, 69, 70
    tips, 80–82
    twist unraveling with, 81–82
    Weston knot, 69, 70
  large tear rehabilitation protocol with, 357–358
  learning curve for, 15–16, 22
  long head of biceps tear rehabilitation protocol with, 360
  massive tear rehabilitation protocol with, 357–358
  medium tear rehabilitation protocol with, 356–357
  positioning for, 17
  postoperative management with, 21–22
  postoperative rehabilitation for, 348–361
  postoperative rehabilitation protocols with, 352–360
  preoperative planning for, 17
  results with, 22–23
  setup for, 17
  small tear rehabilitation protocol with, 352–356
  subscapularis tear rehabilitation protocol with, 358–360
  subscapularis tears with, 174–194
  technique in, 18–21
    assess repair integrity as, 21
    glenohumeral arthroscopy as, 18
    margin convergence as, 19–20
    mobilization/interval release as, 19
    subacromial arthroscopy as, 18
    tear pattern identification as, 19
    tendon preparation as, 19
    tendon-to-bone repair as, 20–21
  transition from mini-open to all, 15–23

Arthroscopic repair (*cont.*)
  pearls in, 22–23
  small crescent-shaped tear as start
    for, 16
Arthroscopic subacromial
    decompression (ASAD),
    83–102
  acromioclavicular controversies
    with, 88–89
  anatomy with, 89–90
    anterior acromial protuberance
      in, 90
    coracoacromial ligament in, 89–
      90
    posterior bursal curtain in, 89
    subacromial bursa in, 89
  complications with, 100–101
    excessive bleeding as, 100
    heterotopic bone formation as,
      100
    inaccurate bone resection as, 100
    incomplete resection as, 101
    muscle injury as, 100
  controversies with, 86–88
  defined, 87
  diagnosis for, 90–91
  etiology of, 84–86
  historical perspective on, 83
  iatrogenic harm to coracoacromial
    arch with, 87
  impingement type with, 84–86
    anterior subcoracoid impingement
      as, 86
    chronic secondary with
      subacromial changes as, 85
    extrinsic impingement as, 85–86
    internal impingement as, 85
    posterior superior impingement
      as, 85
    primary impingement cont as, 85–86
    secondary impingement as, 84–85
  indications for, 86–88
  postoperative management for, 100
  preoperative planning for, 91–92
  surgical procedure for, 92–100
    glenohumeral diagnostic
      arthroscopy in, 92–94
    lateral approach technique in,
      94–95

    limited anterior resection
      technique in, 94–95
    patient positioning in, 92, 93
    setup in, 92
    technique in, 92–100
    two portal cutting block technique
      in, 95–100
Articular avulsion, 144, 147
AS. *See* Anterosuperior portal
ASA. *See* Anterior subacromial portal
ASAD. *See* Arthroscopic subacromial
    decompression
Axial strain, 220

B
Basic fibroblast growth factor (bFGF),
    tendon healing involved with,
    247
Beach chair orientation, 26
  anesthesia with, 26
  padding bony prominences with, 26
Belly press test
  anterosuperior cuff tears evaluation
    with, 230
  subscapularis tears in, 191
bFGF. *See* Basic fibroblast growth
    factor
Biceps pulley, arthroscopy of
    anterosuperior cuff tears
    with, 233–234
Biceps soft tissue tenodesis, 276–288
  anatomy of, 277, 278
  anterosuperior bursectomy for, 279
  diagnostic arthroscopy for, 279
  pathological findings classified for,
    278
  patient positioning with, 279
  postoperative management of,
    286
  setup for, 279
  surgical procedure with, 279–284
  surgical technique for, 280–284
Biceps subpectoral mini-open
    tenodesis, 306–316
  complications with, 312–315
  contraindications for, 307
  implant cost with, 314
  indications for, 307
  instrumentation for, 308

patient demographics for, 312
patient positioning for, 308
postoperative management for, 312
preoperative planning for, 307–308
results with, 312–315
    biceps tendon condition in, 313
    range of motion in, 313
setup for, 308
surgical technique for, 308–311
    anatomy of approach with, 309
    mid-axillary incision in, 311
    schematic for, 310
    skin incision in, 309
Biceps tendon, arthroscopy of
            anterosuperior cuff tears
            with, 233
Biceps tenodesis with interference
            screw, 290–305
complications with, 302–305
    bicipital groove pain as, 304
    deltoid fiber incarceration as, 304
    failure of fixation as, 303
    nerve injury as, 304
contraindications for, 290–291
indications for, 290
instrumentation for, 295–296
patient positioning for, 295
portals for, 295, 296
postoperative management for, 302
preoperative planning for, 291–294
    accordion biceps in, 293
    hourglass biceps in, 291–292
    imaging studies for, 291
    MRI for, 291
results with, 302–305
setup for, 295
surgical procedure with, 294–302
surgical technique for, 296–302
    anterior subdeltoid bursectomy in,
        297
    Beath needle's passage in, 300
    exteriorization/preparation of
        biceps in, 297–298
    interference screw fixation in,
        301–302
    reaming humeral socket in, 299
    tenotomy of LHB in, 296–297
    transhumeral ligament release in,
        297

Biceps tenotomy, 269–275
complications with, 274–275
contraindications for, 270
indications for, 269–270
instrumentation for, 270
patient positioning with, 270
postoperative management for, 271
preoperative planning for, 270
results with, 274
setup with, 270
surgical procedure with, 270–274
surgical technique for, 271–274
    diagnostic arthroscopy with, 271
    stabilizing ligamentous pulley
        with, 271
    tenotomy with, 272
Biceps testing, anterosuperior cuff
            tear evaluation with, 230
Bigliani and Morrison acromial
            classification, 107
Bio-Corkscrew™, 41–43
BioRaptor™, 46, 48–49
BioZip™, 50–52
Bupivacaine, anesthesia with, 26
Bursoscopy, arthroscopy of
            anterosuperior cuff
            tears with, 233, 234

C
CHL. See Coracohumeral ligaments
Chronic secondary impingement with
            subacromial changes, 85
Clavicle resection, partial. See
            Arthroscopic subacromial
            decompression
Concealed tear, 338
Coracohumeral ligaments (CHL), 89–
            90, 175, 333
Coracoplasty, subscapularis tears with,
            185
Crescent-shaped suture hook, 62–63,
            64
Crescent-shaped tears
    arthroscopic repair with, 16
    interval slides v. margin convergence
        for, 218–219
Cuff mobilization, tendon-to
            tuberosity repair with,
            121–122

CuffPatch® Bioengineered Tissue
          Reinforcement, 248, 251
  clinical/human studies on, 263
  comparison of, 253–254
  FDA regulatory status for, 251
  preclinical/animal studies on, 256
  product description for, 251
  tendon augmentation indication
          with, 248
Cutting block technique, ASAD
          surgery with, 95–100

D

Deep surface tear, 338
Degenerative tear, 144, 146
Depuy Mitek, 44–46
Double diameter knot pusher, 72–76
Double row fixation
  advantages with, 128–129
  complications with, 140–141
  contraindications for, 131–132
  delayed repairs with, 130
  disadvantages with, 129–130
  history of, 127–128
  indications for, 131–132
  instrumentation for, 132–133
  load distribution improved with,
          128
  MRI of, 130–131
  patient positioning for, 132
  postoperative management with,
          140
  preoperative planning for, 132
  results with, 140–141
  setup for, 132
  surgical procedure for, 132–140
  surgical technique for, 133–140
    anchor placement controversy in,
            136, 139–140
    assessment in, 133
    decortication in, 133
    double medial mattress
            configuration in, 133, 136
    entry with, 133
    lateral row anchors drilled in, 136,
            137
    medial anchors drilled in, 133,
            134
    preparation in, 133

  suture passing in, 133, 135, 137
  suture shuttle in, 136, 137
  tendon-to tuberosity repair with,
          127–141
Duet™, 46, 47
Duncan loop, 69, 70
Dynema, 38

E

ECM. *See* Extracellular matrix
Electromyogram (EMG)
  suprascapular nerve entrapment
          before/after, 326–329
  suprascapular nerve entrapment
          diagnosis with, 329
EMG. *See* Electromyogram
Endotracheal intubation (GET), 26
ExpresSew suture passer, suture
          anchor repair with, 164–166
Extracellular matrix (ECM), tendon
          with normal, 332–334
Extracellular matrix grafts
  biological enhancement with,
          247–249
  commercial products for, 248,
          250–253
    CuffPatch® Bioengineered Tissue
            Reinforcement, 248, 251, 256,
            263
    GraftJacket® Regenerative Tissue
            Matrix, 248, 251–252, 256,
            262
    Restore® Orthobiologic Implant,
            248, 250–251, 255–262
    TissueMend® Soft Tissue
            Repair Matrix, 248, 253, 257,
            263
    Zimmer® Collagen Repair
            Patch, 248, 252–253, 256,
            262–263
  comparison of, 253–254
  gene therapy with, 247–248
  growth factors with, 247
    bFGF, 247
    IGF-I, 247
    PDGF, 247
    TGF-β, 247
    VEGF, 247
  indications for use of, 249

peer-reviewed studies literature on, 254–263
   clinical/human, 259–263
   preclinical/animal, 255–257
   surgical technique in, 257–259
  regulatory aspects of, 250
  rotator cuff repair with, 246–264
Extrinsic impingement, 85–86

F

Fastin RC, 44–46
FiberWire®, 38
  antegrade suturing with, 58
Fibroblastic phase, healing mechanics with, 341–343
Fixation, subscapularis tears with, 185–187
Fluid dynamics, arthroscopic repair complications with, 367
Footprint, 127, 134. *See also* Medial footprint fixation
  secure reconstruction of, 221

G

GAG. *See* Glycosaminoglycans
GET. *See* Endotracheal intubation
GIRD. *See* Glenohumeral internal rotation deficit
Glenohumeral arthroscopy, 18
Glenohumeral diagnostic arthroscopy, ASAD surgery with, 92–94
Glenohumeral internal rotation deficit (GIRD), 85
Glenohumeral joint
  lateral decubitus orientation with repair of, 25
  suture anchor repair with inspection of, 161–162
  tendon-to tuberosity repair with, 120–121
Glenohumeral stabilization, rotator cuff tears v., 34
Glycosaminoglycans (GAG), 332–333
GraftJacket® Regenerative Tissue Matrix, 248, 251–252
  clinical/human studies on, 262
  comparison of, 253–254

FDA regulatory status for, 252
preclinical/animal studies on, 256
product description for, 252
tendon augmentation indication with, 248

H

Healing mechanics, 332–345
  future directions with, 345
  postoperative rehabilitation with, 344
  repair tension in, 343
  three phases with, 341–343
    fibroblastic, 341–343
    inflammatory, 341–343
    remodeling, 341–343
Hidden lesion, 229
Hourglass biceps, 291–292

I

IGF-I. *See* Insulin-like growth factor-I
Impact™, 46
Infection, arthroscopic repair complications with, 364
Inflammatory phase, healing mechanics with, 341–343
Infraspinatus muscle, 333
Inserters, arthroscopic repair with, 17–18
Insulin-like growth factor-I (IGF-I), tendon healing involved with, 247, 341
Internal impingement, 85
Interscalene regional block (ISB), 26
Interval release, contracted rotator cuff repair, 208–216
  crescent-shaped tear with, 210
  longitudinal tear with, 210
  patient positioning for, 209
  postoperative management for, 216
  range of motion with, 216
  setup for, 209
  special repair considerations for, 215–216
  surgical procedure for, 208–216
  surgical technique for, 209–215
    acromioplasty in, 214
    basket punch in, 214

Interval slides, margin convergence v.,
    218–226
  axial strain with, 220
  crescent-shaped tears with, 218
  L-shaped tears with, 218–219
  massive contracted rotator cuff tears
      with, 220–226
  secure footprint reconstruction with,
      221
  tear pattern recognition with, 218
  U-shaped tears with, 218–219
Intratendinous tear, 338
ISB. *See* Interscalene regional block

K
Knot tying
  arthroscopic repair, 68–82
  cannula use with, 80
  definitions for, 68–69
    post limb, 68
    wrapping limb, 68
  dry land training with, 80
  Duncan loop, 69, 70
  knot types with, 69–70
  loop with, 68–69
  lost suture finding with, 81
  Nicky's knot, 69, 70, 78
  retrieving sutures with, 80–81
  Revo knot, 69–70
  Roeder knot, 69, 70, 76–80
    arthroscopic view with, 79
    defined, 76
    expansion of suture loop with,
        78
    performed, 76–77
  security with, 68
  sliding knot, 69–70, 76–80
  SMC knot, 69, 70
  static knot, 70–76
  surgeon's knot, 70–76
    double diameter knot pusher for,
        72–76
    reversing half hitch in, 70–71
    Surgeon's Sixth Finger™ for,
        72–76
  suture sliding determination with,
      81
  tendon-to tuberosity repair with,
      114, 115, 124

Tennessee slider, 69, 70
tips, 80–82
twist unraveling with, 81–82
Weston knot, 69, 70

L
LA. *See* Lateral acromial portal
Large tear rehabilitation protocol,
    357–358
Laryngeal mask airway (LMA), 26
Lateral acromial portal (LA), 29,
    31
  entry site for, 31
  field of view with, 31
  path with, 31
  structures transgressed with, 31
  uses for, 31
Lateral approach technique, ASAD
    surgery with, 94–95
Lateral decubitus orientation, 25–26
  anesthesia with, 25
  glenohumeral joint with, 25
  mini-open approach with, 26
Lateral fixation
  acromioplasty for, 121
  anchor placement for, 123
  anchor selection for, 122–123
  anesthesia for, 120
  complications with, 124
  contraindications for, 119
  cuff mobilization for, 121–122
  glenohumeral joint in, 120–121
  indications for, 119
  knot tying for, 124
  patient positioning for, 120
  portals for, 120
  postoperative management with,
      124–125
  preoperative planning for, 119–
      120
  repair site preparation for, 122
  results with, 125
  subacromial space with, 121
  suture passing for, 124
  suture placement for, 123–124
  suture selection for, 123
  tear classification for, 121
  tendon-to tuberosity repair with,
      118–126

Lateral subacromial portal (LSA), 29, 30
  entry site for, 30
  field of view with, 30
  path with, 30
  structures transgressed with, 30
  uses for, 30
Lift off testing
  anterosuperior cuff tear evaluation with, 230
  subscapularis tears in, 191
Limited anterior resection technique, ASAD surgery with, 94–95
Linvatec, 46
LMA. See Laryngeal mask airway
Long head of biceps (LHB), 175, 277–288
  anatomy of, 277, 278
  anterosuperior bursectomy for, 279
  diagnostic arthroscopy for, 279
  pathological findings classified for, 278
  patient positioning with, 279
  postoperative management of, 286
  setup for, 279
  surgical procedure with, 279–284
  surgical technique for, 280–284
  tear rehabilitation protocol for, 360
  tendon disorders of, 277–288
LSA. See Lateral subacromial portal
L-shaped tears
  interval slides v. margin convergence for, 218–219
  side-side suturing with, 62

M
MA. See Midanterior portal
Magnetic resonance imaging (MRI)
  Anchors placement in, 39
  anterosuperior cuff tear evaluation with, 230
  bicipital pathology in, 291
  repairability assessed with, 2
  rotator cuff injury diagnosis with, 339
  suprascapular nerve entrapment diagnosis with, 329

tendon-to tuberosity repair with, 107, 120, 130–131
Magnum™, 43–44
Margin convergence, 19–20
  interval slides v., 218–226
    axial strain with, 220
    crescent-shaped tears with, 218
    massive contracted rotator cuff tears with, 220–226
    secure footprint reconstruction with, 221
    tear pattern recognition with, 218
    U-shaped tears with, 218–219
Massive tear rehabilitation protocol, 357–358
Medial footprint fixation, 105–116
  arthroscopic rotator cuff repair steps with, 110–115
    knot tying in, 114, 115
    screw-in suture anchor insertion in, 112
    side-to-side repairs in, 110, 112
    Spectrum 2® needle in, 112
    Spectrum II suture hook in, 111, 112
    Spectrum® suture hook in, 112
    Suture Savers® in, 111, 114
    Suture Shuttle Relay® in, 112
  complications with, 116
  contraindications for, 106
  indications for, 105–106
  instrumentation for, 109–110
  patient positioning for, 108–109
  postoperative management with, 116
  preoperative planning for, 106–107
    active range of motion in, 106
    Bigliani and Morrison classification in, 107
    imaging studies in, 106–107
    MRI in, 107
  results with, 116
  setup for, 108–109
  STaR Quiver® for, 108–109
  surgical procedure for, 108–109
  surgical technique for, 109–115
  ThRevo® anchors for, 110, 112
Medium tear rehabilitation protocol, 356–357

Midanterior portal (MA), 32
Mini-open repair
  lateral decubitus orientation with,
    26
  transition to all-arthroscopic repair
    from, 15–23
    instrumentation for, 17–18
    learning curve for, 15–16, 22
    pearls in, 22–23
    postoperative management with,
      21–22
    preoperative planning for, 17
    small crescent-shaped tear as start
      for, 16
Mobilization/interval release, 19
MRI. See Magnetic resonance imaging

N
Nausea, anesthesia with, 26
Neurological injury, arthroscopic
    repair complications with,
    365–366
Neviaser. See Superomedial portal
Nicky's knot, 69, 70, 78
Nonsteroidal anti-inflammatory drugs
    (NSAID), rotator cuff tears
    with, 5, 10–11
NSAID. See Nonsteroidal anti-
    inflammatory drugs

O
Opus auto cuff, suture anchor repair
    with, 166–167, 170–171

P
P. See Posterior portal
Partial articular-sided tear avulsion
    (PASTA), 143–157
  anterosuperior cuff tears surgery
    with, 234, 236
  controversy with, 144
  etiology of, 143–144
  history of, 143
  patient evaluation for, 145
  postoperative management for, 151
  results with, 151–153
  surgical repair for, 145–151
    conversion to full tear with,
      150–154

percutaneous side-to-side repair
    in, 145–146, 148
  suture anchor repair with, 147–
    150, 152
  treatment classification for, 144–147
    articular avulsion, 144, 147
    degenerative tear, 144, 146
    supraspinatus split tear, 144, 146
    T-crescent tear, 144, 147
Passive external rotation testing,
    anterosuperior cuff tear
    evaluation with, 230
PASTA. See Partial articular-sided
    tear avulsion
Patient positioning, 25–26
  arthroscopic repair with, 17
  ASAD surgery, 92, 93
  beach chair orientation as, 26
  biceps subpectoral mini-open
    tenodesis, 308
  biceps tenodesis with interference
    screw with, 295
  biceps tenotomy with, 270
  interval release, contracted rotator
    cuff repair, 209
  lateral decubitus orientation as,
    25–26
  long head of biceps disorders with,
    277
  subscapularis tears repair, 179–181
  suprascapular nerve entrapment
    with, 329
  tendon mobilization with, 197
  tendon-to tuberosity repair with,
    108–109, 120, 132
PDGF. See Platelet-derived growth
    factor
PDLLA. See Poly L-lactic acid with
    dextro and levo
PDS. See Ariadne guide suture
Penetrator™, 56, 58
  side-side suturing with, 63, 66
Permacol™ scaffolds, comparison of,
    253–254
Physical therapy, 349–350
Platelet-derived growth factor
    (PDGF), tendon healing
    involved with, 247, 341
PLLA. See Poly L-lactic acid

PLSA. *See* Posterolateral subacromial portal
Poly L-lactic acid (PLLA), 38
Poly L-lactic acid with dextro and levo (PDLLA), 38–39
Portals, 28–33
    accessory, 31–33
    anchor, 161
    anterior, 29
    anterior acromioclavicular, 32, 33
    anterior subacromial, 29
    anterolateral, 32
    anterosuperior, 32
    arthroscopic repair complications with, 366
    biceps tenodesis with interference screw using, 295, 296
    lateral acromial, 29, 31
    lateral subacromial, 29, 30
    midanterior, 32
    posterior, 28–29
    posterior subacromial, 29
    posterolateral subacromial, 29, 30–31
    primary, 28–31
    subscapularis tears repair, 179–181
    superomedial, 31–32
    suprascapular nerve entrapment, 329
    suture anchor repair, 160–161
    technique for, 28
    tendon-to tuberosity repair, 120
    viewing, 161
    waiting, 161
    working, 161
Posterior bursal curtain, 89
Posterior portal (P), 28–29
    entry site for, 28
    field of view with, 28
    path with, 28
    structures transgressed with, 28
    uses for, 28
Posterior subacromial portal (PSA), 29
    entry site for, 29
    field of view with, 29
    path with, 29
    structures transgressed with, 29
    uses for, 29

Posterior superior impingement, 85
Posterior tear, 338
Posterior viewing portal, arthroscopy of anterosuperior cuff tears with, 233
Posterolateral subacromial portal (PLSA), 29, 30–31
    entry site for, 30
    field of view with, 30–31
    path with, 30
    structures transgressed with, 30
    uses for, 30
Post limb, 68
Postoperative rehabilitation, 344, 348–361
    physical therapy for, 349–350
    principles of, 348–352
        pain control in, 348–349
        phases/stages of healing in, 350–352
        preoperative beginning for, 348
        ROM exercises in, 351
    protocols for, 352–360
        large tear arthroscopic repair, 357–358
        long head of biceps tear arthroscopic repair, 358–360
        massive tear arthroscopic repair, 357–358
        medium tear arthroscopic repair, 356–357
        small tear arthroscopic repair, 352–356
        subscapularis tear arthroscopic repair, 358–360
    sling worn for, 349
    stages of healing for, 350–352
        phase I/acute/protective stage in, 350
        phase III/functional stage in, 351–352
        phase II/subacute/recovery stage in, 350–351
PSA. *See* Posterior subacromial portal

R
Radiography, rotator cuff injury diagnosis with, 338–339

Range of motion (ROM)
anterosuperior cuff tears evaluation
with, 230
contracted rotator cuff repair with,
216
large tear rehabilitation protocol for,
357–358
long head of biceps tear
rehabilitation protocol for,
360
massive tear rehabilitation protocol
for, 357–358
medium tear rehabilitation protocol
for, 356–357
postoperative rehabilitation
exercises in, 351
postoperative rehabilitation
protocols for, 352–360
small tear rehabilitation protocol
for, 352–356
subscapularis tear rehabilitation
protocol for, 358–360
tendon-to tuberosity repair in test
of, 106
Reduction, subscapularis tears with,
185
Rehabilitation. *See also* Postoperative
rehabilitation
anchors with, 40–41
Remodeling phase, healing mechanics
with, 341–343
Repairability, 1–11
assessing, 2–5
arthrography for, 2, 4
MRI for, 2
ultrasound for, 2–3
double-row anchor fixation for, 9–10
enhancing, 9–11
environmental factors with, 10–11
NSAID influencing, 5, 10–11
postoperative management for, 11
smoking influencing, 5, 10–11
tendon healing potential with, 4–5
Restore® Orthobiologic Implant, 248,
250–251
clinical/human studies on, 259–262
complications in, 260–262
comparison of, 253–254
FDA regulatory status for, 251

preclinical/animal studies on,
255–256
product description for, 250–251
SIS with, 250, 255–256
surgical technique using, 257–259
tendon augmentation indication
with, 248
Retracted L-shaped tear, side-side
suturing with, 62
Retracted U-shaped tear, side-side
suturing with, 62–63
Retrograde suturing, 55–58
advantages of, 56
disadvantages of, 56
Penetrator™ for, 56, 58
technique for, 56, 57
Revo knot, 69–70
Rim tear, 338
Roeder knot, 69, 70, 76–80
arthroscopic view with, 79
defined, 76
expansion of suture loop with, 78
performed, 76–77
ROM. *See* Range of motion
Rotator cuff injury. *See also* Rotator
cuff tears
causes of, 335
diagnosis of, 338–339
MRI in, 339
radiography in, 338–339
ultrasound in, 339
full-thickness tear, 338
healing mechanics of, 332–345
fibroblastic phase in, 341–343
future directions for, 344
inflammatory phase in, 341–343
postoperative rehabilitation in,
344
remodeling phase in, 341–343
repair tension in, 343
three phases with, 341
healthy tendon biology/biochemistry
in, 332–334
incidence of, 334
overuse/exercise in changes with,
337
partial tear, 338
concealed tear, 338
deep surface tear, 338

intratendinous tear, 338
posterior tear, 338
rim tear, 338
severity of, 334–335
tendinitis with, 335
tendinosis with, 335–337
treatment of, 339–341
types of, 334–341
Rotator cuff tears. *See also*
    Anterosuperior cuff tears
biceps tenotomy for irreparable,
    269–275
    complications with, 274–275
    contraindications for, 270
    indications for, 269–270
    instrumentation for, 270
    patient positioning with, 270
    postoperative management for,
        271
    preoperative planning for, 270
    results with, 274
    setup with, 270
    surgical procedure with, 270–274
    surgical technique for, 271–274
complications with, 363–371
    anchor-related, 369–371
    anesthetic-related, 364–365
    fluid dynamics, 367
    infection, 364
    neurological injury, 365–366
    nonspecific surgical, 364–365
    portals, 366
    rates of, 363
    specific shoulder arthroscopy,
        365–367
    stiffness, 367
    subacromial decompression,
        368–369
    vascular, 366
crescent-shaped, 210
environmental factors with, 10–11
extracellular matrix grafts for,
    246–264
    biological enhancement with,
        247–249
    clinical/human studies on,
        259–263
    commercial products for, 248,
        250–253

comparison of, 253–254
CuffPatch® Bioengineered Tissue
    Reinforcement, 248, 251, 256,
    263
gene therapy with, 247–248
GraftJacket® Regenerative Tissue
    Matrix, 248, 251–252, 256,
    262
growth factors with, 247
indications for use of, 249
peer-reviewed studies literature
    on, 254–263
preclinical/animal studies on,
    255–257
regulatory aspects of, 250
Restore® Orthobiologic Implant,
    248, 250–251, 255–262
surgical technique in studies on,
    257–259
TissueMend® Soft Tissue Repair
    Matrix, 248, 253, 257, 263
Zimmer® Collagen Repair Patch,
    248, 252–253, 256, 262–263
full-thickness, 2–4, 338
glenohumeral stabilization v., 34
incidence of, 2–4
interval release for contracted,
    208–216
longitudinal, 210
massive contracted immobile,
    220–226
    interval slide in continuity with,
        222
    release/not release with, 222,
        226
    subscapularis tears associated
        with, 222
natural history of, 2–4
NSAID with, 5, 10–11
partial, 338
    concealed tear, 338
    deep surface tear, 338
    intratendinous tear, 338
    posterior tear, 338
    rim tear, 338
partial-thickness, 2, 4
postoperative management for, 11
postoperative rehabilitation for, 344,
    348–361

Rotator cuff tears (*cont.*)
   prevalence in elderly population of,
      1
   repairability of, 1–11
      assessing, 2–5
      enhancing, 9–11
      risk factors for, 10–11
      smoking with, 5, 10–11
      surgical indications for, 1–11
      tendon healing potential with, 4–5
      tendon mobilization for large,
         195–206
      three categories for, 6–9
         group I, 6, 8
         group II, 6, 8
         group III, 6–7, 9

S
Secondary impingement, 84–85
SGHL. *See* Superior glenohumeral
      ligaments
SGL. *See* Spinoglenoid ligament
Side-side suturing, 62–66
   crescent-shaped suture hook for,
      62–63, 64
   Penetrator™ for, 63, 66
   retracted L-shaped tear with, 62
   retracted U-shaped tear with, 62–
      63
   suture hand-off for, 63, 66
SIS. *See* Small intestine submucosa
Sliding knots, 69–70, 76–80
   Duncan loop, 69, 70
   Nicky's knot, 69, 70, 78
   Roeder knot, 69, 70, 76–80
   SMC knot, 69, 70
   Tennessee slider, 69, 70
   Weston knot, 69, 70
SM. *See* Superomedial portal
Small intestine submucosa (SIS), 250,
      255–256
Small tear rehabilitation protocol,
      352–356
Smartstitch, suture anchor repair with,
      166–167, 170–171
SMC knot, 69, 70
Smith & Nephew Endoscopy, 46–50
Smoking, rotator cuff tears with, 5,
      10–11

Snare retrieval technique, suture
      anchor repair with, 163–
      165
Spectrum II suture hook, 111, 112
Spectrum® suture hook, 112
Spinoglenoid ligament (SGL), 319
SpiraLok™, 44–46
SSN. *See* Suprascapular nerve
STaR Quiver®, 108–109
Stiffness
   arthroscopic repair complications
      with, 367
   supraspinatus tears complications
      with, 172–173
Strength testing, anterosuperior cuff
      tear evaluation with, 230
Stryker Endoscopy, 50–52
Subacromial arthroscopy, 18
Subacromial bursa, 89
Subacromial decompression,
      arthroscopic repair
      complications with, 368–369
Subacromial space, tendon-to-
      tuberosity repair with, 121
Subscapularis tear rehabilitation
      protocol, 358–360
Subscapularis tears, 334
   anatomy of, 174–178
      axillary artery in, 177
      axillary nerve in, 177
      CHL in, 175
      coracoid process in, 176
      LHB in, 175
      SGHL in, 175
   arthroscopic repair of, 174–194
   causes of, 178–179
   classification of, 181–183, 190
      type I, 181
      type II, 181–182
      type III, 181–183
      type IV, 181, 183, 184
      type V, 181, 183, 184
   complications with, 192
   diagnosis/evaluation of, 179
   endoscopy with, 174–178
   indications for, 193–194
   literature v. results comparison for,
      192–193
   patient positioning for, 179–181

patient selection with surgery for, 189
portals for, 179–181
postoperative management with, 187
radiological assessment before/after surgery for, 189
results with surgery for, 189, 190–192
  belly press test with, 191
  Constant score with, 190
  lift off test with, 191
  pain change with, 191
  radiological, 192
  strength change with, 191
  UCLA score with, 190
surgical procedure for, 179–189
surgical technique for, 183–187
  coracoplasty as, 185
  fixation as, 185–188
  lesions associated with, 187
  reduction as, 185
visualization with, 179–181
Superior glenohumeral ligaments (SGHL), 175
Superolateral. See Anterosuperior portal
Superomedial portal (SM), 31–32
  entry site for, 31
  path with, 32
  structures transgressed with, 32
  uses for, 31
Super Revo™, 46, 47
Suprascapular nerve (SSN), anesthesia with, 26
Suprascapular nerve entrapment, 318–330
  anatomy of, 319–320
  diagnosis of, 329
    arthro-CT in, 329
    EMG in, 329
  etiology of, 320
  patient positioning for, 326–329
  patient selection with, 327–330
  portals for, 321–323
    Nevasier nerve, 321
    posterior, 321
    suprascapular nerve, 321

postoperative care after, 326
results with, 326–329
  Constant score evaluation and, 329
  EMG and, 326–329
surgical technique for, 321–328
Supraspinatus, arthroscopy of anterosuperior cuff tears with, 233–234
Supraspinatus muscle, 333
Supraspinatus split tear, 144, 146
Supraspinatus tears, 159–173
  acromioplasty with, 162
  anchor placement with, 162–163
  complications with, 172–173
    pain as, 172
    re-tear as, 172
    stiffness as, 172–173
  contraindications for, 160
  glenohumeral inspection for, 161–162
  indications for, 159–160
  mobilization with, 162
  operating room setup for, 160
  portals for, 160–161
    anchor, 161
    viewing, 161
    waiting, 161
    working, 161
  postoperative management of, 167, 169, 171–172
    week 1, 167
    week 10, 171–172
    weeks 2 to 4, 167
    weeks 5 to 10, 169
  surgical procedure for, 160–171
  suture anchor repair for, 159–173
  suture passing with, 163–171
    ExpresSew suture passer for, 164–166
    Opus auto cuff for, 166–167, 170–171
    procedure completion in, 167
    pulling stitches for, 166, 168–169
    Smartstitch for, 166–167, 170–171
    snare retrieval technique for, 163–165

Surgeon's knot, 70–76
  double diameter knot pusher for,
      72–76
  reversing half hitch in, 70–71
  Surgeon's Sixth Finger™ for, 72–76
Surgeon's Sixth Finger™, 72–76
Surgical repair. *See also* Arthroscopic
      repair
  all-arthroscopic from mini-open
      transition for, 15–23
  assessing repairability in, 2–5
  double-row anchor fixation for,
      9–10
  enhancing repairability in, 9–11
  indications for, 5–9
  NSAID influencing, 5, 10–11
  postoperative management after, 11
  rotator cuff tears, 1–11
  smoking influencing, 5, 10–11
  timing of, 5–9
Suture anchor repair
  acromioplasty with, 162
  anchor placement with, 162–163
  complications with, 172–173
    pain as, 172
    re-tear as, 172
    stiffness as, 172–173
  contraindications for, 160
  glenohumeral inspection for,
      161–162
  indications for, 159–160
  mobilization with, 162
  operating room setup for, 160
  portals for, 160–161
    anchor, 161
    viewing, 161
    waiting, 161
    working, 161
  postoperative management of, 167,
      169, 171–172
    week 1, 167
    week 10, 171–172
    weeks 2 to 4, 167
    weeks 5 to 10, 169
  supraspinatus tears with, 159–173
  surgical procedure for, 160–171
  suture passing with, 163–171
    ExpresSew suture passer for,
        164–166

Opus auto cuff for, 166–167,
    170–171
procedure completion in, 167
pulling stitches for, 166, 168–169
Smartstitch for, 166–167, 170–171
snare retrieval technique for,
    163–165
Suture hand-off technique, 63, 66
Suture hook retrograde shuttle
    technique, 56, 57
Suture passing devices, arthroscopic
    repair with, 18
Sutures
  anchor options with, 34–52
    anchor material/removal in, 38–39
    Arthrex, 41–43
    Arthrocure, 43–44
    Bio-Corkscrew™, 41–43
    BioRaptor™, 46, 48–49
    BioZip™, 50–52
    Depuy Mitek, 44–46
    developments in, 41–52
    Duet™, 46, 47
    evaluation for, 35–36
    eyelet in, 37–38
    failure in, 40
    Fastin RC, 44–46
    glenohumeral stabilization v.
        rotator cuff in, 34
    history of, 34
    Impact™, 46
    Linvatec, 46
    Magnum™, 43–44
    placement in, 39–40
    rehabilitation in, 40–41
    shape of, 36–37
    size of, 36
    Smith & Nephew Endoscopy,
        46–50
    SpiraLok™, 44–46
    Stryker Endoscopy, 50–52
    Super Revo™, 46, 47
    suture material in, 38
    Twinfix™ AB, 47–49
    Twinfix™ Quick T, 49–50
    Twinfix™ Ti, 49
  antegrade, 58–62
    advantages of, 58
    cost awareness with, 61–62

disadvantages of, 58
FiberWire® for, 58
instruments for, 58–60
long-needle technique for, 58–60
Scorpion™ for, 58–60
suture hook with, 61
arthroscopic repair with, 17–18
management, 55–67
passage, 55–67
retrograde, 55–58
advantages of, 56
disadvantages of, 56
Penetrator™ for, 56, 58
technique for, 56, 57
side-side, 62–66
crescent-shaped suture hook for, 62–63, 64
Penetrator™ for, 63, 66
retracted L-shaped tear with, 62
retracted U-shaped tear with, 62–63
suture hand-off for, 63, 66
tendon-to tuberosity repair
passing in, 133, 135, 137
placement for, 123–124
selection for, 123
Suture Savers®, 111, 114
Suture Shuttle Relay®, 112

T
T-crescent tear, 144, 147
Tear pattern identification, 19
Tendinitis, 335
Tendinosis, 335–337
Tendon
ECM of, 332–334
GAG with, 332–334
healthy biology/biochemistry of, 332–334
supraspinatus, 334
Tendon mobilization, large rotator cuff tears with, 195–206
anatomy with, 196–197
contraindications for, 196
indications for, 195–196
instrumentation for, 197
patient positioning for, 197
preoperative planning for, 196–197
release techniques for, 204–206

setup for, 197
surgical technique for, 197–204
acromion post-bursa release arthroscopic view in, 202
anterior capsule arthroscopic view in, 198
coracacromial ligament arthroscopic view in, 200
coracoid arthroscopic view in, 198
posterior portal arthroscopic view in, 204
posterior release arthroscopic view in, 199
scapular spine arthroscopic view in, 203
subacromial bursa arthroscopic view in, 201
subdeltoid bursa contractures view in, 200
venous plexus arthroscopic view in, 201
Tendon preparation, 19
Tendon-to-bone repair, 20–21
Tendon-to tuberosity repair
arthroscopic rotator cuff repair steps with, 110–115
knot tying in, 114, 115
screw-in suture anchor insertion in, 112
side-to-side repairs in, 110, 112
Spectrum 2® needle in, 112
Spectrum II suture hook in, 111, 112
Spectrum® suture hook in, 112
Suture Savers® in, 111, 114
Suture Shuttle Relay® in, 112
double row fixation, 127–141
advantages with, 128–129
complications with, 140–141
contraindications for, 131–132
delayed repairs with, 130
disadvantages with, 129–130
history of, 127–128
indications for, 131–132
instrumentation for, 132–133
load distribution improved with, 128
MRI of, 130–131

Tendon-to tuberosity repair (*cont.*)
   patient positioning for, 132
   postoperative management with, 140
   preoperative planning for, 132
   results with, 140–141
   setup for, 132
   surgical procedure for, 132–140
   surgical technique for, 133–140
  lateral fixation, 118–126
   acromioplasty for, 121
   anchor placement for, 123
   anchor selection for, 122–123
   anesthesia for, 120
   complications with, 124
   contraindications for, 119
   cuff mobilization for, 121–122
   glenohumeral joint in, 120–121
   indications for, 119
   knot tying for, 124
   patient positioning for, 120
   portals for, 120
   postoperative management with, 124–125
   preoperative planning for, 119–120
   repair site preparation for, 122
   results with, 125
   subacromial space with, 121
   suture passing for, 124
   suture placement for, 123–124
   suture selection for, 123
   tear classification for, 121
  medial footprint fixation, 105–116
   arthroscopic rotator cuff repair steps with, 110–115
   complications with, 116
   contraindications for, 106
   indications for, 105–106
   instrumentation for, 109–110
   patient positioning for, 108–109
   postoperative management with, 116
   preoperative planning for, 106–107
   results with, 116
   setup for, 108–109
   STaR Quiver® for, 108–109
   surgical procedure for, 108–109
   surgical technique for, 109–115
   ThRevo® anchors for, 110, 112
   preoperative planning for, 106–107, 119–120, 132
   active range of motion in, 106
   Bigliani and Morrison classification in, 107
   imaging studies in, 106–107
   MRI in, 107, 120
Tennessee slider, 69, 70
Tenotomy, 314
TGF-β. *See* Transforming growth factor beta
ThRevo® anchors, 110, 112
Tissue grasper, arthroscopic repair with, 17
TissueMend® Soft Tissue Repair Matrix, 248, 253
  clinical/human studies on, 263
  comparison of, 254
  FDA regulatory status for, 253
  preclinical/animal studies on, 256
  product description for, 253
Transforming growth factor beta (TGF-β), tendon healing involved with, 247, 341
Twinfix™ AB, 47–49
Twinfix™ Quick T, 49–50
Twinfix™ Ti, 49
Two portal cutting block technique, ASAD surgery with, 95–100

U

UHMW. *See* Ultra-high molecular weight polyethylene
Ultra-high molecular weight (UHMW) polyethylene, 38
Ultrasound
  repairability assessed with, 2–3
  rotator cuff injury diagnosis with, 339
U-shaped tears
  interval slides v. margin convergence for, 218–219
  side-side suturing with, 62–63

V

Vascular endothelial growth factor (VEGF), tendon healing involved with, 247

Vascular system, arthroscopic repair
    complications with, 366
VEGF. *See* Vascular endothelial
    growth factor
Viewing portal, suture anchor repair
    with, 161

W
Waiting portal, suture anchor repair
    with, 161
Weston knot, 69, 70
Working portal, suture anchor repair
    with, 161
Wrapping limb, 68

Z
ZCR. *See* Zimmer® Collagen Repair
    Patch
Zimmer® Collagen Repair Patch
    (ZCR), 248, 252–253
    clinical/human studies on, 262–
        263
    complications using, 262–263
    FDA regulatory status for, 253
    preclinical/animal studies on,
        256
    product description for, 252–253
    tendon augmentation indication
        with, 248

Printed in China

Springer